Clinical Reasoning in the Health Professions

Clinical Reasoning in the Health Professions

Second edition

Edited by

Joy Higgs BSc, Grad Dip Phty, MHPEd, PhD
Professor, Faculty of Health Sciences, The University of Sydney, New South Wales, Australia

and

Mark Jones BSc (Psych), PT, M App Sc
Coordinator, Senior Lecturer, Graduate Programs in Manipulative Physiotherapy, School of
Physiotherapy, University of South Australia, South Australia, Australia

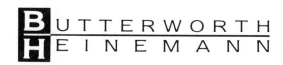

OXFORD   AUCKLAND   BOSTON   JOHANNESBURG   MELBOURNE   NEW DELHI

Butterworth-Heinemann
Linacre House, Jordan Hill, Oxford OX2 8DP
225 Wildwood Avenue, Woburn, MA 01801–2041
A division of Reed Educational and Professional Publishing Ltd

A member of the Reed Elsevier plc group

First edition 1995
Reprinted 1995
Second edition 2000

British Library Cataloguing in Publication Data
Clinical reasoning in the health professions. – 2nd ed.
  1. Clinical medicine   2. Medical logic
  I. Higgs, Joy   II. Jones, Mark A.
  610

Library of Congress Cataloguing in Publication Data
Clinical reasoning in the health professions/edited by Joy Higgs and Mark Jones – 2nd ed.
  p. cm.
  Includes bibliographical references and index.
  ISBN 0 7506 3907 5
  1. Medical logic.   I. Higgs, Joy.   II. Jones, Mark A.
  [DNLM: 1 Decision Making.   2. Health Occupations.   3. Clinical Competence.
  4. Problem Solving.   5. Teaching – methods. W 21 C641]
  R723.C57
  610–dc21   99–051959

ISBN 0 7506 3907 5

Composition by Genesis Typesetting, Laser Quay, Rochester, Kent
Printed and bound in Great Britain by the Bath Press, Somerset

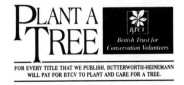

Contents

Acknowledgements

We wish to acknowledge and thank Joan Rosenthal for her invaluable assistance in the production of this book. The participation of the authors in creating this exciting work and the support of our families is much appreciated.

Production of the book

The production of this book has been supported by funding from the Centre for Professional Education Advancement of the Faculty of Health Sciences, The University of Sydney. The following chapters were written by affiliates and honorary research associates of the Centre: 1, 2, 3, 5, 7, 8, 12, 14, 15, 17, 21, 22, 24, 27, 29, 30, 33, 34, 35, 36.

Clinical Reasoning: An Introduction

Joy Higgs and Mark Jones

In this second edition of *Clinical Reasoning in the Health Professions* we have further developed the orientation of clinical reasoning as a patient or client-centred process where the interaction between the clinical task or problem and its context is considered integral to the broader understanding of the problem. These issues are reflected in our new cover design and the revised model in Chapter 1, which focus attention on the place of clients, their care givers and the task–context relationship in the process and outcomes of clinical reasoning. These themes are also highlighted in three of the nine new chapters in this edition. In Chapter 6 Fleming and Mattingly explore the action and narrative dynamics of clinical reasoning; in Chapter 8 Ersser and Atkins examine clinical reasoning and patient-centred care and in Chapter 29 Henley and Twible examine intercultural issues in clinical reasoning practice and education. Clinical reasoning is presented as occurring within a system comprising numerous participants (client, care givers, clinicians, and agents in the larger health care context) all contributing to an understanding of the clinical problem and seeking to implement collaboratively sound, high quality strategies to achieve problem resolution.

Clinical reasoning is the foundation of professional clinical practice. In the absence of sound clinical reasoning, clinical practice becomes a technical operation requiring direction from a decision maker. It is the role of professional health care practitioners to practise in a manner which demonstrates professional autonomy, competence and accountability, to engage in lifelong learning and to contribute to the development of the knowledge base of their discipline (Higgs, 1993). In order to achieve these outcomes health professionals need to be able to reason effectively, to make sound and defensible clinical decisions and to learn through their clinical experience and other avenues in order to continually develop their knowledge, as the basis for making effective clinical decisions and useful contributions to the knowledge of the field.

In this multidisciplinary text written for the health professions we have brought together many of the world's leading and emerging scholars and educators in the field of clinical reasoning. Throughout the text, international scholars, researchers and teachers have contributed their ideas, research findings and experi-ences to promote discussion on the nature and teaching of clinical reasoning. We have focused our 'state of the art' of clinical reasoning chapters on four professions: medicine, nursing, physiotherapy and occupational therapy. Each of these chapters has been updated since the first edition, reflecting the dynamic nature of this topic area.

In the process of updating the book we have acquired twenty new authors. Some of these people have been co-opted by authors from the first edition to add new insights and research or teaching developments to existing chapters. Others have contributed to the new chapters: namely Chapters 6, 7, 8, 19, 22, 29, 33, 34 and 35. These new chapters have strengthened exploration of clinical reasoning teaching and learning discussions in speech–language pathology, medicine, nursing, occupational therapy and physiotherapy. A number of new teaching–learning strategies (e.g. peer coaching – Chapter 33, and case-based learning – Chapter 34) and learning contexts (e.g. intercultural clinical education – Chapter 29, and critical care nursing – Chapter 35) have been added.

This book clearly supports the argument that not only can clinical reasoning be learned, but that teachers, mentors and experienced clinicians can help others, both novices and peers to develop their clinical reasoning expertise. In reflecting on these assumptions, we present several arguments: the regularities of human experience are more unpredictable and multi-faceted than those of the physical sciences. This makes reasoning in human contexts both complex and challenging. Experience is a profound source of learning. This has long been the foundation of educational systems. In clinical reasoning there is no one method to be learned. Rather, alternative methods or more general strategies can be learned, or indeed created, to suit the client, the context and the clinician. There may be several viable paths to a successful outcome for a clinical problem; at the same time the skill of clinical reasoning lies in matching the reasoning strategy to the variables in the given situation.

Throughout this book Harris' (1993) argument that professional practice involves science/technology, art and craft and the use of the corresponding forms of knowledge (propositional, reflective and practical) is strongly supported. We argue that teaching clinical reasoning can involve many approaches (e.g. explanations, providing opportunities for experience and prompting reflection and self-directed learning). Each of these activities would be aimed at enhancing the learner's understanding and ability to perform clinical reasoning. We contend that effective teaching of a cognitive skill such as clinical reasoning involves enhancing learners' abilities to perform clinical reasoning as well as their understanding of this phenomenon (with the latter often being achieved through the former).

Clinical reasoning is a highly complex phenomenon. This is evident in examining the growing body of literature in this field of study. There is no one accepted theoretical or research-based model of clinical reasoning. Indeed this text encourages readers to construct their personal interpretation of clinical reasoning from the spectrum of ideas and perspectives that are presented, and invites clinicians, scholars and researchers to take today's literature and ideas and turn them into tomorrow's visions and explorations. At the same time, in the midst of this complexity, and mindful of the need for clinical reasoning to operate within a context and rules of the relevant disciplinary paradigm, we consider that clinical reasoning also has an essential simplicity. We have defined clinical reasoning as the thinking and decision making processes which are integral to clinical practice. Reasoning may also be described as 'judgement in action' leading to 'action based upon judgement' (Fleming and Mattingly, 1994, p. 342).

The book is divided into four sections. The nature and operation of clinical reasoning is explored in Section One, with chapters on the process of clinical reasoning, the relationships between knowledge, reasoning, critical thinking and expertise, the relationships between action and narrative in reasoning, the goal of clinical reasoning to facilitate patient-centred care and methods of studying clinical reasoning.

Section Two examines clinical reasoning in the practice of medicine, nursing, physiotherapy and occupational therapy. As well as indicating developments in the individual professions, these chapters combine to present the image of a rapidly developing field of literature with a growing emphasis on the interdependence between clinical knowledge and clinical reasoning and on the importance of higher level cognitive functions in the effective operation of clinical reasoning. The four disciplines examined here, along with others discussed in Section Three, approach clinical reasoning in unique as well as related ways. This illustrates the existence of common or core features of clinical reasoning (such as the role of clinical knowledge) and the context-dependent nature of clinical reasoning which is created by such factors as the conceptual framework of the discipline and the role these professions play in health care. For instance, the dominance of the 'illness model' or the 'wellness model', or the relative emphasis on diagnostic and management decisions in a given profession, can significantly influence the nature of clinical reasoning within that profession.

Section Three deals with teaching clinical reasoning. Here twenty-two chapters explore discipline-specific as well as interdisciplinary teaching and learning programs to promote the development of clinical reasoning skills. A wide variety of issues (e.g. the context of learning), strategies (including internet, simulated and case-based learning), venues (including clinics, classrooms and cyberspace) and challenges (including assessing clinical reasoning and promoting self-assessment) are posed in these chapters. These chapters emphasize an adult learning approach to teaching clinical reasoning. The adult learning approach, through its emphasis on such elements as learning through experience, the search for personal meaning, learner responsibility, empowerment of the learner, an internal motivation to solve problems and the autonomy of self-reward through enquiry, is highly compatible with the nature of the phenomenon (clinical reasoning) which is to be learned. These cognitive and humanist perspectives and strategies which underpin adult learning are evident in clinical reasoning education literature. They are highlighted in the essentially cognitive nature of clinical reasoning and the particularly human and humanistic context of health care. A further link between both clinical reasoning and adult learning is the notion of higher level cognitive processes. In both situations the quality of the cognition, decision making and resulting action will be enhanced through the application of such higher level cognitive processes as reflection (both after and during action), metacognition (or the processing of cognition) and evaluation.

The final chapter in Section Four looks to the future of clinical reasoning within the context of evidence-based practice. It asks, 'Will evidence-based practice take the reasoning out of practice?' and argues strongly that professionalism will always require reasoning. In essence, both evidence in its broadest sense and reasoning as a process of applying sound knowledge and evidence to the challenge of complex human health problems and situations, are and will remain essential elements of professional clinical practice.

References

Fleming, M. H. and Mattingly, C. (1994) Action and inquiry: reasoned action and active reasoning. In *Clinical Reasoning: Forms of Inquiry in a Therapeutic Practice* (C. Mattingly and M. H. Fleming, eds), pp. 316–342, Philadelphia: F.A. Davis Co.

Harris, I. B. (1993) New expectations for professional competence. In *Educating Professionals: Responding to New Expectations for Competence and Accountability* (L. Curry and J. Wergin, eds), pp. 17–52, San Francisco: Jossey-Bass.

Higgs J. (1993) Physiotherapy, professionalism and self-directed learning, *Journal of the Singapore Physiotherapy Association*, **14**, 8–11.

Process-oriented perspective

Process-oriented research into clinical reasoning can be closely linked to the field of psychology. Much of the early clinical reasoning research of the 1950s and 1960s focused on attempting to analyse the behaviours (and steps) involved in problem solving, within the psychometric paradigm (e.g. Rimoldi, 1961). The focus of these studies was the assessment of physician/student performance. The research of this era supported the notion of the generic nature and transferability of effective problem-solving skills (Grant, 1992).

Along with the rise of cognitive psychology, research into clinical reasoning also adopted a cognitive (rather than behavioural) focus with an emphasis on understanding the nature of clinical reasoning and on the development of clinical reasoning expertise. This cognitive psychology approach to clinical reasoning research led to information processing, simulation, decision theory and categorization studies. In each of these approaches, use of knowledge derived from the clinical knowledge base of the individual was an important factor, as well as the active processing of received data, in enabling interpretation and solution of the clinical problem. Examples of research in this area include work by Elstein *et al.* (1978), Bordage and Zacks (1984), Feltovich and Barrows (1984), Payton (1985), Putzier *et al.* (1985) and Corcoran (1986). Recent developments in the cognitive tradition have included the use of propositional analysis (e.g. Patel and Groen, 1986; Schmidt *et al.*, 1988).

For some time in nursing and occupational therapy, and more recently in physiotherapy, clinical reasoning research has challenged the domination of this field by the empirico-analytical research paradigm (to which much of the above research belongs). Newer research models are being adopted which operate within the interpretive and critical research paradigms.[1] (See below.)

The interpretive and critical paradigms add an important dimension to the search for (and use of) knowledge in the human sciences. The empirico-analytical research paradigm relies on rules and causal laws more appropriate to the natural sciences, and the knowledge produced is insufficient for operation within human contexts (Barnett, 1990; Manley, 1991; Schön, 1983). The human sciences need a view of knowledge that accords validity to both propositional (theoretical/scientific) knowledge and non-propositional knowledge (e.g. professional craft knowledge and personal knowledge/knowledge of self), that seeks both personal and public validation, and that recognizes that knowledge is a dynamic phenomenon.[2]

Content (knowledge)-oriented perspective

It is now well accepted that clinical reasoning and clinical knowledge are interdependent, rather than being factors that can be learned separately. Norman (1990), for instance, writes that in an endeavour to deal effectively with the knowledge explosion, many educational programs over the last few decades adopted the goal of developing problem-solving skills, simultaneously diminishing their curricular emphasis on knowledge acquisition. In doing so they neglected to recognize that effective problem solving requires a large store of relevant knowledge. This argument is supported in the model of clinical reasoning expertise developed by Boshuizen and Schmidt (1992),[3] in which expertise is linked to depth and organization of clinical knowledge.

Interpretations of clinical reasoning in the literature

Various models have been used to interpret and explain the process of clinical reasoning. These include hypothetico-deductive reasoning (Elstein *et al.*, 1978), pattern recognition (Barrows and Feltovich, 1987), knowledge reasoning integration (Schmidt *et al.*, 1990), and reasoning as a process of integrating knowledge, cognition and meta-cognition (Higgs and Jones, 1995).

Hypothetico-deductive reasoning

Hypothetico-deductive reasoning as a model of clinical reasoning originated in medical research (Barrows *et al.*, 1978; Elstein *et al.*, 1978; Feltovich *et al.*, 1984; Gale, 1982). This reasoning approach involves the generation of hypotheses based on clinical data and knowledge, and testing of these hypotheses through further inquiry. The approach has also been identified in physiotherapy (Jones, 1992), and has been identified as one of the

---

[1] Refer to Chapter 3 for further discussion of these paradigms.

[2] Refer to Chapter 3 for exploration of these forms of knowledge.

[3] Refer to Chapter 2.

modes of reasoning in occupational therapy (where it is linked to the concept of 'procedural reasoning') (Fleming, 1991a), and as an approach used by nurses as part of diagnostic reasoning (Padrick *et al.*, 1987).

Hypothesis generation and testing involves both inductive reasoning (moving from a set of specific observations to a generalization) and deductive reasoning (moving from a generalization to a conclusion in relation to a specific case) (Ridderikhoff, 1989). Induction is used to generate hypotheses and deduction to test hypotheses. Albert *et al.* (1988) describe inductive reasoning as probabilistic reasoning, since a conclusion is reached (e.g. concerning a diagnostic hypothesis) on the basis of the probability of that conclusion in relation to the evidence available. This evidence is evaluated in relation to existing knowledge. Deductive reasoning is widely used in the health sciences in the presentation of arguments to defend decisions and actions. Such reasoning follows the 'if ... then' mode, with the 'if' referring to an implicit or explicit premise (or supporting statement) and the 'then' to the conclusion that is derived from that premise in relation to the situation and evidence in question.

Pattern recognition

Pattern recognition or inductive reasoning, as an interpretation of the clinical reasoning process (in particular, diagnostic reasoning), has been supported by a number of researchers (e.g. Gorry, 1970; Hamilton, 1966; Scadding, 1967). Groen and Patel (1985) identified that expert reasoning in non-problematic situations resembles pattern recognition or direct automatic retrieval of information from a well-structured knowledge base. Elstein *et al.* (1990, p. 10) argue, however, that experts 'clearly do consider and evaluate alternatives when confronted with problematic situations'.

Inductive reasoning has both strengths and weaknesses. While it lacks certainty, inductive reasoning enables conclusions to be reached in the face of imprecise data and limited premises. Albert *et al.* (1988, p. 100) comment, 'Of course we would all prefer to deal with certainties rather than probabilities. Unfortunately, in most instances in medicine and science, sufficient information for correct deductive arguments from acceptable premises is lacking. We must then rely on inductive inferences from premises accepted as true.'

Patel and Groen (1986) and Arocha *et al.* (1993) have used the terms *backward reasoning* where the re-interpretation of data or the acquisition of new clarifying data is invoked in order to test a hypothesis and *forward reasoning* to describe inductive reasoning in which data analysis results in hypothesis generation or diagnosis, utilizing a sound knowledge base. Forward reasoning is more likely to occur in familiar cases with experienced clinicians, and backward reasoning with inexperienced clinicians or in atypical or difficult cases (Patel and Groen, 1986).

Pattern recognition could be thought of as pattern interpretation. Through the use of inductive reasoning, pattern recognition/interpretation is a process characterized by speed and efficiency (Arocha *et al.*, 1993; Ridderikhoff, 1989). By comparison, hypothetico-deductive reasoning, particularly the phase of backward/deductive reasoning, is generally regarded as being a slower, more demanding and more detailed process (Arocha *et al.*, 1993; Patel and Groen, 1986, 1991).

Explanations of pattern recognition include categorization and the use of prototypes. *Categorization* involves grouping of objects or events. It can be related to the process of recognizing the similarity between a set of signs and symptoms or treatment options and outcomes from a previously experienced clinical case. The new case is placed in the same category as the past case(s) and is given the same label (diagnosis) (Brooks *et al.*, 1991; Schmidt *et al.*, 1990). An important aspect of the use of categorization in clinical reasoning is the link made by the clinician between the context of the condition, events or situation and previous cases. In the prototype model, experience results in the construction of abstract associations which convey the meanings assigned to symptoms and signs (Bordage and Zacks, 1984) or semantic relationships consisting of links between clinical features (e.g. local versus general location of pain) (Elstein *et al.*, 1990). The use of *prototypes* enhances the ability of clinicians to interpret clinical data, since the recognition of the clinical pattern is matched against learned abstractions rather than specific instances which may be difficult to match clearly.

Knowledge–reasoning integration

Recent research in the health sciences has demonstrated that clinical reasoning is not a separate skill that can be developed independently of relevant professional knowledge and other clinical skills, such as investigative skills (e.g. Schmidt *et al.*, 1990). There is increasing evidence to support the importance of domain-specific knowledge and an organized knowledge base in clinical problem-solving expertise (Elstein *et al.*, 1990; Hassebrock *et al.*, 1993; Patel and Groen, 1986; Patel *et al.*, 1990; Schmidt *et al.*, 1990). However, it is the interaction between such knowledge and skills in reasoning which lies at the heart of clinical reasoning expertise. Domain-specific knowledge and skills in cognition (critical, creative, reflective and logical/analytical thinking) and metacognition are essential for effective thinking and problem solving (Alexander and Judy, 1988).

Boshuizen and Schmidt (1992, 1995) propose a stage theory of the development of expertise, which emphasizes the parallel development of knowledge acquisition and clinical reasoning expertise. This model is based upon the notion and observation that developing knowledge and the resultant reasoning expertise are largely the result of changes in knowledge structure. The progress from medical student to expert clinician is accompanied by a transition from biomedical knowledge, through encapsulation of knowledge into concept clusters with clinically relevant foci, to structuring of knowledge around *illness scripts* and finally to *instantiated scripts* (actual detailed cases/specific instances). This development in knowledge is accompanied by increasing expertise in reasoning.

Patel and Kaufman (1995) regard the above interpretation as idealized, and cite biomedical misconceptions held by physicians and the different structure of the biomedical and clinical sciences as evidence that the biomedical sciences and clinical medicine constitute two distinct and not fully compatible worlds, with distinct modes of reasoning and knowledge. They suggest that the key role played by basic sciences may be in facilitating explanation and coherent communication rather than in facilitating clinical reasoning itself. In our model of clinical reasoning, the roles of knowledge in clinical reasoning are numerous and the use of various forms of knowledge is closely linked to the context (of the client, profession, situation) in which the knowledge is being utilized.

Recent interpretive models

In a number of health professions, other models of clinical reasoning, many based upon interpretive paradigm research studies, are gaining prominence. Work in the interpretive paradigm has been conducted by Benner (1984) in nursing (with an emphasis on seeking understanding of behaviours and context), by Crepeau (1991) and Fleming (1991b) in occupational therapy (with an emphasis on structuring meaning and interpreting the problem from the patient's perspective), and by Jensen *et al.* (1992) in physiotherapy (with a focus on elucidating the complex and unknown processes that occur during therapeutic interventions). The clinical reasoning processes which such approaches describe focus on strategies which seek a deep understanding of the client's perspective and the influence of contextual factors, in addition to the more traditional and 'clinical' understanding of the patient's condition. The relevance of this broader perspective is evident in the growing body of research demonstrating that the meaning patients give to their problem (including their understanding of and feelings about their problem) can significantly influence their levels of pain tolerance, disability and eventual outcome (Borkan *et al.*, 1991; Feuerstein and Beattie, 1995; Malt and Olafson, 1995). As the volume and depth of research into clinical reasoning grows, it is becoming more and more apparent that traditional clinical reasoning models do not encompass the varying dimensions or reflect the diverse discipline-specific practice paradigms which exist across the health professions.

In nursing, a number of studies (Agan, 1987; Pyles and Stern, 1983; Rew and Barrow, 1987; Rew, 1990) have emphasized the role of intuitive skills in clinical reasoning, linking intuitive knowledge to past experience with specific patient cases. In this sense 'intuitive knowledge' could be another way of describing 'instance scripts' which can be used unconsciously in inductive reasoning. Fonteyn and Fisher (1992) have linked nurses' experience and associated intuition to the use of advanced reasoning strategies or heuristics. Such heuristics include pattern matching and listing (or listing items relevant to the working plan) (Fonteyn and Grobe, 1993).

In occupational therapy, Fleming (1991a) proposes a reasoning theory of an occupational therapist with a 'three track mind'. In this model clinical reasoning involves an integration of three reasoning strategies, procedural, conditional (projected) and interactive reasoning.

In physiotherapy, recent investigators (Edwards *et al.*, 1998)[4] have identified the value and use of a number of the reasoning strategies arising from interpretive paradigm research within physio-

---

[4] See also Chapter 12.

therapy practice. They found that expert physio-therapists in three different fields of physiotherapy (manipulative/orthopaedic, neurological and domiciliary care) consistently used these recently identified clinical reasoning strategies. Educationally, these clinical reasoning strategies can be regarded as an application of clinical reasoning principles to the tasks of clinical practice.

Interpretive models of clinical reasoning include:

- *Diagnostic reasoning* is that reasoning which aims to reveal the client's impairment(s), disability(ies) and handicap(s), and the underlying pathobiological mechanisms. While diagnostic reasoning is the most familiar reasoning strategy, in clinical practice it is combined with other strategies to establish patient rapport and to educate and promote patient self-efficacy and responsibility.
- *Interactive reasoning* occurs when dialogue in the form of social exchange is used deliberately to enhance or facilitate the assessment/management process. This reasoning provides an effective means of better understanding the context in which the patient's problem(s) exist while creating a relationship of interest and trust.
- *Narrative reasoning* involves the use of stories regarding past or present patients to further understand and manage a clinical situation. Such real-life scenarios bring credibility to the advice or explanation which they are used to support and can be strategically employed by practitioners to strengthen their message.
- *Collaborative reasoning* refers to the shared decision making that ideally occurs between practitioner and patient. Here the patient's opinions as well as information about the problem are actively sought and utilized.
- *Predictive* or *conditional reasoning* is part of the practitioner's thinking directed to estimating patient responses to treatment and likely outcomes of management, based on information obtained through the patient interview, physical examination and response to management.
- *Ethical/pragmatic reasoning* alludes to those less recognized, but frequently made decisions regarding moral, political and economic dilemmas which clinicians regularly confront, such as deciding how long to continue treatment.
- *Teaching as reasoning* occurs when practitioners consciously use advice, instruction and guidance for the purpose of promoting change in the patient's understanding, feelings and behaviour.

Clinical reasoning expertise

The attainment of clinical reasoning and clinical practice expertise is a target of clinicians and an expectation of health care consumers. What then is this expertise and how is it developed?

Glaser and Chi (1988, pp. xvii–xx) have identified seven characteristics of experts:

- Experts excel mainly in their own domains.
- Experts perceive large meaningful patterns in their domain.
- Experts are fast: they are faster than novices at performing the skills of their domain and they quickly solve problems with little error.
- Experts have superior short-term and long-term memory.
- Experts see and represent a problem in their domain at a deeper (more principled) level than novices; novices tend to represent a problem at a superficial level.
- Experts spend a great deal of time analysing a problem qualitatively.
- Experts have strong self-monitoring skills.

In addition to these generic skills of experts which are applicable to clinical reasoning expertise, there are particular characteristics of experts which are pertinent to the health professions.

Expertise and shared decision making

Experts are expected to achieve better clinical results, based on reasoning which is 'accurate' and relevant (to the client and the situation), and on effective technical competence. However, other outcome dimensions, particularly as viewed from the patient's perspective, may be lacking in some peer-judged experts. The clinical reasoning behind clinical performance encompasses not only diagnostic and management-oriented problem solving but also deals with clients' unique personal experience of their problems (the specific meaning and influences of their clinical problems). Recipients of health care may regain their health or function yet still feel that the clinician's performance was inadequate. A premise of this chapter, and indeed of many chapters throughout this book, is that clinical reasoning cannot be fully understood when only the clinician's perspective is considered. Shared decision making between client and clinician is important if 'success' is to be realized from the client's perspective.

Expertise and metacognition

Alexander and Judy (1988) argue that cognitive research over the last 20 years has indisputably found that, in addition to a greater domain-specific knowledge base, expertise is demonstrated by those people who monitor and regulate their cognitive processing (i.e. use metacognition) during task performance. Metacognition refers to being aware of one's cognitive processes and exerting control over these processes, and the cognitive skills that are necessary for the management of knowledge and other cognitive skills (Biggs, 1988). Biggs (1986, p. 143) argues that 'high quality human performance inevitably requires metacognitive as well as cognitive components. To perform well, one needs to be aware not only of the knowledge and algorithms required for the task, but of one's own motives and resources, the contextual constraints, and to plan strategically on that knowledge'.

Expertise and the critical use of knowledge in several forms

Nickerson *et al.* (1985, p. 68) identify two key features of expertise, 'the ability to manage one's intellectual resources and to use whatever domain-specific knowledge one has most efficiently' and the presence of a wealth of domain-specific knowledge. Three forms of knowledge are necessary for clinical expertise: propositional knowledge, professional craft knowledge and personal knowledge (Higgs and Titchen, 1995). The critical use of knowledge, based on the ability to be self-aware and self-critical, and to reflect on one's decision making, is essential for effective professional decision making, critical self-evaluation and responsible practice (Higgs and Titchen, 1995). Critical thinking relies on continual updating of knowledge in the professional domain and within the individual clinician's knowledge base, and on the use of professional judgement to appraise the relevance, worth and currency of knowledge in application to clinical reasoning.

Expertise and skilled companionship: the expert and patient-centred practice

The forces of accountability, cost-efficiency and consumerism have led a number of health professionals to call for a return to patient-centred care and to a recognition of the importance of patient-centred practice as the hallmark of an expert clinician. In occupational therapy, for instance, considerable emphasis is placed on the utilization of a client-centred approach in which the focus is on people's rights to develop the skills and habits required for a balanced, wholesome life (Shannon, 1977).

One way of conceptualizing the skilled or expert clinician is as a skilled companion. Titchen (1998) uses the metaphor *skilled companionship* to mean accompanying patients during their journey toward health. This approach, she argues, is the essence of the helping relationship between a health professional and a patient. Similarly, Ersser (1996) contends that our capacity to understand and respond appropriately to the patient's experience of care is essential to patient-centred practice.

Expertise and critical companionship: the expert as mentor and guide

Titchen (1998, p. 1) also describes the expert as a *critical companion*. Critical companions accompany 'less experienced practitioners on their own very personal, experiential learning journeys'. At the core of this process is the relationship between the critical companion and the practitioner. This relationship involves four processes: mutuality (working together), reciprocity (valued exchange), particularity (knowing the particulars of the situation) and graceful care. Practical rational-intuitive tools of intentionality, saliency and temporality help to create the learning relationship. Facilitation of learning is based on four concepts, consciousness raising, problematization, self-reflection and critique, and these concepts are translated into learning facilitation strategies such as *articulation of craft knowledge* and *critical dialogue*. The overarching dimension of the critical companion's expertise is *the facilitative use of self*. This dimension involves bringing together the human and situational aspects of the learning context, blending craft and theoretical knowledge, intuitive and rational thinking, self-awareness and professional artistry.

Expertise and communication

Higgs and Titchen (1995) argue that the capacity to justify clinical decisions articulately is essential for effective professional practice. The expert is expected to communicate effectively with clients, colleagues and families, to listen as well as to explain, educate and negotiate, and to use language appropriate to the people and situation involved. Professionals are expected to communicate effectively across language, cultural and situational barriers (Josebury *et al.*, 1990).

Expertise and cultural competence

To perform clinical reasoning expertly clinicians need cultural competence. They need to reason in a manner which is culturally sensitive and appropriate for their clients. (Chapter 29 explores this topic further.)

Clinical expertise

From the above considerations, we would add to Glaser and Chi's (1988) seven characteristics of experts the following points, pertinent to health professional experts:

- Experts value the participation of relevant others (clients, caregivers, team members) in the decision-making process.
- Experts utilize high levels of metacognition in their reasoning.
- Experts recognize the value of different forms of knowledge in their reasoning and use this knowledge critically.
- Experts are patient-centred.
- Experts share their expertise to help develop expertise in others.
- Experts are able to communicate their reasoning well and in a manner appropriate to their audience.
- Experts demonstrate cultural competence in their reasoning and communication.

We propose that clinical expertise, of which clinical reasoning is a critical component, be viewed as a continuum along multiple dimensions. These dimensions include clinical outcomes, personal attributes such as professional judgement, technical clinical skills, communication and interpersonal skills (to involve the client and others in decision making and to consider the client's perspectives), a sound knowledge base, as well as cognitive and metacognitive proficiency.

An integrated, patient-centred model of clinical reasoning

The interpretation of clinical reasoning we presented in the first edition of this book (Higgs and Jones, 1995) involved three core elements of clinical reasoning (knowledge, cognition or thinking and metacognition). These elements interact throughout the process of receiving, interpreting, processing and utilizing clinical information during decision making, clinical intervention, and reflection on actions and outcomes. Clinical reasoning was described as a process of reflective inquiry, involving the client if possible, which seeks to promote a deep and contextually relevant understanding of the clinical problem, in order to provide a sound basis for clinical intervention.

In our revised model we retain the three dimensions as above:

- Cognition or reflective inquiry.
- A strong discipline-specific knowledge base.
- Metacognition, which provides the integrative element between cognition and knowledge.
    To these dimensions we add:
- Mutual decision making, or the role of the client or patient in the decision-making process.
- Contextual interaction, or the interactivity between the decision makers and the situation or environment of the reasoning process.
- Task impact, or the influence of the nature of the clinical problem or task on the reasoning process.

The basis for the inclusion of these new dimensions is the growing expectation by and of consumers that they play an active role in their own health care. The image of compliant, dependent patients is replaced by one of informed health care consumers who expect their needs and preferences to be listened to, who increasingly want to participate in decision making about their health, and who expect to take action to enhance their health. Alongside this health rather than illness focus on the part of the consumer there are also economic factors such as an increasing reliance on 'user-pays' funding strategies, which mean that consumers are indeed purchasing health care, and their expectations of service, quality and ownership of health programs are therefore increasing. Similarly, caregivers need and wish to play a greater role in health management and decision making.

The increasing participation by, and dependence upon, clients and caregivers in health care management also highlights the need to pay greater attention to the client's environment. This includes the physical home and work environment, clients' personal circumstances (e.g. culture, family, finances), and their access to health care. Access involves considerations such as location of health care facilities, transportation options, language and cultural factors, and economic provisions for health care.

Many of these situational factors also interact with the nature of the clinical problem or task facing the health care team and the client (and caregivers). Clinical problems facing clients and health professionals can be difficult, changeable, uncertain and multi-dimensional. They involve human and non-human elements. They are affected by local and global contexts, and occur in the context of uncertainty, changeability and the indeterminate knowledge base of the health sciences.

The model of the interactional health professional (Higgs and Hunt, 1999) is particularly pertinent to these three added dimensions. Such individuals have the capacity to interact effectively (both proactively and responsively) with the many elements (people, task, situation) of the work environment. They seek and value the input of others, particularly clients, caregivers and other health care team members, in the reasoning and decision-making processes, to achieve the goal of providing quality, appropriate and acceptable (to the client) health care.

In our revised model (Figure 1.1), clinical reasoning is defined as a process in which the clinician, interacting with significant others (client, caregivers, health care team members), structures meaning, goals and health management strategies based on clinical data, client choices, and professional judgement and knowledge. This process is centred on the client and the client's clinical problem(s) and the related environment. The major function of clinical reasoning is to enhance understanding (by clinician and client) of the clinical

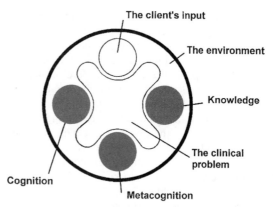

Figure 1.1 Client centred clinical reasoning

problem, in order to provide the basis for sound health management.

The process of clinical reasoning is represented by an upward and outward spiral. This image is intended to demonstrate clinical reasoning as both a cyclical and a developing process. Each loop of the spiral incorporates data input, data interpretation (or re-interpretation) and problem formulation (or re-formulation) to achieve a progressively broader and deeper understanding of the clinical problem (Figure 1.2). Based on this deepening understanding, decisions are made concerning intervention, and actions are taken. For instance, the clinician can decide to refrain from intervention, to collect further data or to provide care, etc. The efficacy of the clinical reasoning process relies on the clinician's reasoning proficiency and the client's capacity and willingness to participate in clinical decision making. The combined process can be represented by parameters

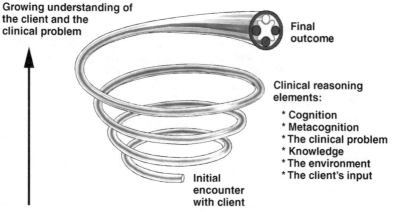

Figure 1.2 Clinical reasoning – overview

such as the speed of decision making (i.e. the speed of 'ascending the spiral'), the depth of understanding of the clinical problem that is achieved, and the validity and relevance of the management approach adopted. These outcomes are influenced by internal factors relating to the health professional (e.g. knowledge base, familiarity and experience with this type of case, reasoning skills), factors relating to the client (e.g. needs, communication skills, circumstances, choices) and external factors (e.g. institutional expectations, profession-specific frameworks of operation, complexity of the case).

Throughout the reasoning process the core elements of task impact, knowledge, cognition and metacognition interact in a process of mutual decision making and context interaction. That is, cognitive or thinking skills (such as analysis, synthesis and evaluation of data collected) are utilized to process clinical data against the clinician's existing discipline-specific and personal knowledge base in consideration of the client's needs and the clinical problem. At the same time, metacognition is employed to monitor the clinician's thinking processes and conclusions, in order to detect links or inconsistencies between clinical data and existing clinical patterns or expectations based upon prior learning, to reflect on the soundness (accuracy, reliability, validity) of observations and conclusions, and to critique the reasoning process itself (for logic, scope, client relevance, efficiency, creativity, etc.). The process of clinical reasoning occurs throughout the clinician's interaction with the client, each decision or action producing a clearer picture of the clinical problem and context influences or targets, which in turn generates further information and/or questions in the continuing process of data interpretation and mutual decision making.

Our model supports the interpretive and critical paradigms, not only for the relevance of these approaches to the clinical context, but also because we emphasize that clinical reasoning, and the understanding or interpretation which results from this process in a given situation, is unique to the clinician (and client) involved. This argument rests on the following premises: that clinical reasoning occurs within the frame of reference of the participating individuals; that the knowledge base of the clinician is unmatched, being derived from personal and professional experiences as well as from the learning of propositional knowledge; and that the engagement of individual clinicians (within their particular frame of reference and knowledge base) with clients in their specific contexts must result in a unique understanding of and proposed solution to client's clinical problem. We recognize that many human problems can have multiple interpretations and solutions. The key to effective and accountable clinical practice, we contend, is that the clinician's understanding of the problem should be substantial in order to avoid potential harmful or ineffective intervention outcomes, and that management should be justifiable in terms of sound arguments based upon the propositional, professional and personal knowledge of the clinician and (as appropriate) the personal knowledge of the client.

Conclusion

In this chapter we have argued that clinical reasoning is central to clinical practice, and have explored the nature of clinical reasoning and criteria for demonstrating expertise in clinical practice and reasoning. An integrated, patient-centred model of clinical reasoning is presented, incorporating the key elements of knowledge, cognition, metacognition and task impact interacting in a process of mutual decision making and context interaction. This process occurs within the frame of reference of the clinician, the context of the client and the complex, variable world of health care, and seeks to achieve a growing understanding of the clinical problem with which to provide the basis for sound clinical management.

References

Agan, R. (1987) Intuitive knowing as a dimension of nursing. *Advances in Nursing Science*, 10, 63–70.

Albert, A. D., Munson, R. and Resnik, M. D. (eds) (1988) *Reasoning in Medicine: An Introduction to Clinical Inference*. Baltimore, MD: Johns Hopkins University Press.

Alexander, P. A. and Judy, J. E. (1988) The interaction of domain-specific and strategic knowledge in academic performance. *Review of Educational Research*, **58**, 375–404.

Arocha, J. F., Patel, V. L. and Patel, Y. C. (1993) Hypothesis generation and the coordination of theory and evidence in novice diagnostic reasoning. *Medical Decision Making*, **13**, 198–211.

Barnett, R. (1990) *The Idea of Higher Education*. Buckingham: The Society for Research into Higher Education and Open University Press.

Barrows, H. S., Feightner, J. W., Neufield V. R. and Norman G. R. (1978) *An Analysis of the Clinical Methods of Medical Students and Physicians*. Report to the Province of Ontario Department of Health, McMaster University, Hamilton, Ontario.

Barrows, H. S. and Feltovich P. J. (1987) The clinical reasoning process. *Medical Education*, **21**, 86–91.

Benner, P. (1984) *From Novice to Expert: Excellence and Power in Clinical Nursing Practice*. London: Addison-Wesley.

Biggs, J. (1988) The role of metacognition in enhancing learning. *Australian Journal of Education*, **32**, 127–138.

Biggs, J. B. (1986) Enhancing learning skills: The role of metacognition. In *Student Learning: Research Into Practice – The Marysville Symposium* (J. A. Bowden, ed.), pp. 131–148. The University of Melbourne: Centre for the Study of Higher Education.

Bordage, G. and Zacks, R. (1984) The structure of medical knowledge in the memories of medical students and general practitioners: Categories and prototypes. *Medical Education*, **18**, 406–416.

Borkan, J. M., Quirk, M. and Sullivan, M. (1991) Finding meaning after the fall: Injury narratives from elderly hip fracture patients. *Social Science and Medicine*, **33**, 947–957.

Boshuizen, H. P. A. and Schmidt, H. G. (1992) On the role of biomedical knowledge in clinical reasoning by experts, intermediates and novices. *Cognitive Science*, **16**, 153–184.

Bordage, G. and Zacks, R. (1984) The structure of medical knowledge in the memories of medical students and general practitioners: Categories and prototypes. *Medical Education*, **18**, 406–416.

Bransford, J., Sherwood, R., Vye, N. and Rieser, J. (1986) Teaching thinking and problem solving: Research foundations. *American Psychologist*, **41**, 1078–1089.

Brooks, L. R., Norman, G. R. and Allen, S. W. (1991) Role of specific similarity in a medical diagnostic task. *Journal of Experimental Psychology, General*, **120**, 278–287.

Cervero, R. M. (1988) *Effective Continuing Education for Professionals*. San Francisco: Jossey-Bass.

Checkland, P. B. (1981) *Systems Thinking: Systems Practice*. New York: Wiley.

Corcoran, S. (1986) Planning by expert and novice nurses in cases of varying complexity. *Research in Nursing and Health*, **9**, 155–162.

Crepeau, E. B. (1991) Achieving intersubjective understanding: Examples from an occupational therapy treatment session. *American Journal of Occupational Therapy*, **45**, 1016–1025.

Edwards, I. C., Jones, M. A., Carr, J. and Jensen, G. M. (1998) Clinical reasoning in three different fields of physiotherapy – A qualitative study. In *Proceedings Fifth International Congress* pp. 298–300. Melbourne: Australian Physiotherapy Association.

Elstein, A. S., Shulman, L. S. and Sprafka, S. A. (1978) *Medical Problem Solving: An Analysis of Clinical Reasoning*. Cambridge, MA: Harvard University Press.

Elstein, A. S., Shulman, L. S. and Sprafka, S. A. (1990) Medical problem solving: a ten year retrospective. *Evaluation and the Health Professions*, **13**, 5–36.

Ersser, S. (1996) Ethnography and the development of patient-centred nursing. In *Essential Practice in Patient-Centred Care* (K. W. M. Fulford, S. Ersser and T. Hope, eds), pp. 53–63. Oxford: Blackwell Science.

Feltovich, P. J. (1983) Expertise: Reorganizing and refining knowledge for use. *Professions Education Researcher Notes*, **4**, 5–9.

Feltovich, P. J. and Barrows, H. S. (1984) Issues of generality in medical problem solving. In *Tutorials in Problem-Based Learning: A New Direction in Teaching the Health Professions* (H. G. Schmidt and M. L. De Volder, eds), pp. 128–141. Assen: Van Gorcum.

Feltovich, P. J., Johnson, P. E., Moller, J. H. and Swanson, D. B. (1984) LCS: The role and development of medical knowledge in diagnostic expertise. In *Readings in Medical Artificial Intelligence: The First Decade* (W. J. Clancey and E. H. Shortliffe, eds), pp. 275–319. Reading, MA: Addison-Wesley.

Feuerstein, M. and Beattie, P. (1995) Biobehavioral factors affecting pain and disability in low back pain: Mechanisms and assessment. *Physical Therapy*, **75**, 267–280.

Fleming, M. H. (1991a) The therapist with the three track mind. *American Journal of Occupational Therapy*, **45**, 1007–1014.

Fleming, M. H. (1991b) Clinical reasoning in medicine compared with clinical reasoning in occupational therapy. *American Journal of Occupational Therapy*, **45**, 988–996.

Fonteyn, M. and Fisher, S. (1992) The study of expert nurses in practice. Paper presented at *Transformation Through Unity: Decision-Making and Informatics in Nursing*, University of Oregon Health Science Centre, Portland, OR, October 17, 1992.

Fonteyn, M. and Grobe, S. (1993) Expert critical care nurses' clinical reasoning under uncertainty: Representation, structure and process. In *Sixteenth Annual Symposium on Computer Applications in Medical Care* (M. Frisse, ed.), pp. 405–409. New York: McGraw-Hill.

Gale, J. (1982) Some cognitive components of the diagnostic thinking process. *British Journal of Educational Psychology*, **52**, 64–76.

Glaser, R. and Chi, M. T. H. (1988) Overview. In *The Nature of Expertise* (M. T. H. Chi, R. Glaser and M. J. Farr, eds), pp. xvi–xxviii. Hillsdale, NJ: Lawrence Erlbaum.

Gorry, G. A. (1970) Modelling the diagnostic process. *Journal of Medical Education*, **45**, 293–302.

Grant, R. (1992) Obsolescence or lifelong education: Choices and challenges. *Physiotherapy*, **78**, 167–171.

Groen, G. J. and Patel, V. L. (1985) Medical problem-solving: Some questionable assumptions. *Medical Education*, **19**, 95–100.

Hamilton, M. (1966) *Clinicians and Decisions*. Leeds: Leeds University Press.

Harris, I. B. (1993) New expectations for professional competence. In *Educating Professionals: Responding to New Expectations for Competence and Accountability* (L. Curry, and J. Wergin *et al.*, eds), pp. 17–52. San Francisco: Jossey-Bass.

Hassebrock, F. and Johnson, P. E. (1986) Medical knowledge and cognitive effort in diagnostic reasoning. Paper presented at the *Annual Meeting of the American Educational Research Association*, San Francisco.

Hassebrock, F., Johnson, P. E., Bullemer, P., Fox, P. W. and Moller, J. H. (1993) When less is more: Representation and selective memory in expert problem solving. *American Journal of Psychology*, **106**, 155–189.

Higgs, C., Neubauer, D. and Higgs, J. (1999) The changing health care context: globalization and social ecology. In *Educating Beginning Practitioners: Challenges for Health Professional Education* (J. Higgs and H. Edwards, eds), pp. 30–37. Oxford: Butterworth-Heinemann.

Higgs, J. (1993) Physiotherapy, professionalism and self-directed learning. *Journal of the Singapore Physiotherapy Association*, **14**, 8–11.

Higgs, J. and Hunt, A. 1999, Rethinking the beginning practitioner: 'the Interactional Professional'. In *Educating Beginning Practitioners: Challenges for Health Professional Education*, (J. Higgs and H. Edwards, eds), pp. 10–18. Oxford: Butterworth-Heinemann.

Higgs, J. and Jones, M. (1995) Clinical reasoning. In *Clinical Reasoning in the Health Professions* (J. Higgs and M. Jones, eds), pp. 3–23. Oxford: Butterworth-Heinemann.

Higgs, J. and Titchen, A. (1995) Propositional, professional and personal knowledge in clinical reasoning. In *Clinical Reasoning in the Health Professions* (J. Higgs and M. Jones, eds), pp. 129–146. Oxford: Butterworth-Heinemann.

Jensen, G. M., Shepard, K. F. and Hack, L. M. (1992) Attribute dimensions that distinguish master and novice physical therapy clinicians in orthopedic settings. *Physical Therapy*, **72**, 711–722.

Jones, M. A. (1992) Clinical reasoning in manual therapy. *Physical Therapy*, **72**, 875–884.

Josebury, H. E., Bax, N. D. S. and Hannay, D. R. (1990) Communication skills and clinical methods: A new introductory course. *Medical Education*, **24**, 433–437.

Jungermann, H. (1986) The two camps on rationality. In *Judgment and Decision Making: An Interdisciplinary Reader* (H. R. Arkes and K. R. Hammond, eds), pp. 627–641. New York: Cambridge University Press.

Kassirer, J. P. and Kopelman, R. I. (1991) *Learning Clinical Reasoning*. Baltimore, MD: Williams & Wilkins.

Kennedy, M. (1987) Inexact sciences: Professional education and the development of expertise. *Review of Research in Education*, **14**, 133–168.

Malt, U. F. and Olafson, O. M. (1995) Psychological appraisal and emotional response to physical injury: A clinical, phenomenological study of 109 adults. *Psychiatric Medicine*, **10**, 117–134.

Manley, K. (1991) Knowledge for nursing practice. In *Nursing: A Knowledge Base for Practice* (A. Perry and M. Jolley, eds), pp. 1–27. London: Edward Arnold.

Newell, A. and Simon, H. A. (1972) *Human Problem Solving*. Englewood Cliffs, NJ: Prentice-Hall.

Nickerson, R. S., Perkins, D. N. and Smith, E. E. (1985) *The Teaching of Thinking*. Hillsdale, NJ: Lawrence Erlbaum.

Norman, G. R. (1990) Editorial: Problem-solving skills and problem-based learning. *Physiotherapy Theory and Practice*, **6**, 53–54.

Padrick, K., Tanner, C., Putzier, D. and Westfall, U. (1987) Hypothesis evaluation: A component of diagnostic reasoning. In *Classification of Nursing Diagnosis: Proceedings of the Seventh Conference* (A. McClane, ed.), pp. 299–305. Toronto: Mosby.

Patel, V. L. and Groen, G. J. (1986) Knowledge-based solution strategies in medical reasoning. *Cognitive Science*, **10**, 91–116.

Patel, V. L. and Groen, G. J. (1991) The general and specific nature of medical expertise: A critical look. In *Toward a General Theory of Expertise: Prospects and Limits* (A. Ericsson and J. Smith, eds), pp. 93–125. New York: Cambridge University Press.

Patel, V. L., Groen, G. J. and Arocha, J. F. (1990) Medical expertise as a function of task difficulty. *Memory and Cognition*, **18**, 394–406.

Patel, V. L. and Kaufman, D. R. (1995) Clinical reasoning and biomedical knowledge: Implications for teaching. In *Clinical Reasoning in the Health Professions* (J. Higgs and M. Jones, eds), pp. 117–128. Oxford: Butterworth-Heinemann.

Payton, O. D. (1985) Clinical reasoning process in physical therapy. *Physical Therapy*, **65**, 924–928.

Payton, O. D., Nelson, C. E. and Ozer, M. N. (1990) *Patient Participation in Program Planning: A Manual for Therapists*. Philadelphia, PA: F. A. Davis.

Putzier, D., Padrick, K., Westfall, U. and Tanner, C. (1985) Diagnostic reasoning in critical care nursing. *Heart and Lung*, **14**, 430–436.

Pyles, S. and Stern, P. (1983) Discovery of nursing gestalt in critical care nursing: The importance of the grey gorilla syndrome. *Image: The Journal of Nursing Scholarship*, **15**, 51–57.

Rew, L. (1990) Intuition in critical care nursing practice. *Dimensions of Critical Care Nursing*, **9**, 30–37.

Rew, L. and Barrow, E. (1987) Intuition: a neglected hallmark of nursing knowledge. *Advances in Nursing Science*, **10**, 49–62.

Ridderikhoff, J. (1989) *Methods in Medicine: A Descriptive Study of Physicians' Behaviour*. Dordrecht: Kluwer.

Rimoldi, H. J. A. (1961) The test of diagnostic skills. *Journal of Medical Education*, **36**, 73–79.

Scadding, J. G. (1967) Diagnosis: The clinician and the computer. *Lancet*, **i**, 877–882.

Schmidt, H., Boshuizen, H. P. A. and Hobus, P. P. M. (1988) Transitory stages in the development of medical expertise: The 'intermediate effect' in clinical case representation studies. In *Proceedings of the Tenth Annual Conference of the Cognitive Science Society* (V. L. Patel and G. J. Groen, eds), pp. 139–145. Hillsdale, NJ: Lawrence Erlbaum.

Schmidt, H. G., Norman, G. R. and Boshuizen, H. P. A. (1990) A cognitive perspective on medical expertise: Theory and implications. *Academic Medicine*, **65**, 611–621.

Schön, D. A. (1983) *The Reflective Practitioner: How Professionals Think in Action*. London: Temple Smith.

Shannon, P. (1977) The derailment of occupational therapy. *American Journal of Occupational Therapy*, **31**, 229–234.

Titchen, A. (1998) *A Conceptual Framework for Facilitating Learning in Clinical Practice*. Occasional Paper No. 2. Sydney: Centre for Professional Education Advancement, The University of Sydney.

2

The development of clinical reasoning expertise

Henny P. A. Boshuizen and Henk G. Schmidt

The main objective of medical schools is to turn relative novices into knowledgeable and skilled professionals. Despite all the efforts of teachers and students, clinical teachers are not always content with the outcomes. One complaint is that students might have knowledge about subjects X or Y, but that they do not demonstrate that knowledge in contexts where it has to be applied. Another complaint is that students are not able to solve clinical problems, especially in practical settings. Over the years, these observations have been made by many teachers, inspiring a great deal of research (e.g. Barrows *et al.*, 1978; Elstein *et al.*, 1978) and the introduction of new approaches to teaching medicine, such as problem-based learning (Norman and Schmidt, 1992), aiming at the improvement of clinical reasoning in medicine.

This chapter seeks to answer the question of whether clinical reasoning can be taught to medical students. It starts by describing the development from novice in medicine to expert, providing a theoretical framework. Several approaches to clinical-reasoning skills training are then described and the implications are considered of this theory for the way medical education can improve students' clinical reasoning.

A theory on the development of medical expertise

For a long time, it has been thought that the human mind can be trained in logical thinking, problem solving or creativity. For that purpose children are

encouraged to play chess or to learn Latin in school. Polya's (1957) problem-solving training program also cherishes this general idea about the human mind. In the same vein, it was thought that experts in an arbitrary domain had trained their minds and had developed general problem-solving and thinking skills. This opinion has, however, been superseded, since research outcomes have shown that experts in a specific domain have not developed separate problem-solving skills that can be applied across domains. Instead, domain knowledge and associated skills to use this knowledge in problem solving develop simultaneously. This phenomenon has been observed in very different domains (chess: De Groot, 1965; engineering: Ackermann and Barbichon, 1963; statistics: Allwood and Montgomery, 1981, 1982; mathematics: Bloom and Broder, 1950; physics: Chi *et al.*, 1981).

In medicine, research has shown that clinical reasoning is not a separate skill acquired independently of medical knowledge and other diagnostic skills. Instead, it suggests a stage theory on the development of medical expertise, in which knowledge acquisition and clinical reasoning go hand in hand (see Boshuizen and Schmidt, 1992; Schmidt and Boshuizen, 1992; Schmidt *et al.*, 1990, 1992).

This theory of medical diagnosis is essentially a theory of the acquisition and development of knowledge structures upon which a student or a physician operates diagnosing a case. Structural changes in knowledge result in dramatic changes in problem solving or clinical reasoning.

During the first stage, medical students acquire large amounts of knowledge about the biomedical, basic sciences. They acquire concepts linked together in a knowledge network. By and by, more concepts are added and refined, and more and better connections are made. Knowledge accretion and validation are the students' main concerns in this period of their study. This process takes much more time than teachers might expect. Especially the integration and integrated use of knowledge from different domains (e.g. the clinical sciences, biochemistry, pathophysiology and microanatomy) is not self-evident (see Boshuizen and Van de Wiel, 1998; Groothuis *et al.*, 1998). During this stage the clinical reasoning process is characterized by lines of reasoning consisting of chains of small steps commonly based on detailed, biomedical concepts.

An example of detailed reasoning is given in Table 2.1. It has been taken from a longer protocol in which a fourth year medical student is dealing with a case of pancreatitis. His initial hypothesis set contained gall bladder and pancreas disease. Apparently, this student is entertaining the hypothesis of biliary tract obstruction. First, he reasons whether the new finding about the patient's stools affects this hypothesis and decides that this is not the case. Next, three items later, he combines the information acquired and concludes that there is no inflammation (causing this obstruction) [step 1], hence, no cholecystitis [step 2], hence the biliary tract must be obstructed by something else, a stone for instance [step 3], or a carcinoma [step 4], which

might be the case because the patient has lost weight [step 5].

By the end of the first stage of knowledge acquisition, students have a knowledge network that allows them to make direct lines of reasoning between different concepts within that network. The more often these direct lines are activated the more these concepts cluster together and students become able to make direct links between the first and last concept in such a line of reasoning, skipping intermediate concepts. We have labelled this process 'knowledge encapsulation', a term that refers to the clustering aspect of the process and can account for the automatization involved (e.g. Boshuizen and Schmidt, 1992; Schmidt and Boshuizen, 1993). Many of these concept clusters have (semi-) clinical names, such as micro-embolism, aorta-insufficiency, forward failure or extra-hepatic icterus, providing a powerful reasoning tool.

Encapsulation of biomedical knowledge results in the next stage of development of clinical-reasoning skills, in which biomedical knowledge has been integrated into clinical knowledge. At this stage, students' clinical reasoning processes no longer involve many biomedical concepts. Students tend to make direct links between patient findings and clinical concepts that have the status of hypotheses or diagnoses in their reasoning process. However, if needed, this encapsulated biomedical knowledge can be unfolded again, e.g. when dealing with a very complicated problem.

At the same time, a transition takes place from a network-type of knowledge organization to another

Table 2.1 Lines of reasoning by a fourth medical student

Case item (number and text)	Think-aloud protocol

31 (History)
    Defecation: paler and more malodorous
    stools according to the patient
	. . . not so much undermines that idea . . . er . . . their frequency . . . and their pattern compared with colour and the like . . . their smell . . . er . . . yes . . . no problems with defecation, that means in any case no constipation, which you wouldn't expect with an obstruction of the biliary tract . . . well yes

32 (History) Last bowel movement was yesterday	. . .
32 (History) Temperature: 37°C at 6 p.m.	So no temperature
33 (Physical examination) Pulse rate: regular, 72/min	. . . er . . . yes . . . the past two . . . together . . . means that there's . . . er . . . no inflammation . . . and that would eliminate an . . . er . . . an . . . er . . . cholecystitis . . . and would rather mean an . . . er . . . obstruction of the biliary tract . . . caused by a stone, for instance . . . or, what may be the case too, by a carcinoma, but I wouldn't . . . although, it might be possible, lost 5 kilograms in weight . . .

Note. Protocol fragment obtained from a fourth year medical student working on a pancreatitis case showing detailed reasoning steps. See Boshuizen and Schmidt (1992) for a detailed description of the experiment.

type of structure, which we refer to as 'illness scripts'. Illness scripts have three components. The first component refers to Enabling Conditions of disease, i.e. the conditions or constraints under which a disease occurs. These are the personal, social, medical, hereditary and environmental factors that affect health in a positive or a negative way, or which affect the course of a specific disease. The second component is the Fault, i.e. the pathophysiological process that is taking place in a specific disease, represented in encapsulated form. The third component consists of the Consequences of the Fault, i.e. the signs and symptoms of a specific disease (also see Feltovich and Barrows, 1984, who introduced this theoretical notion).

Contrary to (advanced) novice knowledge networks, illness scripts are activated as a whole. After an illness script has been activated, no active, small-step search within that script is required; the other elements of the script are activated immediately and automatically. Therefore, people whose knowledge is organized in illness scripts have an advantage over those who have only semantic networks at their disposal. While solving a problem, a physician activates one or a few illness scripts. Subsequently the illness script elements (Enabling Conditions and Consequences) are matched to the information provided by the patient. Illness scripts not only incorporate matching information volunteered by the patient, they also generate expectations about other signs and symptoms the patient might have. Activated illness scripts provide a list of phenomena to seek in history taking and in physical examination. In the course of this verification process the script is instantiated; expected values are substituted by real findings, while scripts that fail in this respect will de-activate. The instantiated script yields a diagnosis or a differential diagnosis when a few competing scripts remain active.

An example of script activation by an experienced physician, dealing with the same clinical case as the student in Table 2.1, is given in Table 2.2. The information he heard about the patient's medical past and psycho-social circumstances (summarized in the protocol) are combined with the presenting complaint, and activate a few competing illness scripts: pancreatic disease, liver disease and abdominal malignancy (which he considers implausible due to the patient's age), and stomach perforation. In addition, he thinks of cardiomyopathy as an effect of excessive drinking. In the course of the think-aloud protocol he seemed to monitor the level of instantiation of every illness script. Except for gall bladder disease, no new scripts were activated.

So far we have seen that expert and novice knowledge structures differ in many respects. As a consequence, their clinical reasoning differs as well. Medical experts, who have large numbers of ready-made illness scripts that organize many enabling conditions and consequences associated with a specific disease, will activate one or more of these illness scripts when dealing with a case.

Table 2.2 Illness script activation by a family physician

Case item (number and text)	Think-aloud protocol
8 Complaint: Continuous pain in the upper part of the abdomen, radiating to the back	. . . well, when I am visiting someone who is suffering an acute . . . continuous – since when? – pain in his upper abdomen, radiating to the back, who had pancreatitis a year before . . . of whom I don't know for sure if he still drinks or not after that course of Refusal, but of whom I do know that he still has mental problems, so still receives a disability benefit, then I think that the first thing to cross my mind will be: well, what about that pancreas, . . . how's his liver . . . and also that – considering his age – eh . . . it is not very likely that there will be other things wrong in his abdomen . . . eh . . . of a malign thing . . . er . . . nature . . . of course . . . eh . . . if he's taking huge amounts of alcohol there's always the additional possibility of a stomach . . . eh . . . problem, a stomach perforation . . . . . . excessive drinking can also cause . . . eh . . . serious cardiomyopathy, which . . . eh . . . may cause heart defects . . . mm I can't . . . er . . . judge the word continuous very well yet in this context

Note. Protocol fragment obtained from an experienced family physician working on a pancreatitis case. Earlier, he had received information about enabling conditions such as mental problems and alcohol abuse. See Boshuizen and Schmidt (1992) for a detailed description of the experiment.

Table 2.3 Knowledge restructuring and clinical reasoning at subsequent levels of expertise level

Expertise level	Knowledge representation	Knowledge acquisition and (re)structuring	Clinical reasoning	Control required in clinical reasoning	Demand on cognitive capacity
Novice	Networks	Knowledge accretion and validation	Long chains of detailed reasoning steps through pre-encapsulated networks	Active monitoring of each reasoning step	High
Intermediate	Networks	Encapsulation	Reasoning through encapsulated network	Active monitoring of each reasoning step	Medium
Expert	Illness scripts	Illness script formation (instantiated scripts)	Illness script activation and instantiation	Monitoring of the level of script instantiation	Low

Activation will be triggered by information concerning enabling conditions and/or consequences. Expert hypothesis activation and testing can be seen as an epiphenomenon of illness script activation and instantiation. These are generally automatic and 'unconscious' processes. As long as new information matches an active illness script, no active reasoning is required. Only in case of severe mismatch or conflict does the expert engage in active clinical reasoning. During this process either illness-script-based expectations are adjusted based on specific features of the patient or the expert reverts to pure biomedical reasoning, drawing on de-encapsulated biomedical knowledge.

An example of the first process is given by Lesgold *et al.* (1988), who describe expert radiologist interpretations of an enlarged heart shadow on an X-ray screen. These experts took into consideration the marked scoliosis of the patient's thoracic spine, affecting the position of his heart relative to the slide. Hence, they concluded that the heart was not actually enlarged.

Students, on the other hand, can rely only on knowledge networks, which are less rich and less easily activated than experts' illness scripts. For that reason they will require more information before a specific hypothesis will be generated, only because the disease labels in the network are linked to a very limited number of Enabling Conditions or Consequences. Semantic networks must be reasoned through, step by step. This is a time consuming process and often requires active monitoring. Hence, contrary to illness scripts, the knowledge structures which students activate do not automatically generate a list of signs and symptoms that are expected. Active search through their networks is needed in order to generate such a list of symptoms that might verify or falsify the

hypotheses entertained. In general, students' clinical reasoning is less orderly, less goal oriented and more time consuming, but most importantly, it is based on less plausible hypotheses resulting in less accurate diagnoses than those of experts.

Table 2.3 summarizes these differences between novices, intermediates and experts. The picture that emerges here is that novices and intermediates are handicapped in two ways: Their knowledge is insufficient and requires extra cognitive capacity when solving problems. Both aspects negatively influence clinical problem solving. Teaching should be organized in such a way that both aspects, knowledge structure and control required, improve.

Teaching clinical reasoning

Traditional approaches to enhancing clinical reasoning in students are based on the assumption that clinical reasoning or problem solving is a skill, separate from content knowledge. A typical example is described by Elstein *et al.* (1978). In this training program, students were taught a few heuristics that had been derived from analysis of the reported and observed errors of diagnostic reasoning committed by medical students. For instance as the planning heuristic, students were taught that each piece of information they requested should be related to a plan for solving the problem. They were also taught that they should have at least two or three competing hypotheses under consideration and that each piece of information should be evaluated with respect to all hypotheses presently considered.

It was found, however, that this training program had no significant effects on the students' diagnostic accuracy and cost. Furthermore, it was found that students varied widely in their ability to apply the heuristics recommended in different cases. This finding and outcomes of comparisons of experts and weaker problem solvers suggested to the investigators that differences are more to be found in the repertory of individuals' experiences organized in long-term memory than in differences in the planning and problem-solving heuristics employed.

Until this moment we have avoided defining the concepts of clinical reasoning and clinical-reasoning skills, first giving attention to the knowledge structures upon which these reasoning processes operate. Nor have we addressed the question of whether clinical reasoning can be taught. Generally, clinical reasoning equals the thinking process occurring while dealing with a clinical case. Most researchers differentiate between different stages in the clinical reasoning process: beginning with hypothesis generation, inquiry strategy, data analysis, problem synthesis or diagnosis, and finally ending with diagnostic and treatment decision making. Most often these different stages are thought to require different skills: hypothesis generation skills, inquiry skills, data analysis skills, etc.

Experts, performing better, are supposed to have better skills than novices and intermediates. Barrows and Pickell (1991) take this position. They assume that the clinical reasoning process itself can be improved. From the description of our theory, it will be evident that we take a different position. Despite these differences, there are many correspondences as well. Therefore, in order to picture our position most clearly, we will compare our approach with and differentiate it from that of Barrows and Pickell.

In their book entitled *Developing Clinical Problem Solving Skills: A Guide to More Effective Diagnosis and Treatment*, Barrows and Pickell (1991, pp. xii–xiii) emphasize:

> There are two components of expert clinical problem-solving that need to be considered separately, even though they can not be separated in practice. One is content, the rich, extensive knowledge base about medicine that resides in the long-term memory of the expert. The other is process, the method of knowledge manipulation the expert uses to apply that knowledge to the patient's problem. In expert performance these components are inexorably intertwined. Both are required; a well developed reasoning process appropriately bringing accurate knowledge to bear on a problem in a most effective manner . . . This book should

help you *perfect the process of clinical reasoning* (italics added by Boshuizen and Schmidt) to best deliver the knowledge that you now have (and will acquire in the future) to the care of your patients . . . To develop these skills you must practise, analyse, and repractise them until they are automatic. More important, if you associate your medical-school learning with this regime, your knowledge will be organized for effective recollection in your clinical work.

Their advice focuses the different stages of clinical reasoning and associated skills, e.g. hypothesis generation and testing. For instance, they suggest that students should practise their scientific clinical-reasoning skills at every opportunity. They provide the following advice (Barrows and Pickell, 1991, pp. 215–216):

> To develop an accurate initial concept,[1] look carefully for important initial information as the patient encounter begins.

> Generate a complete set of hypotheses in every patient encounter, carefully watching their degree of specificity and their complementarity. Be sure to watch out for hidden biases.

> Use your creativity, and your inductive skills, to develop these hypotheses.

> Use your critical deductive skills to inquire in a manner that will establish the more likely hypothesis.

> Generate new hypotheses whenever your inquiries become unproductive or new data make your present hypotheses less likely.

> In both your hypothesis generation and in inquiry strategy, be guided by an awareness of the basic pathophysiologic mechanism that may be operative in your patient's problem.

Superficially, the advice given suggests many correspondences with our theory. For instance, the authors' suggestion to look for important initial information as the patient encounter begins, agrees with our emphasis on the role of enabling conditions in script activation. But what if a student does not have any scripts? Furthermore, their proposition to be aware of the basic pathophysiologic mechanism that might play a role corresponds with our conceptions of Fault. In our theory, applying biomedical knowledge would be helpful if a diagnostician cannot activate a matching illness script.

---

[1] The term 'initial concept' refers to the first interpretation and representation of a patient's problem constructed by the doctor or student.

However, the difference between our approach and that of Barrows and Pickell is that these authors suggest that every student and physician, independent of level of expertise, should always apply these skills, while our theory suggests that applying information about enabling conditions or activating basic science knowledge are not skills, but are phenomena associated with a person's knowledge structure. More importantly, as long as the student does not have the relevant knowledge, many of the suggestions given can only be counterproductive.

This analysis generates the question of whether clinical-reasoning skills can be taught and trained as such or whether other educational measures will be needed in order to improve a student's clinical reasoning. It might be evident that our theory and previous experiences with direct training programs suggest that other measures are needed, as far as the cognitive, the reasoning component of the diagnostic process is concerned. What is more important, our theory suggests that in order to improve clinical reasoning, education must focus on the development of adequate knowledge structures. Hence, teaching, training, coaching, modelling or supervising should adapt to the actual knowledge organization of the student.

During the first stage in which knowledge accretion and validation take place, students should be given ample opportunity to test the knowledge they have acquired for its consistency and connectedness, and to correct concepts and their connections and to fill the gaps they have detected. Students will do many of these things by themselves if they are provided with stimuli for thinking and with appropriate feedback. This stuff for thinking does not necessarily have to consist of patient problems. One could also think of short descriptions of physiological phenomena (e.g. jet lag) that have to be explained.

During the following stage of knowledge encapsulation, students should deal with (more elaborate) patient problems. As the student goes through the process of diagnosing a patient and afterwards explaining the diagnosis to a peer or a supervisor, biomedical knowledge will become encapsulated into higher level concepts. For instance, diagnosing a patient with acute bacterial endocarditis will first require detailed reasoning about infection, fever reaction, temperature regulation, circulation, haemodynamics, etc. Later on, a similar case will be explained in terms of bacterial infection, sepsis, microembolisms and aortic insufficiency (Boshuizen, 1989).

These problems are not necessarily presented by real patients in real settings. Paper cases and simulated patients will serve the same goal, sometimes even better. Especially during the earlier stage of knowledge encapsulation, when students have to do a great deal of reasoning, it might be more helpful to work with paper cases that present all relevant information. Reasoning through their knowledge networks in order to build a coherent explanation of the information available, students need not be concerned whether the information on which they work is complete and valid. Later in this stage, when knowledge has been restructured into a more tightly connected format, greater uncertainty can be allowed.

Finally, the stage of illness script acquisition requires experience with real patients in real settings. Research by Custers *et al.* (1993) suggests that at this stage, practical experience with typical patients (i.e. patients whose disease manifestations resemble the textbooks) should be preferred over experiences with atypical patients. There are no empirical data that can help to answer the question of whether illness script formation requires active dealing with the patient, or whether observing a doctor–patient contact could serve the same goal. On the other hand, since encapsulation and script formation go hand in hand, especially earlier on in this stage, it is probable that 'hands on' experience is to be preferred. Having to reason about the patient would result in further knowledge encapsulation, while direct interaction with the patient provides the opportunity for perceptual learning, adding 'reality' to the symbolic concepts learned from textbooks.

During this phase students might initially be overwhelmed by the information available in reality. They can easily overlook information when they do not know its relevance. This will especially affect their perception of Enabling Conditions. Therefore, it might be helpful to draw the student's attention to the Enabling Conditions operating in specific patients, to make sure that their illness scripts are completed with this kind of information. Boshuizen *et al.* (1992) emphasize that in this stage of training a mix of practical experience and theoretical education is needed. They have found that during clinical rotations students tend to shift toward the application of clinical knowledge although it is not yet fully integrated in their knowledge base. A combination of the two ways of learning can help students to build a robust and flexible knowledge base.

Thus we see that working on problems and diagnosing and explaining patient cases, applying biomedical knowledge and providing feedback on the student's thinking might help them to form a knowledge system that enables efficient and accurate clinical reasoning that does not require all control capacity available (monitoring of reasoning on encapsulated concepts in a network requires less control than monitoring of reasoning on pre-encapsulated, detailed concepts; see Table 2.3). However, in practice, clinical reasoning must be performed in a context of real patients.

In the end, students should be able to collect information through history taking, physical examination and laboratory, guided by their clinical reasoning process, and to find a (preliminary) diagnosis in the time available. A well-organized knowledge base is a first requirement, along with well-trained social, perceptual and psychomotor skills.[2] Hence, students must learn to do their clinical reasoning and to perform these skills in a coordinated way. This again necessitates training and practice (Patrick, 1992).

The same discussion as occurred earlier in this chapter concerning the possibility of separating knowledge acquisition and the acquisition of clinical reasoning can be repeated regarding the question of whether a well-organized knowledge base and well-trained social, perceptual and psychomotor skills could be acquired independently. Van Merri'nboer (1997) has shown that a good planning and design of the learning process, such that integration and automatization are fostered, is very important. A good combination of learning environments like part-task practise, timely presentation of information, whole task practise, and elaboration and understanding might be the key to success.

The reader might have observed a similarity between what has been proposed in this chapter and problem-based curricula. This similarity is not incidental. However, our suggestions for learning with cases and from practical experience do not necessarily require a problem-based curriculum. They can be applied in traditional course-based curricula as well. On the other hand, not every problem-based curriculum is structured in the way we have proposed. For example, a program that uses problems as a starting point for learning may neglect the encapsulation function of working with cases. In our opinion it is essential that students do not work with problems and cases only. They also need an educational program, based on an insight into the different obstacles that students experience at successive stages of development toward expertise.

The question remains, whether the phases in knowledge structure development should be translated into a curriculum in which a complete, coherent and well-integrated knowledge base is first required, followed by a term in which knowledge is encapsulated, and completed by a period in which illness scripts are formed. As far as our theory and the available empirical evidence are concerned, there is no need at all for such a strict separation. Intuitively we say, 'better not'. If students have developed a complete knowledge base of a specific subject, e.g. the effects of vitamin B12 deficiency on the cellular and organic level, there is no need to prevent encapsulation as long as students remain willing and able to adjust their knowledge base and re-encapsulate when new knowledge is acquired. For motivational reasons it would be preferable to construct a curriculum in which different phases overlap.

Acknowledgements

Preparation of this chapter was enabled by a grant to the first author by the Spencer Foundation, National Academy of Education, USA.

References

Ackermann, W. and Barbichon, G. (1963) Conduites intellectuelles et activité technique. *Bulletin CERP*, **12**, 1–16.

Allwood, C. M. and Montgomery, H. (1981) Knowledge and technique in statistical problem solving. *European Journal of Science Education*, **3**, 431–450.

Allwood, C. M. and Montgomery, H. (1982) Detection of errors in statistical problem solving. *Scandinavian Journal of Psychology*, **23**, 131–140.

Barrows, H. S., Feightner, J. W., Neufeld, V. R. and Norman, G. R. (1978) *An Analysis of the Clinical Method of Medical Students and Physicians*. Hamilton, Ontario: McMaster University.

Barrows, H. S. and Pickell, G. C. (1991) *Developing Clinical Problem-Solving Skills: A Guide to More Effective Diagnosis and Treatment*. New York: Norton.

Bloom, B. S. and Broder, L. J. (1950) *Problem Solving Processes of College Students*. Chicago: University of Chicago Press.

Boshuizen, H. P. A. (1989) De ontwikkeling van medische expertise; een cognitief-psychologische benadering (The development of medical expertise; a cognitive-psychological approach). *PhD thesis*. University of Limburg, Maastricht.

---

[2] These skills have a knowledge component, which makes it quite difficult to train them in isolation, separate from knowledge acquisition

Boshuizen, H. P. A., Hobus, P. P. M., Custers, E. J. F. M. and Schmidt, H. G. (1992) Cognitive effects of practical experience. In *Advanced Models of Cognition for Medical Training and Practice* (A. E. Evans and V. L. Patel, eds). New York: Springer.

Boshuizen, H. P. A. and Schmidt, H. G. (1992) On the role of biomedical knowledge in clinical reasoning by experts, intermediates and novices. *Cognitive Science*, **16**, 153–184.

Boshuizen, H. P. A. and Wiel, M. W. J. van den (1998) Multiple representations in medicine: How students struggle with it. In *Learning with Multiple Representations* (M. W. van Someren, P. Reimann, H. P. A. Boshuizen and T. de Jong, eds). Amsterdam: Elsevier, in press.

Chi, M. T. H., Feltovich, P. J. and Glaser, R. (1981) Categorization and representation of physics problems by experts and novices. *Cognitive Science*, **5**, 121–152.

Custers, E. J. F. M., Boshuizen, H. P. A. and Schmidt, H. G. (1993) The influence of typicality of case descriptions on subjective disease probability estimations. Paper presented at the *Annual Meeting of the American Educational Research Association*, Atlanta, GA.

De Groot, A. D. (1965) *Thought and Choice in Chess*. The Hague: Mouton.

Elstein, A. S., Shulman, L. S. and Sprafka, S. A. (1978) *Medical Problem Solving: An Analysis of Clinical Reasoning*. Cambridge, MA: Harvard University Press.

Feltovich, P. J. and Barrows, H. S. (1984) Issues of generality in medical problem solving. In *Tutorials in Problem-Based Learning: A New Direction in Teaching the Health Professions* (H. G. Schmidt and M. L. De Volder, eds), pp. 128–142. Assen: Van Gorcum.

Groothuis, S., Boshuizen, H. P. A. and Talmon, J. L. (1998) Analysis of the conceptual difficulties of the endocrinology domain and an empirical analysis of student and expert understanding of that domain. *Teaching and Learning in Medicine*, **10**, 207–216.

Lesgold, A, Rubinson, H., Feltovich, P. J., Glaser, R. and Klopfer, D. (1988) Expertise in a complex skill: Diagnosing X-ray pictures. In *The Nature of Expertise* (M. T. H. Chi, R. Glaser and M. Farr, eds), pp. 311–342. Hillsdale, NJ: Lawrence Erlbaum.

Merri'nboer, J. J. G. van (1997) *Training Complex Cognitive Skills: A Four-Component Instructional Design Model for Technical Training*. Englewood Cliffs, NJ: Educational Technology Publications.

Norman, G. R. and Schmidt, H. G. (1992) The psychological basis of problem-based learning: A review of the evidence. *Academic Medicine*, **67**, 557–565.

Patrick, J. (1992) *Training: Theory and Practice*. London: Academic Press.

Polya, G. (1957) *How to Solve it*. Garden City, NY: Doubleday.

Schmidt, H. G. and Boshuizen, H. P. A. (1992) Encapsulation of biomedical knowledge. In *Advanced Models of Cognition for Medical Training and Practice* (A. E. Evans and V. L. Patel, eds). New York: Springer.

Schmidt, H. G. and Boshuizen, H. P. A. (1993) On acquiring expertise in medicine. *Educational Psychology Review*, **5**, 205–221.

Schmidt, H. G., Boshuizen, H. P. A. and Norman, G. R. (1992) Reflections on the nature of expertise in medicine. In *Deep Models for Medical Knowledge Engineering* (E. Keravnou, ed.), pp. 231–248. Amsterdam: Elsevier.

Schmidt, H. G., Norman, G. R. and Boshuizen, H. P. A. (1990) A cognitive perspective on medical expertise: Theory and implications. *Academic Medicine*, **65**, 611–621.

3

Knowledge and reasoning[1]

Joy Higgs and Angie Titchen

Knowledge is a fundamental element in the definition and operation of a profession. Firstly, the body of knowledge of a profession is a key to delineating and describing the profession, and the generation of knowledge by the profession is a charter of being a profession. Secondly, knowledge is essential for reasoning and decision making which are central to professional practice. In the health professions, clinical reasoning provides the vehicle for knowledge use in clinical practice as well as for knowledge generation. Thus, knowledge and clinical reasoning are interdependent phenomena.

Approaches to generating knowledge

Health professionals have a responsibility to contribute to the development of their profession's knowledge base as well as to continually expand and critique their own knowledge. In addition, they are charged with employing strategies (including research) with a clear understanding of the expected outcomes (e.g. the type of knowledge they could produce), and of the assumptions, conditions and rules of using these tools and strategies.

The qualitative and quantitative research approaches, the scientific method, and the constructivist and critical science research approaches are different paths to knowledge and different practices. These paths are 'shaped by different aims, standards, values, and social and political realities' and thus 'are rooted not simply in matters of epistemology but in relations of power, influence, and control in communities of inquirers' (Eisner, 1988). To dismiss the various research paradigms/approaches as just so many methodological dogmas is to reduce social inquiry to matters of technique, separating the means of inquiry from the issues of purpose, value and assumptions that shape the very act of inquiry itself (Schwandt, 1989). 'To focus solely on techniques and procedures produces certain limitations to the conduct of inquiry ... the lack of situating concepts and techniques within their social and philosophical contexts produces knowledge that is often trivial and socially conservative' (Popkewitz, 1984, p. 3).

Research paradigms provide frameworks for generating knowledge. The term *paradigm* is used in science to describe the model within which a community of scientists generates knowledge. Within a paradigm, assumptions, problems, research strategies, criteria and techniques are shared and accepted by the community. To claim that we are working within a particular research paradigm, then, requires us to understand the principal assumptions and conventions of that paradigm. In particular, researchers who are knowledgeably and informedly working within a particular paradigm have chosen to accept the common understanding of that paradigm in relation to the following questions.

[1] This chapter is written from the perspective of a researcher and practitioner (and not that of a philosopher) in an attempt to understand ontology and epistemology in ways that inform both practice and research.

What can we know? What is reality?

A defining feature of a research paradigm is the ontological assumptions of that paradigm. Ontology is defined as 'the theory of existence or, more narrowly, of what really exists, as opposed to that which appears to exist but does not' (Bullock and Trombley, 1988, p. 605).

How can what exists be known?

Strongly related to ontology (which deals with what exists, what is reality, what is the nature of the world) is epistemology (which deals with how what exists may be known) or 'the philosophical theory of knowledge which seeks to define it, distinguish its principal varieties, identify its sources, and establish its limits' (Bullock and Trombley, 1988, p. 279).

What kinds of knowledge exist? What is true knowledge?

We support a view of knowledge in which both personal and public validation are sought, where both propositional (theoretical/scientific) and non-propositional knowledge are accorded validity, and where knowledge is regarded as a dynamic phenomenon undergoing constant change and testing. We distinguish between knowledge of the individual and knowledge of the field. The former refers to the knowledge base constructed by the individual through learning, discovery, processing of experience and testing of emerging knowledge claims. The latter refers to knowledge claims by a particular group which currently have general acceptance within the field, discipline or paradigm in question. Again such knowledge claims imply the need for both conviction and testing.

This interpretation of knowledge is largely based on a constructivist perspective which contends that all knowledge is 'a deliberate construction of human beings striving to know about nature and experience' (Gowin, 1981, p. 27). The key elements of this definition are that knowledge is constructed not discovered, that individuals create unique constructions or interpretations of nature and of their own experiences, and that knowledge is the product of a dynamic and indeed difficult process of knowing, or striving to understand. In such striving, the individual's depth and certainty of knowledge grows. In addition, what is being learned and the relationships between elements of such knowledge are tested and refined, both against the individual's prior knowledge and experience, and also against

external knowledge (including the knowledge and experiences of others and the established knowledge of the field).

The nature of the evidence which validates knowledge is an important element of knowledge interpretation. In particular, it is important to note that as well as being individually constructed, reality and knowledge are socially constructed. That is, reality exists because we give meaning to it (Berger and Luckmann, 1985). Thus, the individual's perceptions of reality, truth and knowledge have subjective dimensions or interpretations, as well as objective dimensions (reflecting the *world out there*). What is termed 'objective reality', although it is a socially constructed interpretation of the world out there, gains an objective character or is seen as evidence, because of its testing in the public domain and because it 'transcends the domain of subjective or private experience' (Wildemeersch, 1989, p. 63).

Despite the importance of knowledge validation it is essential also to see knowledge as a developing or dynamic phenomenon. Perkins (1986, p. xiii), for instance, presents the concept of 'active knowledge that one thinks critically and creatively about and with, not just passive knowledge that does little but await the final exam'. Similarly, Kleinig (1982, p. 152) argues 'the knowing subject must continually reflect on and test what is presented to it'. Ayer (1956, p. 222) takes the argument further by contending that when seeking to verify knowledge claims we should take scepticism of these claims seriously, since it will enable us to learn 'to distinguish the different levels at which our claims to knowledge stand'. Thus, knowing is a continual process of generating, refining and understanding knowledge. Clinicians need to develop an appreciation of the reliability of their knowledge; to be able to defend their knowledge, but at the same time, acknowledge that much of the range and depth of their knowledge has conditional certainty in terms of contextual relevance and durability.

What kinds of knowledge will be recognized in a paradigm?

Many writers have emphasized that the type of knowledge obtained from research will be dependent on the paradigm adopted (Habermas, 1972; Domholdt, 1993; Guba and Lincoln, 1994). Conversely, the type of knowledge desired (how the research question is posed) will be a major factor in determining which paradigm is adopted. Powers and Knapp (1995, p. 133) contend that quantitative research reflects a realist view of the world (philosophy) which asserts that physical reality exists independently of being perceived. Realist philosophy supports the *received view* of what counts as knowledge. In this perspective, 'the purpose of research is to describe, explain, and predict subsequent occurrences of objectifiable phenomena in order to produce or control desired outcomes'. In comparison, Powers and Knapp (1995, p. 133) argue that the collection of research methods labelled 'qualitative' reflect an idealist philosophy which 'questions the possibility of a mind-independent world, insisting that the external material world is known through the perceptions and subjectivity of humans'.

Research paradigms

Three research paradigms will be considered in this discussion: the empirico-analytical paradigm, the interpretive paradigm and the critical research paradigm.

The empirico-analytical paradigm

The scientific method (as adopted in the natural sciences) belongs to the empirico-analytical paradigm. It is based on positivist philosophy and dominated the philosophy of science from the 1920s to the 1960s (Manley, 1991). The scientific paradigm or empiricist model of knowledge relies on observation and experiment in the empirical world, resulting in generalizations about the content and events of the world, which can be used to predict future experience (Moore, 1982). Knowledge is discovered (i.e. universal and external truths are grasped) and justified on the basis of empirical processes which are reductionist, value-neutral, quantifiable, objective and operationalizable. Only statements publicly verifiable by sense data are valid. This paradigm is the basis for the medical model and for the development of technical knowledge which is used, for example, when diagnosing the cause of a patient's symptoms and determining the most effective intervention for treating the cause.

In many of the health professions it is questioned whether the medical model and its underlying paradigm is a sufficient or indeed preferred model for the health sciences. The medical model is increasingly being regarded as inappropriate for the study of people by other health professions and

for holistic care which balances biological, behavioural and spiritual aspects of human functioning. This questioning is evident in nursing (Doering, 1992; Holmes, 1990), in physiotherapy (Parry, 1991, 1997; Shepard, 1987) and in occupational therapy (Breines, 1990; Mattingly, 1991). Practitioners in these fields identify a dissonance between the philosophical bases for practice and research (Holmes, 1990; Manley, 1991). There is a greater emphasis, in nursing and occupational therapy in particular, on the humanistic movement and on knowledge generated within the interpretive and critical paradigms. Humanistic psychology has derived much of its theoretical support from the existential-phenomenological approach to the understanding of human events (Holmes, 1990). In this approach, knowledge relates to the individual's consciousness and feelings arising from his/her experiences (Kneller, 1958), and knowledge is generated through a search for meaning, beliefs and values, and through looking for wholes and relationships with other wholes. This way of knowing is different to that in the medical model where facts are described and phenomena are reduced to component parts to describe, explain and predict how, when and where these parts work.

Skinner (1985, p. 6) argues that the empirico-analytical paradigm relies on the 'fundamentally misconceived' argument that 'all successful explanations must conform to the same deductive model' and fails to recognize that 'the explanation of human behaviour and the explanation of natural events are logically distinct undertakings'. Psychologists argue that the normative presuppositions of positivism and the desire to analyse behaviour by causal laws fails to recognize the individual's ability to choose and to act strategically, rather than simply responsively (Skinner, 1985). Similarly, Habermas (1974) argues that in trying to model the social sciences on the natural sciences, 'positivism' fails to recognize one of the significant features which makes us human, the capacity for 'self-reflection' or 'reflexivity' and the consequent ability to change our future (in Giddens, 1985). The scientific method is also criticized for its rejection of the effects of the nature and uniqueness of the contexts in which human beings exist (Manley, 1991).

The interpretive paradigm

We suggest that the interpretive paradigm is often more suited to the generation of knowledge in the human sciences, in both its philosophical stance and the methods utilized. Ontologically, the interpretive paradigm acknowledges relativism and local, multiple and specific constructed realities. Interpretive paradigm research seeks to interpret phenomena, particularly human phenomena, and thereby to generate knowledge of these phenomena. The various approaches do not look for cause–effect relationships or use the experimental method; rather they look at the whole phenomenon under investigation and take account of the context of the situation, the timings, the subjective meanings and intentions within the particular situation. They also seek to uncover the meanings and significant aspects of the situation from the perspective of the actor. Methodologically this paradigm includes a variety of research traditions originating in such fields as philosophy, psychology, sociology and anthropology, as follows:

- *Hermeneutic inquiry* refers to the theory and practice of interpretation. Writing in this tradition, Gadamer (1975) contends that to understand human behaviour we need to seek to understand the reasons behind that behaviour or the unarticulated questions to which the text (qualitative data in some form) is the answer. He also states that understanding is a holistic process, seeking the relationship of the individual phenomenon to our conception of the totality in question.
- *Constructivist philosophy* is 'concerned with how people individually make sense of their worlds and how they create personal systems of meaning that guide them throughout their lives' (Candy, 1991, p. xv).
- *Ethnography* describes a phenomenon from a given societal or cultural focus (Omery, 1988).
- *Phenomenology* (Benner, 1994; Heidegger, 1962; Schutz, 1962) provides another valuable alternative. It strives 'to understand and describe lived experiences' (Swanson-Kauffman and Schonwald, 1988, p. 97) and to bring to the surface phenomena which usually remain hidden in practice itself due their ordinariness or taken-for-grantedness. These approaches generate practical knowledge. Such knowledge would inform practitioners' understanding of, for example, patients' and families' responses to illness and disability. These kinds of understanding would contribute to clinical reasoning and could help practitioners to develop skill in making clinical decisions in partnership with patients and families.

The critical paradigm

The critical paradigm generates emancipatory knowledge which enhances awareness of how our thinking is socially and historically constructed, and how this limits our actions, in order to enable us to challenge these learned restrictions, compulsions or dictates of habit, and to transform current structures, relationships and conditions which constrain development and reform (Freire, 1970). This tradition of generating emancipatory knowledge was established in the early 19th century in German universities. In this epistemology, knowledge is not grasped or discovered but is acquired through critical debate (Barnett, 1990). The emancipatory tradition also focuses on the development of the individual, assuming that the process of becoming an adult requires critical thinking, reflecting upon the assumptions which underlie ideas and actions, and considering alternative ways of thinking (Brookfield, 1987). The continuous development of the individual is described by Mezirow (1981) as 'perspective transformation'. He uses the term 'transformation learning' to describe 'the process of learning through critical self-reflection, which results in the reformulation of a meaning perspective to allow a more inclusive, discriminating, and integrative understanding of one's experience' and a greater capacity to act on those insights (Mezirow, 1990, p. xvi). The research traditions used in this paradigm include action research and collaborative or participative inquiry. Emancipatory knowledge is useful in clinical reasoning when seeking solutions to problems that seem inevitable because of seemingly unchangeable organizational structures, relations and social conditions.

Ways of knowing

In addition to exploring research paradigms to identify methods of generating knowledge, it is valuable to consider other fields of study, particularly education, which have examined a broader concept, 'ways of knowing'. Four frameworks for categorizing ways of knowing are:

- Habermas (1972) proposes three forms of empirical knowledge, technical, practical and emancipatory, derived from the empirico-analytical paradigm, interpretive paradigm and critical paradigm respectively.
- Reason and Heron's (1986) framework comprises experiential knowledge (gained through direct encounter with persons, places or things),

practical knowledge (gained through activity and related to skills or competencies) and propositional knowledge (knowledge of things, gained through conversation/reading, etc.).

- Carper (1978) identifies four fundamental patterns of knowing: empirics (science), aesthetics (art), personal knowledge and ethics (moral knowledge), and proposes that none of them alone should be considered sufficient or mutually exclusive. Building on Carper's work, Sarter (1988) adds a fifth way of knowing called 'intellectual/interpretive', which includes gaining knowledge through philosophical analysis, metaphysical analysis or hermeneutics.
- Kolb (1984) argues that new knowledge is generated through confrontation among four modes of experiential learning: concrete experience, reflective observations, abstract conceptualization and active experimentation. To make sense of learning experiences, the learner needs abilities in each of these four areas.

In clinical practice we need various forms of knowledge, such as those identified above. Restricting ourselves to any single paradigm or way of knowing can result in a limitation to the range of knowledge and the depth of understanding which can be applied to a given problem situation. Schön (1987, p. 13) concludes that professional practice requires a combination of the different paradigms. He argues that, 'in the terrain of professional practice, applied science and research-based technique occupy a critically important though limited territory, bounded on several sides by artistry' which is 'an exercise in intelligence, a kind of knowing [that is] . . . inherent in the practice of professionals'. For effective clinical reasoning, we consider that health professionals rely upon the scientific knowledge of human behaviour and body responses in health and illness, the aesthetic perception of significant human experiences, a personal understanding of the uniqueness of the self and others, and the ability to make decisions within concrete situations involving particular moral judgements. Each way of knowing, therefore, has a place in the education of health science students and in the practice of clinical reasoning.

Types of knowledge

In Western philosophy, knowledge has been commonly classified into two categories, propositional knowledge (or 'knowing that') and non-propositional knowledge (or 'knowing how') (Polanyi, 1958). Propositional knowledge is derived through research and scholarship, with an attempt to generalize findings. Non-propositional knowledge is derived primarily through practice, without an attempt to generalize beyond the practitioner's own experience. A perceptible hierarchical relationship has developed between propositional and non-propositional knowledge, with the former having a higher status. However, we support Barnett's (1990) argument that modern society is unreasonably dominated by the cognitive framework of science, to the extent that other forms of knowledge are downgraded and not even regarded as real knowledge. He argues that in a world where problems are not discrete nor solutions definite, we need knowledge beyond science.

In this chapter we present three overlapping and interactive types of knowledge. We use the label *propositional knowledge* to refer to theoretical or research knowledge which has been ratified or supported by the field; and we describe two forms of non-propositional knowledge, *professional craft knowledge* which incorporates 'knowing how' and tacit knowledge of the profession, and *personal knowledge* or knowledge which is tied to the individual's reality or experience.

Propositional knowledge

Propositional knowledge is public, objective knowledge of the field and knowledge of the external world. It encompasses book knowledge and the presentation of the abstract, logical and formal relationships between concepts or constructs, and formal statements concerning interactional and causal relationships between events (Benner, 1984). Heron (1981, p. 27) states that 'the outcome of research is stated in propositions, which claim to be assertions of facts or truths, a contribution to the corpus of knowledge statements'. Propositional knowledge can be generated in any research paradigm, whether empirico-analytical, interpretive or critical. Related terms are discursive knowledge (rational knowledge resulting from discourse) and declarative knowledge ['knowing about a topic so that one may declare that knowledge; an aspect of espoused knowledge' (Biggs and Telfer, 1987, p. 543)].

Professional craft knowledge

According to Schön (1987, p. 10) there is increasing concern about the growing gap between the research-based (propositional) knowledge taught in professional schools and the practical knowledge and 'actual competencies required of practitioners in the field'. Schön argues that in order to deal with the crisis of professional knowledge and education we need to recognize that outstanding practitioners do not have more professional knowledge but more 'wisdom', 'talent', 'intuition' or 'artistry'. We need to assimilate such knowledge into the dominant model of (propositional) professional knowledge and to give this artistic knowledge recognition in an environment which supports the hegemony of technical knowledge.[2]

Procedural (Biggs and Telfer, 1987) or practical (Benner, 1984; Heron, 1981) knowledge encompasses practical expertise and skills. It guides everyday activities of caring for patients and underpins the practitioner's rapid and fluent response to a situation. Short-term, taken-for-granted goals are achieved by strategies which take account of, and show sensitivity to a multiplicity of situational variables. The practitioner reacts to the whole situation and makes highly skilled judgements without being conscious of a deliberate way of acting. Such knowledge is often tacit in nature and may remain hidden if practitioners do not reflect upon or document their everyday practice.

The ability of health practitioners to interpret incomplete and ambiguous data and to identify implications which are not directly deducible from explicit data depends upon clinical knowledge or judgement which can be likened to intuitive knowledge (as described by Agan, 1987; McCormack, 1992). Such knowledge or judgement can be considered a learned awareness or contextual receptivity, as compared to the more innate idea of intuition as an inherent individual and idiosyncratic phenomenon. Clinical intuition or clinical judgement is compatible with analytical clinical reasoning, and is often used in a complementary manner (Benner and Tanner, 1987). The depth of clinical judgement or intuition demonstrated by an expert clinician is, we argue, born of a wealth of personal experience of clinical practice in combination with a processing of prior learning.

An alternative term or metaphor, 'professional craft knowledge',[3] has been introduced which combines these different types of non-propositional knowledge (Brown and McIntyre, 1993; Titchen, 1996, 1998a). In this chapter we use this metaphor to refer to knowledge within the professional domain which has both public and individual forms. This term incorporates the notions of (clinical) intuitive knowledge or professional judgement and the cognitive aspects of practical knowledge and experiential knowledge as described here. We use the term 'professional craft knowledge' because it is rhetorically useful in that it gives a sense of the aesthetic and of knowing what and when, as well as how. Along with empirical knowledge (technical, practical and emancipatory knowledge) a practitioner uses this tacit and individual professional craft knowledge in problem solving and in making clinical judgements (Carroll, 1988).

Personal knowledge

Personal knowledge is a category of knowledge with particular relevance to clinical reasoning in the health professions. It is defined here as the unique frame of reference and knowledge of self which is central to the individual's sense of self. It is the result of the individual's personal experiences and reflections on these experiences (Butt *et al.*, 1982). Our use of this term incorporates but extends Carper's (1978) concept of personal knowledge as knowing oneself.

The individual's internal frame of reference and store of personal knowledge shape the architecture of the self and the individual's construction of reality, and create what could be termed the individual's unique personal intentionality (Butt, 1985). Weiser (1987) uses the term 'consciousness' to refer to the primary frames of meaning we use to interpret our own life and the world. The individual's behaviour is highly influenced by his/her frame of reference. Within this frame of reference, scientific knowledge and professional knowledge are translated into decisions for practice which are influenced by the individual's convictions and judgements about the worth of this knowledge and its relevance to the current situation. New knowledge is compared

---

[2] We are aware that some curriculum developers and educators in nursing and the health care professions are beginning to value non-propositional knowledge and to reshape professional knowledge maps in their curricula, but we suspect that these cases are in a minority and that the majority of health systems still place more value on propositional knowledge and on technical knowledge in particular.

[3] Titchen (1998a) includes personal knowledge in her description and analysis of professional craft knowledge, but in this chapter we make a distinction between professional craft knowledge and personal knowledge.

with the individual's existing system of beliefs and values. If new knowledge or ideas are incongruent with their belief system, individuals may reject the new information. Barnett (1990) argues that the generation of knowledge by the individual is a developmental process which occurs within a value system and that these values provide an important influence on the knowledge which develops.

Within the health professions it is the well-being of the whole person which lies at the heart of health care. Clinicians need to develop a personal knowledge base, including a depth of self-understanding which will enable them to understand complex human desires for dignity, independence and support, to appreciate the concerns, needs and frames of reference of their patients or clients, to learn to cope with pain, frailty and human endeavour, and to learn to deal with ethical dilemmas within the clinical situation. According to Hundert (1987) this is achieved through the development of a dynamic 'reflective equilibrium'. Personal knowledge needs to incorporate affective (feelings), conative (purposefulness, will) and spiritual elements of self, to look beyond the limits of cognition. In considering personal knowledge and its place in clinical reasoning, we encourage educators to adopt an approach which values and focuses on personal experience and which does not diminish or lose the 'humanness' of a relationship.

The importance of developing and testing knowledge

Because of continual changes in health and illness phenomena and related sciences and technologies, propositional knowledge in the health fields will continue to face rapid growth as well as rapid obsolescence. Ongoing research and theoretical development conducted within the three research paradigms is required, particularly in developing professions. Professional craft knowledge possibly provides a deeper and more practical basis for coping with the uncertainties of health care contexts.

At the same time, professional craft knowledge is faced with demands for public verification and accountability, and methods of making it accessible and available for public scrutiny need to be found. Research conducted in the interpretive paradigm is now bringing this knowledge into the public domain (e.g. Benner, 1984; Lawler, 1991). Building on the methods of such research, one of us (A. T.) conducted a study which suggests that critical

companionship[4] is an effective way of accessing this knowledge, scrutinizing it publicly and enabling its transformation into propositional knowledge (see Titchen, 1998a,b). Using facilitation methods derived from qualitative research methods and educational theories, the critical companion helps expert practitioners to surface, articulate and then reflect critically upon their professional craft knowledge. Once these practitioners are able to make this knowledge available to other expert practitioners (in the same field) and compare, debate and critique it, then consensual validation and verification could be sought. A. T. suggests that groups of expert practitioners could be assisted by critical companions at local, regional, national and international levels to test this consensual knowledge through critical dialogue and debate. Thus professional craft knowledge could become propositional knowledge through the methods of the critical research paradigm without necessarily accepting all its assumptions.

Personal knowledge is an essential element in the ability to deal with the interpersonal, ethical, emotional and spiritual aspects of human interactions and the clinician's choices and dilemmas, and needs to be validated. This knowledge should work in harmony with each of the two other areas of knowledge to provide the depth of understanding which is needed to underpin effective clinical reasoning. Self-evaluation and an understanding of the need to test and re-test one's individual knowledge base to justify knowledge claims are also essential. We propose that critical companionship can help practitioners to achieve this harmony, self-evaluation and testing.

Knowledge and clinical reasoning

Knowledge and thinking are interdependent, since the development of knowledge requires thinking, and thinking can be defined as the ability to apply knowledge (Nickerson *et al.*, 1985). According to Rumelhart and Ortony (1977, p. 99) people 'process and reprocess information, imposing on it and producing from it knowledge which has structure' and creating a human memory system which is 'a vast repository of such knowledge'. The value of the individuals' existing cognitive

---

[4] *Critical companionship* is a metaphor for a helping relationship in which the critical companion accompanies practitioners on their personal, experiential learning journey – in this case, learning to articulate and critique professional craft knowledge.

structure to their cognition and their generation of knowledge was identified by Ausubel (1977, p. 94), who stressed the importance of 'the availability in cognitive structure of specifically relevant anchoring ideas'.

The nature of knowledge structures and their use in reasoning is illustrated in the study of *schemata* (abstractions or representations of previous experience). 'Schema theory attempts to describe how acquired knowledge is organized and represented and how such cognitive structures facilitate the use of knowledge in particular ways' (Glaser, 1984, p. 100). Schemata are particularly valuable in that they provide background knowledge (often tacit knowledge) which helps people interpret new information. New events are labelled 'instantiations' of these schemata (Howard, 1987). As new instances are interpreted, the prior knowledge constructions or schemata are tested. The process of categorization also provides a means (and theory) for the structuring of knowledge. Medin (1989, p. 1469) emphasizes the importance of categorization, saying that 'clinicians need some way to bring their knowledge and experience to bear on the problem under consideration, and that requires the appreciation of some similarity or relationship between the current situation and what has gone before'.

The importance of domain-specific knowledge in problem-solving expertise is widely supported (Bordage and Lemieux, 1986; Grant and Marsden, 1987). Baron and Sternberg (1987, p. 28), however, argue that 'although domain-specific knowledge is essential to good thinking within a domain, it is not sufficient to assure that good thinking will occur'. As well as relevant knowledge, skills in cognition (critical, creative, reflective and dialectical thinking) and metacognition are essential for effective thinking and problem solving. Similarly, Alexander and Judy (1988) conclude that 'there are at any rate two undisputed findings from cognitive research over the last 20 years. One is that those who know more about a particular domain generally understand and remember better; the other is that those who regulate and monitor their cognitive processing (i.e. use metacognition) during task performance do better' (cited in Radford, 1991, p. 10). Metacognitive skills can be thought of as cognitive skills that are necessary for the management of knowledge and other cognitive skills (Biggs, 1988).

To reason effectively, clinicians need different forms of knowledge, including conceptual and procedural knowledge (Glaser, 1984). They also need personal knowledge to support their caring relationship with others. Mezirow (1990, p. xvi), for instance, contends that knowledge structure also refers to the individual's 'meaning perspective' or a 'structure of assumptions that constitutes a frame of reference for interpreting the meaning of an experience'.

Conclusion

The accumulated propositional, professional and personal knowledge of the individual constitutes his/her unique knowledge base. Such knowledge bases have contextual influences generated by the societal, professional, paradigmatic and experiential situations in which the individual's knowledge was generated. The relevance of the individual's knowledge base to the task in hand is important (Feltovich *et al.*, 1984) and the effective use of this knowledge in the reasoning process is an essential element in quality health care.

Beyond the notions of clinical expert, clinician scientist or competent professional, we present the need for the health professional to be a skilled companion.[5] Titchen (1998a) describes this person as accompanying and assisting a patient on a journey from pain to comfort, from distress to coping, from fear to confidence or from loss to adjustment. Her skilled companionship model and the parallel framework of critical companionship draw together several of the key arguments presented in this chapter: the need for the clinician to have a sound knowledge base comprising propositional, professional and personal knowledge, the need for this knowledge base to be continually critiqued and updated, and the need for sound reasoning, metacognitive and self-evaluative skills to provide the vehicle for use of this knowledge in clinical decision making. In addition, this model shows the need for self-knowledge and self-awareness on the part of practitioners so that they can be attuned to patients and their concerns, experiences and interpretations of their illnesses and develop, sustain and close relationships therapeutically. From a stance of concern, engagement and care, and by accessing patients' and families' concerns and taking these into account when reasoning , intuiting, diagnosing and designing care or interventions, the skilled companion achieves the goal of providing patient-centred care.

[5] This term was first used by Campbell (1984).

References

Agan, R. D. (1987) Intuitive knowing as a dimension of nursing. *Advances in Nursing Science*, **10**, 63–70.

Alexander, P. A. and Judy, J. E. (1988) The interaction of domain-specific and strategic knowledge in academic performance. *Review of Educational Research*, **58**, 375–404.

Ausubel, D. P. (1977) Cognitive structure and transfer. In *How Students Learn* (N. Entwistle and D. Hounsell, eds), pp. 93–103. Lancaster: Institute for Research and Development in Post-Compulsory Education, University of Lancaster.

Ayer, A. J. (1956) *The Problem Of Knowledge*. London: Penguin Books.

Barnett, R. (1990) *The Idea of Higher Education*. Buckingham: The Society for Research into Higher Education and Open University Press.

Baron, J. B. and Sternberg, R. J. (1987) *Teaching Thinking Skills: Theory and Practice*. New York: Freeman.

Benner, P. (1984) *From Novice to Expert: Excellence and Power in Clinical Nursing Practice*. London: Addison-Wesley.

Benner P. (1994) The tradition and skill of interpretive phenomenology in studying health, illness, and caring practices. In *Interpretive Phenomenology: Embodiment, Caring, and Ethics in Health and Illness* (P. Benner, ed.), pp. 99–127. London: Sage.

Benner, P. and Tanner, C. (1987) Clinical judgment: How expert nurses use intuition. *American Journal of Nursing*, **87**, 23–31.

Berger, P. and Luckmann, T. (1985) *The Social Construction of Reality*. Harmondsworth: Penguin.

Biggs, J. (1988) The role of metacognition in enhancing learning. *Australian Journal of Education*, **32**, 127–138.

Biggs, J. B. and Telfer, R. (1987) *The Process of Learning*. Sydney: Prentice-Hall.

Bordage, G. and Lemieux, M. (1986) Some cognitive characteristics of medical students with and without diagnostic reasoning difficulties. In *Proceedings of the 25th Annual Conference of Research in Medical Education of the American Association of Medical Colleges*, pp. 185–190. New Orleans, LA: American Association of Medical Colleges.

Breines, E. (1990) Genesis of occupation: A philosophical model for therapy and theory. *Australian Occupational Therapy Journal*, **37**, 45–49.

Brookfield, S. D. (1987) *Developing Critical Thinkers*. Milton Keynes: Open University Press.

Brown, S. and McIntyre, D. (1993) *Making Sense of Teaching*. Milton Keynes: Open University Press.

Bullock, A. and Trombley, S. (1988) *The Fontana Dictionary of Modern Thought*, 2nd edn. London: Fontana Press.

Butt, R. (1985), Curriculum: Metatheoretical horizons and emancipatory action. *Journal of Curriculum Theorizing*, **6**, 7–21.

Butt, R., Raymond, D. and Yamaguishi, L. (1982) Autobiographic praxis: Studying the formation of teacher's knowledge. *Journal of Curriculum Theorizing*, **7**, 87–164.

Campbell A. V. (1984) *Moderated Love*. London: SPCK.

Candy, P. C. (1991) *Self-direction for Lifelong Learning*. San Francisco: Jossey-Bass.

Carper, B. A. (1978) Fundamental patterns of knowing. *Advances in Nursing Science*, **1**, 13–23.

Carroll, E. (1988) The role of tacit knowledge in problem solving in the clinical setting. *Nurse Education Today*, **8**, 140–147.

Doering, L. (1992) Power and knowledge in nursing: A feminist poststructuralist view. *Advances in Nursing Science*, **14**, 24–33.

Domholdt, E. (1993) *Physical Therapy Research: Principles and Applications*. Philadelphia, PA: Saunders.

Eisner, E. (1988) The primacy of experience and the politics of method. *Educational Researcher*, **17**, 15–20.

Feltovich, P. J., Johnson, P. E., Moller, J. H. and Swanson, D. B. (1984) LCS: The role and development of medical knowledge in diagnostic expertise. In *Readings in Medical Artificial Intelligence: The First Decade* (W. J. Clancey and E. H. Shortliffe, eds), pp. 275–319. Reading, MA: Addison-Wesley.

Freire, P. (1970) *Cultural Action for Freedom*. Harvard Educational Review. Cambridge, MA: Centre for the Study of Social Change.

Gadamer, H. G. (1975) Hermeneutics and social science. *Cultural Hermeneutics*, **2**, 307–316.

Giddens, A. (1985) Jurgen Habermas. In *The Return of Grand Theory in the Human Sciences* (Q. Skinner, ed.), pp. 121–140. Cambridge: Cambridge University Press.

Glaser, R. (1984) Education and thinking: The role of knowledge. *American Psychologist*, **39**, 93–104.

Gowin, D. B. (1981) *Educating*. Ithaca, NY: Cornell University Press.

Grant, J. and Marsden, P. (1987) The structure of memorized knowledge in students and clinicians: An explanation for diagnostic expertise. *Medical Education*, **21**, 92–98.

Guba, E. G. and Lincoln, Y. S. (1994) Competing paradigms in qualitative research. In *Handbook of Qualitative Research* (N. K. Denzin and Y. S. Lincoln, eds), pp. 105–117. London: Sage.

Habermas, J. (1972) *Knowledge and Human Interest*. London: Heinemann.

Habermas, J. (1974) *Theory and Practice* (translated by J. Viertel). London: Heinemann.

Heidegger, M. (1962) *Being and Time*. New York: Harper & Row.

Heron, J. (1981) Philosophical basis for a new paradigm. In *Human Inquiry: A Sourcebook of New Paradigm Research* (P. Reason and J. Rowan, eds), pp. 19–35. Chichester: Wiley.

Holmes, C. A. (1990) Alternatives to natural science foundations for nursing. *International Journal of Nursing Studies*, **27**, 187–198.

Howard, R. W. (1987) *Concepts and Schemata: An Introduction*. London: Cassell Education.

Hundert, E. M. (1987) A model for ethical problem solving in medicine, with practical applications. *American Journal of Psychiatry*, **144**, 839–849.

Kleinig, J. (1982) *Philosophical Issues in Education*. London: Routledge.

Kneller, G. F. (1958) *Existentialism and Education*. Science Editions. New York: Wiley.

Kolb, D. A. (1984) *Experiential Learning: Experience as the Source of Learning and Development*. Englewood Cliffs, NJ: Prentice-Hall.

Lawler, J. (1991) *Behind the Screens: Nursing, Somology and the Problem of the Body*. Edinburgh: Churchill Livingstone.

Manley, K. (1991) Knowledge for nursing practice. In *Nursing: A Knowledge Base for Practice* (A. Perry and M. Jolley, eds), pp. 1–27. London: Edward Arnold.

Mattingly, C. (1991) The narrative nature of clinical reasoning. *American Journal of Occupational Therapy*, **45**, 998–1005.

McCormack, B. (1992) Intuition: Concept analysis and application to curriculum development. 1. Concept analysis. *Journal of Clinical Nursing*, **1**, 339–344.

Medin, D. L. (1989) Concepts and conceptual structure. *American Psychologist*, **44**, 1469–1481.

Mezirow, J. (1981) A critical theory of adult learning and education. *Adult Education*, **32**, 3–24.

Mezirow, J. (1990) Preface. In *Fostering Critical Reflection in Adulthood: A Guide to Transformative and Emancipatory Learning* (J. Mezirow and Associates, eds), pp. xiii–xxi. San Francisco: Jossey-Bass.

Moore, T. W. (1982) *Philosophy of Education: An Introduction*. London: Routledge & Kegan Paul.

Nickerson, R. S., Perkins, D. N. and Smith, E. E. (1985) *The Teaching of Thinking*. Hillsdale, NJ: Lawrence Erlbaum.

Omery, A. (1988) Ethnography. In *Paths to Knowledge: Innovative Research Methods for Nursing* (B. Sarter, ed.), pp. 17–32. New York: National League for Nursing.

Parry, A. (1991) Physiotherapy and methods of inquiry: Conflict and reconciliation. *Physiotherapy*, **77**, 435–438.

Parry, A. (1997) New paradigms for old: musings on the shape of clouds. *Physiotherapy*, **83**, 423–433.

Perkins, D. N. (1986) *Knowledge as Design*. Hillsdale, NJ: Lawrence Erlbaum.

Polanyi, M. (1958) *Personal Knowledge: Towards a Post-Critical Philosophy*. London: Routledge & Kegan Paul.

Popkewitz, T. S. (1984) *Paradigm and Ideology in Educational Research*, London: Falmer Press.

Powers, B. A. and Knapp, T. R. (1995) *A Dictionary of Nursing Theory and Research*, 2nd edn, Thousand Oaks, CA: Sage.

Radford, J. (1991) Teaching and learning: A selective review. In *Helping Students to Learn: Teaching, Counselling, Research* (K. Raaheim, J. Wankowski and J. Radford, eds), pp. 1–15. Buckingham: The Society for Research into Higher Education and Open University Press.

Reason, P. and Heron, J. (1986) Research with people: The paradigm of cooperative experiential enquiry. *Person-Centred Review*, **1**, 457–476.

Rumelhart, D. E. and Ortony, A. (1977) The representation of knowledge in memory. In *Schooling and the Acquisition of Knowledge* (R. C. Anderson, R. J. Spiro and W. E. Montague, eds), pp. 99–135. Hillsdale, NJ: Lawrence Erlbaum.

Sarter, B. (ed.) (1988) *Paths to Knowledge: Innovative Research Methods for Nursing*. New York: National League for Nursing.

Schön, D. A. (1987) *Educating the Reflective Practitioner*. San Francisco: Jossey-Bass.

Schutz, A. (1962) *Collected Papers*, Vols 1–3. Dordrecht: Kluwer.

Schwandt, T. (1989) Solutions to the paradigm conflict: Coping with uncertainty. *Journal of Contemporary Ethnography*, **17**, 379–407.

Shepard, K. F. (1987) Qualitative and quantitative research in clinical practice. *Physical Therapy*, **67**, 1891–1894.

Skinner, Q. (1985) Introduction: The return of grand theory. In *The Return of Grand Theory in the Human Sciences* (Q. Skinner, ed.), pp. 1–20. Cambridge: Cambridge University Press.Swanson-Kauffman, K. and Schonwald, E. (1988) Phenomenology. In *Paths to Knowledge: Innovative Research Methods for Nursing* (B. Sarter, ed.), pp. 97–110. New York: National League for Nursing.

Titchen A. (1996) A case study of a patient-centred nurse. In *Essential Practice in Patient-Centred Care*. (K. W. M. Fulford, S. Ersser and T. Hope, eds.), pp. 182–193. Oxford: Blackwell Science.

Titchen A. (1998a) Professional craft knowledge in patient-centred nursing and the facilitation of its development. *DPhil thesis*. University of Oxford.

Titchen A. (1998b) *A Conceptual Framework for Facilitating Learning in Clinical Practice*. Occasional Paper 2. Centre for Professional Education Advancement, The University of Sydney.

Weiser, J. (1987) Learning from the perspective of growth of consciousness. In *Appreciating Adults' Learning: From the Learners' Perspective*. (D. Boud, and V. Griffin, eds.), pp. 99–111. London: Kogan Page.

Wildemeersch, D. (1989) The principal meaning of dialogue for the construction and transformation of reality. In *Making Sense of Experiential Learning: Diversity in Theory and Practice* (S. W. Weil and I. McGill, eds), pp. 60–69. Milton Keynes: The Society for Research into Higher Education and Open University Press.

4

Clinical reasoning and biomedical knowledge: Implications for teaching

Vimla L. Patel and David R. Kaufman

We are entering a period of time in which health science curricula world-wide are undergoing dramatic transformations and experiencing significant structural changes. These changes are likely to shape the practice of the health sciences for decades to come. The role of biomedical knowledge in clinical medicine is one of the focal issues in this transformation. Basic science knowledge reflects a subset of biomedical knowledge, although at points in the chapter the two terms are used interchangeably. There are many competing views and assumptions concerning the role of biomedical knowledge and its proper place in a health science curriculum. In this chapter, we consider some of these arguments in the context of empirical evidence from cognitive studies in medicine. The role of basic science knowledge is a subject of considerable debate in medical education. It is generally accepted that basic science or biomedical knowledge provides a foundation upon which clinical knowledge can be built. However, its precise role in medical reasoning is controversial (Clancey, 1988; Patel *et al.*, 1989). Biomedical knowledge has undergone a dramatic transformation over the past couple of decades, presenting unique and formidable challenges to medical education. There is considerable uncertainty concerning the relationship between basic science conceptual knowledge of subject matter and the practice of physicians (e.g. Dawson-Saunders *et al.*, 1990). In recent years, there has been a dramatic increase in the volume of medical knowledge, especially in cellular and molecular biology (Friedman and Purcell, 1983). Medical schools have typically responded by adding the

new content to existing courses, increasing the number of classroom lectures and assigning more textbook readings (Stritter and Mattern, 1983), with a dramatic decrease in laboratory time and small group teaching during the pre-clinical years. The basic science courses are increasingly taught by PhD research scientists from diverse departments (e.g. anatomy) with minimal background in clinical medicine. There is also a lack of coordination between the different basic science departments affiliated with each medical school.

The future role of basic science knowledge

There have been increasing expressions of dissatisfaction with basic science teaching in medicine. It has been argued that substantial parts of the basic science in medical schools are irrelevant to the future needs of practitioners and that the biomedical concepts are presented at a time when students are not prepared to grasp their significance (Neame, 1984). This argument could be extended to cover other health science disciplines as well. Furthermore, the method of presenting information in a didactic lecture format and with text readings that do not usually include clinical reasoning exercises encourages passivity and rote learning, which inhibits the development of understanding. Neame (1984) argues that pre-clinical courses fail to achieve their objectives of imparting useful and relevant knowledge to the future clinical practitioner. In addition, the primary evaluations of students are based on multiple choice examinations that emphasize recall of factual information rather than conceptual understanding and integration of concepts. Serious concerns have been raised about whether future health science practitioners will require the kinds of scientific training that their predecessors received. One of the arguments suggests that technical innovations, in particular the computer, will render much of basic science training unnecessary. Cavazos (1984) expresses this point of view clearly:

> Medical education should not be designed to develop scientists nor students who are encyclopedias of scientific trivia, no matter how vital that trivia might be in pursuit of pure science. We have no need to teach medical students vast quantities of information which results in memorization when such information can be computer-stored and retrieved in seconds. We do have a need to graduate ethical and compassionate students with high level skills in data analysis and independent critical thinking.

This quote underscores a particular cynicism towards the teaching of basic knowledge, and the view that the training of medical scientists and humane medical practitioners are competing goals. The proposal offered by Cavazos, which very likely captures the sentiment of some medical educators, demonstrates a significant misunderstanding about the nature of knowledge acquisition. The view expressed equates understanding with the accumulation of facts; since computers can store facts better than humans, why not take advantage of it? Cavazos fails to appreciate that storing information is not the same as structuring useful and accessible knowledge (Cruess *et al.*, 1985). Even if a practitioner could access information so effortlessly, it would be of relatively little value without some prior knowledge to interpret it. In our view it is unlikely that ethical, compassionate and highly skilled technicians would be a suitable replacement for today's clinical practitioners. The issue of technological change and its relationship to a scientific foundation for medical practitioners is a source of considerable debate (Patel and Kaufman, 1998a; Stead, 1998). The issue is whether technological innovation will require that physicians master an ever expanding body of scientific knowledge or whether future technology will render such knowledge superfluous. Recent advances in information and decision technologies are beginning to transform clinical practice, with the potential to improve patient care substantially. However, the ways in which these changes should affect clinical training

is the subject of ongoing debate in medical informatics (Patel and Kaufman, 1998b). According to Prokop (1992), there are clear historical trends that are likely to continue. New discoveries in science will continue to provide physicians with increasingly powerful investigative tools with which to see the workings of the human body and through which to prevent disease. When we consider the historical precedents, it seems likely that the best clinical judgement will require a broader understanding of both biology and medicine than ever before (Prokop, 1992).

Epistemological and curricular issues

Medical knowledge consists of two types of knowledge: clinical knowledge, including knowledge of disease entities and associated findings, and basic science knowledge, incorporating subject matter such as biochemistry, anatomy and physiology. Basic science or biomedical knowledge is supposed to provide a scientific foundation for clinical reasoning.

It had been widely accepted that biomedical and clinical knowledge could be seamlessly integrated into a coherent knowledge structure that supported all cognitive aspects of medical practice, such as diagnostic and therapeutic reasoning (Feinstein, 1973). From this perspective, clinical and biomedical knowledge become intricately intertwined, providing medical practice with a sound scientific basis. These assumptions have increasingly been called into question (Neame, 1984; Patel *et al.*, 1999). Since the Flexner (1910) report at the beginning of this century, medical schools have made a strong commitment to this epistemological framework. The medical curricula at most medical schools are partitioned into pre-clinical courses which predominantly teach the basic sciences during the first and second years of medical school. The remaining 2 years of medical school and further postgraduate training consist of clinical courses and practicums. The content of a basic curriculum covers a great expanse of knowledge in a relatively short period of time. To illustrate the depth and breadth of content coverage, Figure 4.1 presents a partial model of the biomedical science courses taught in the medical school of McGill University *circa* 1995, within a conventional medical curriculum. Medical students are required to take courses in six major biomedical domains during their first 18 months of medical school. The physiology courses are taught

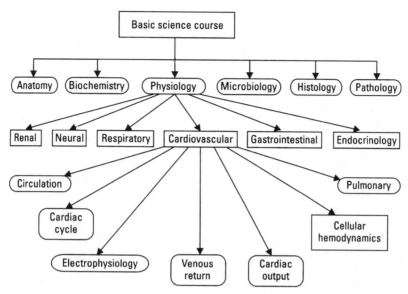

Figure 4.1 A partial model of basic science courses in the medical curriculum at McGill University

for a total of 205 hours, more than any of the other core courses. We can further partition the physiology course into major subsections, of which Figure 4.1 illustrates only six. Cardiovascular physiology is the subject matter that receives the most time within the physiology courses, being taught over 28 hours. This course covers a range of complex topics, such as cardiac output and cellular haemodynamics. Each of these topics receives at most a few hours of lecture time. In these brief periods of time, a lecturer must, at minimum, cover the basic concepts in each topic, explain its relationship to other parts of the system (and the course) and provide some demonstration of its relevance in a clinical context. Although the McGill curriculum has, in recent years, increasingly gravitated towards small group teaching and more intensive focus on important concepts, the essential challenge of balancing depth of understanding with breadth of coverage remains.

As discussed previously, the purpose of basic science teaching is to provide a scientific foundation for tasks of clinical practice, such as diagnosis and therapeutics. Medical problem solving can be characterized as ill-structured, in the sense that the initial states, the definite goal state and the necessary constraints are unknown at the beginning of the problem-solving process. In a diagnostic situation, the problem space of potential findings and associated diagnoses is enormous. The problem space becomes defined through the imposition of a set of plausible constraints that

facilitate the application of specific decision strategies (Pople, 1982). For example, a physician when faced with a multi-system problem such as hypokalemic periodic paralysis associated with hyperthyroidism may need to confirm the more common disorder of hyperthyroidism before solving the more vexing problem of hypokalemia. Once this is confirmed, there is a set of constraints in place such that there are classes of disorders that co-occur with hyperthyroidism, and there is a set of symptoms that have not yet been accounted for by this disorder and are consistent with hypokalemic periodic paralysis. As expertise develops, the disease knowledge of a clinician becomes more dependent on clinical experience, and clinical problem solving is increasingly guided by the use of exemplars and analogy, becoming less dependent on a functional understanding of the system in question. Biomedical knowledge, by comparison, is of a qualitatively different nature, embodying elements of causal mechanisms and characterizing patterns of perturbation in function and structure.

Schaffner (1986) characterizes biomedical science as a series of overlapping inter-level temporal models. Temporal models include collections of entities that undergo a process of change and can be represented as a sequence of events. For example, acute left ventricular failure can produce a disequilibrium in which the output of blood on the right side of the heart temporarily exceeds the output of the left side of the heart. The process by which the output from the left and right sides of the heart equilibrates can be understood in terms of a sequence of events in which there is a change in the pressure–volume relationships in different segments of the circulatory system which will affect the flow dynamics and restore the equilibrium over repeated cardiac cycles. In the physical sciences, time is usually embodied in differential equations. The explicit temporal sequence is of considerably greater significance in biomedical theories (Schaffner, 1986). The term inter-level refers to the fact that entities grouped within a biomedical theory are at different levels of aggregation.

This multi-levelled knowledge can be arranged in a hierarchical schema of scientific sources. Blois (1988) illustrates the inter-level reasoning process in the context of Wilson's disease, a central nervous system disorder caused by a metabolic defect in which the body cannot properly eliminate copper from the blood. At each higher level in the hierarchy, there are newly emergent properties not entirely predictable from lower levels. Blois identifies seven levels of hierarchy in Wilson's disease, from the atomic level findings such as decreased serum copper to 'patient as a whole abnormalities' such as malaise and labile affect. Each new level has different conceptual entities and a unique language of description. The lower-level abnormalities are revealed by laboratory tests and the higher-level attributes come from patient reports and physical examinations. Each higher level introduces a greater degree of inexactness in ascribing causality. For example, it is difficult to precisely account for the patient's altered emotional states. This problem is rather atypical. Few diseases can be traced across aggregate levels in this manner. However, biomedical research is increasingly building these vertical connections that provide medical science with a deeper understanding of biomedical disorders. The example serves to highlight the challenge of synthesizing information from different levels of aggregation.

It should be noted that not all biomedical disciplines can be characterized by having explicitly causal or temporal components. In particular, anatomy and histology are predominantly concerned with aspects of structure. At the clinical level, models of disease are commonly described in terms of associations between clinical findings and diagnoses.

The focus of the instructional approach for the biomedical curriculum is necessarily on the extensive coverage of a broad corpus of knowledge as opposed to in-depth conceptual understanding.

Each domain and even each subdomain represents a unique ontology with distinct conceptual entities and relations between entities. The volume of information in any one of these disciplines or subdisciplines is now so large that it cannot be completely mastered even by a full-time graduate student pursuing doctoral studies for 5 years (Prokop, 1992). It is unreasonable to expect that medical students can master five or more fields in the first 18 months of medical school. The degree of conceptual integration, from a horizontal perspective (across subject domains) and vertical perspective (in terms of the depth within subject matters) is immense. In our view it is not tenable, given a finite time frame and finite psychological resources, to coordinate these multiple sources of knowledge and harmonize all biomedical knowledge with a clinical body of knowledge of disease entities and associated findings.

Research in clinical reasoning

In this section, we review some of the pertinent research in medical reasoning, particularly research that addresses the role of basic science knowledge in clinical medicine. Studies in medical clinical reasoning encompass different domains of knowledge (e.g. cardiology and radiology) and a wide range of performance tasks. Lesgold *et al.* (1988) investigated the abilities of radiologists, at different levels of training and expertise, to interpret chest X-ray pictures and provide a diagnosis. The results revealed that the experts were able to initially detect a general pattern of disease with a gross anatomical localization, serving to constrain the possible interpretations. Novices had greater difficulty focusing on the important structures, being more likely to maintain inappropriate interpretations despite discrepant findings in the patient history. The authors concluded that the knowledge that underlies expertise in radiology includes the mental representation of anatomy, a theory of anatomical perturbation and the constructive capacity to transform the visual image into a three-dimensional representation. The less expert subjects had greater difficulty in building and maintaining a rich anatomical representation of the patient.

Norman *et al.* (1989) compared subjects' performance at various levels of expertise in tasks that required them to diagnose and sort dermatological slides according to the type of skin lesion present. The results indicated that experts were more accurate in their diagnoses and took significantly less time to respond than novices. The sorting task revealed that each group sorted the slides according to different category types. Expert dermatologists grouped the slides into superordinate categories such as viral infections, which reflected the underlying pathophysiological structure. Novices tended to classify lesions according to their surface features such as scaly lesions. The implication is that expert knowledge is organized around domain principles, which facilitate the rapid recognition of significant problem features. This is referred to as domain knowledge.

Clinical reasoning strategies and expertise

In recent years, a considerable amount of research has been undertaken comparing the comprehension and problem solving of experts, intermediates and novices in domains of knowledge, such as chess (Charness, 1991) and physics (Chi *et al.*, 1981). The picture that emerges from this research is that experts use a quite different pattern of reasoning from that used by novices or intermediates and organize their knowledge differently. Three important aspects are that experts (a) have a greater ability to organize information into semantically meaningful, interrelated chunks, (b) do not process irrelevant information and (c) in routine situations, tend to use highly specific knowledge-based problem-solving strategies (Ericsson and Smith, 1991). The use of knowledge-based strategies has given rise to an important distinction between data-driven strategy (forward reasoning), in which hypotheses are generated from data, and hypothesis-driven strategy (backward reasoning), in which one reasons backward from a hypothesis and attempts to find data that elucidate it. Forward reasoning is based on domain knowledge and thus is highly error-prone in the absence of adequate domain knowledge. Backward reasoning is slower and may make heavy demands on working memory (because one has to keep track of such things as goals and hypotheses). It is most likely to be used when domain knowledge is inadequate.

In experiments with expert physicians, clinicians showed little tendency to use basic science in explaining cases, whereas medical researchers showed preference for detailed, basic scientific explanations, without developing clinical descriptions (Patel *et al.*, 1989). In medicine, the pathophysiological explanation task has been used to examine clinical reasoning (Feltovich and Barrows, 1984; Patel and Groen, 1986). Pathophysiology

refers to the physiology of disordered function. This task requires subjects to explain the causal pattern underlying a set of clinical symptoms. Protocols from this task can be used to investigate the ability of clinicians to apply basic science concepts in diagnosing a clinical problem. In one study (Patel and Groen, 1986), expert practitioners (cardiologists) were asked to solve problems within their domain of expertise. Their explanations of the underlying pathophysiology of the cases, whether correctly or incorrectly diagnosed, made virtually no use of basic science knowledge. In another study (Patel *et al.*, 1990b), cardiologists and endocrinologists were asked to read both endocrinology and cardiology cases, recall case information, and explain the underlying pathophysiology of the problems. Subjects thus were operating both within and outside their domains of expertise. The clinicians did not appeal to principles from basic biomedical science, even when they were working outside their own domain of expertise; rather, they relied on clinical associations and classifications to formulate solutions. The results suggest that basic science does not contribute directly to reasoning in clinical problem solving for experienced clinicians.

However, it should be noted that biomedical information was used by practitioners when the task was difficult or when they were uncertain about their diagnosis (Joseph and Patel, 1990; Patel *et al.*, 1990b). In these cases, biomedical information was used in a backward-directed causal reasoning manner, providing some kind of coherence to the explanation of clinical cues that could not be easily accounted for by the primary diagnostic hypothesis that was being considered.

Basic science in students' explanations of clinical cases

We developed a series of experiments in our laboratory designed to elucidate the precise role of basic science in clinical reasoning (Patel *et al.*, 1988, 1990a,b). Our purpose was to determine to what extent basic sciences and clinical knowledge are complementary. One study made use of a standard paradigm in research relating comprehension to clinical reasoning. The authors presented medical students at McGill University with basic science material immediately prior to presenting a clinical case (Patel *et al.*, 1988). Such a procedure is designed to maximize the likelihood that subjects will use related information from separate knowledge sources. Specifically, we prepared a clinical text on acute bacterial endocarditis and three related basic science texts on the physiology of fever, haemodynamics and microcirculation. Subjects were grouped according to their level of medical school training: students in their first year of medical school; second-year medical students who had completed all basic medical sciences but had not begun any clinical work; and final-year medical students 3 months before graduation. The subjects were asked to read the four texts, recall in writing what they had read and then explain the clinical problem in terms of the basic science texts. In our analysis, we coded subjects' statements into propositions and relations among propositions, to establish as precisely as possible what information and inferences subjects employed in performing their tasks. This type of analysis follows a well-developed paradigm in cognitive science for the interpretation of verbal data.

In general, subjects' recall of the basic science texts was poor, indicating a lack of well-developed knowledge structures in which to organize this information. Recall of the clinical text appeared to be a function of clinical experience, but there was no similar correlation between basic science and experience. In the explanation of the problem, the second-year students made extensive use of basic science knowledge. Fourth-year students gave explanations that resembled those of expert physicians outside their domain of specialization, except that the students made more extensive use of basic science information than we find in experts' explanations. It is interesting to note that their greater use of basic science actually resulted in more consistent inferences. Our results can be interpreted as indicating that basic science knowledge is used differently by the three groups of subjects.

In a second experiment, using the same number of subjects at similar levels of training, we asked for recall and explanation of cases when basic science information was provided after the clinical problem (Patel *et al.*, 1990a). We can characterize reasoning as a two-stage process: diagnostic reasoning is characterized by inference from observation to hypothesis and predictive reasoning is characterized by inference from hypothesis to observations. The fourth-year students were able to use the basic science information in a highly effective manner, thus facilitating both diagnostic and predictive reasoning. The second-year students were also able to use this information effectively, but diagnostic reasoning was not facilitated. The first-year students were not able to use basic

science information any more effectively when it was given after the clinical problem than when it was given before the clinical problem. These results suggest that reasoning toward a diagnosis from the facts of a case is frustrated by attempting to use basic science knowledge unless the student has already developed a strong diagnostic hypothesis. Thus, the addition of basic science knowledge seems to improve the accuracy of diagnoses offered by final-year medical students, but does not improve the accuracy of diagnoses by first- and second-year students. The most straightforward explanation is that final-year students, who have had some clinical experience, rely on clinically relevant features in a case to classify the diagnosis (if broadly) and make selective predictions of features that are susceptible to analysis in terms of the basic science facts they have read (Patel *et al.*, 1989). This tendency of clinical solutions to subordinate basic scientific ones and for basic science not to support the clinical organization of facts in a case, was evident among expert physicians as discussed earlier.

Arocha *et al.* (1993) presented medical trainees with cases where they had to generate an initial hypothesis and then were presented evidence disconfirming the initial suggestion. In a manner similar to expert physicians, the novices in this study used little basic science information during the diagnostic process. The strategy that the subjects followed was more like a search through a space of findings based on the weighting of these findings against the possible diagnostic hypothesis they were entertaining at the time. Recourse to pathophysiological information happened only in special situations when the problem-solving process broke down and the subjects had to tie 'loose ends' or unaccounted information in the case. The results of this study are consistent with previously described findings as most students did not use basic science information to evaluate competing diagnoses. These results are also consistent with other reported findings that suggest that unprompted use of biomedical concepts in clinical reasoning decreases as a function of expertise (Boshuizen *et al.*, 1988).

Reasoning and biomedical knowledge in different medical curricula

Patel *et al.* (1991a, 1993) attempted to replicate the above studies in an established problem-based learning (PBL) medical school at McMaster University.

Employing the same methods and procedures used in the studies described earlier, students at three equivalent levels of training were tested in the McMaster medical curriculum. The results showed that when basic science information was provided before the clinical problem, there was again a lack of integration of basic science into the clinical context. This resulted in (a) lack of global coherence in their knowledge structures, (b) errors of scientific fact and (c) disruption of the process of diagnostic reasoning.

When basic science was given after the clinical problem, there was again integration of basic science into the clinical context. It is concluded that clinical problems cannot be easily embedded into a basic science context, but basic science can be more naturally embedded within a clinical context. However, this phenomenon is observed as a short-term effect in the undergraduate medical curricula; the long-term effects of this kind of integration process are not known. It is our belief that when one is attempting to learn two unknown domains, it is better to learn one well, so it can be used as an 'anchor' for the new domain. We also know that basic science knowledge has a causal underlying structure that can be remembered as a story, and clinical knowledge has a classificatory structure of patient signs and symptoms. In our opinion, basic science knowledge would make a better anchor than clinical knowledge. Our earlier finding that basic science cannot be easily integrated into clinical structure, and the suggestion that basic science forms a better anchor, gives rise to a paradox. It appears that a compromise may be needed, such that there is some core basic science taught at the beginning of the curriculum, followed by an early introduction of clinical problems, where early basic science will produce some form of anchor and early clinical problems will provide the structure support.

The results of our study (Patel *et al.*, 1991a, 1993) suggest that in the conventional curriculum (a) basic science and clinical knowledge are generally kept separate, (b) clinical reasoning may not require basic science knowledge, (c) basic science is spontaneously used only when students get into difficulty with the patient problem, and (d) basic science serves to generate globally coherent explanations of the patient problem with connections between various components of the clinical problem. It is proposed that in a conventional curriculum, the clinical aspect of the problem is viewed as separate from the biomedical science aspect, the two having different functions. In the PBL curriculum, basic science and clinical knowledge are spontaneously integrated. However, this integration results in students' inability to decontextualize the problem, in that the basic science is so tightly tied to the clinical context that students appear unable to detach it even when the clinical situation demands it. In addition, a greater number of elaborations are made when students think about problem features using basic science and clinical information. However, these greater elaborations result in fragmentation of knowledge structures resulting in the lack of global coherence (various parts of the problem are not connected). Finally, within PBL such elaborations result in factual errors that persist from first-year students responses to the final year. These differences could conceivably be due to the emphasis on detailed causal reasoning and elaboration, which might be assumed to generate more load on working memory. There are multiple competencies involved in the practice of medicine, some of which are best fostered in the context of real world practice and others best acquired through a process of formal learning. It has become more apparent that the extent to which aspects of a domain are best learned in context is determined jointly by the nature of domain knowledge and the kinds of tasks that are performed by practitioners (Patel *et al.*, 1999).

Progressions in understanding of biomedical concepts

In the preceding studies, we examined the role of basic science knowledge in a clinical context. Evidence emerged to suggest that the biomedical concepts were not, in and of themselves, well understood by most students. In this section, we focus on a study related to students' understanding of important biomedical concepts. Our investigations of medical problem solving indicate that biomedical knowledge is not used optimally in clinical contexts (Patel *et al.*, 1989). These research findings suggest that basic science is used differentially in different tasks and in different medical domains, that experts and novices differ in their use of basic science and that, in many instances, basic science knowledge may actually interfere with clinical reasoning. The evidence also suggests that students possess substantial inert knowledge that frustrates their ability to apply specific biomedical concepts to clinical problem-solving tasks. As discussed previously, the problems appear to be at least equally pervasive in problem-based medical schools with integrated curricula. The results also suggest that, when used appropriately, biomedical knowledge can facilitate explanation (Patel *et al.*, 1989).

Patel *et al.* (1991b) examined medical students' understanding of complex biomedical concepts in the domain of cardio-pulmonary physiology. In particular, the study focused on the concepts related to ventilation–perfusion matching. The concept of ventilation–perfusion matching is a fundamental one, whose understanding is integral to diverse domains of medicine. It has applications in both diagnostic and therapeutic contexts. It was found that students at the end of first year of the medical school exhibited significant misconceptions in reasoning about ventilation–perfusion matching in the context of a clinical problem. Specifically, students had considerable difficulty in conceptualizing the cardio-pulmonary system as a closed mechanistic system. Students' explanations revealed that they reasoned about each lung as if it were semi-autonomous and did not impose constraints on the other lung's functioning. It was also observed that students were not able to map clinical findings onto pathophysiological manifestations. This can partly be explained by the fact that the pulmonary physiology course that preceded the study did not make these relationships sufficiently explicit.

The results of this study are consistent with other research (*cf.* Patel *et al.*, 1989) that indicates that students' oversimplified representations of biomedical phenomena fail to support clinical reasoning. The research of Feltovich *et al.* (1989) in the related domain of congestive heart failure documented widespread misconceptions in students' understanding of the structure and function of the cardiovascular system. Congestive heart failure is a syndrome in which the heart's effectiveness as a pump can diminish greatly and as a result the rate of blood flow slows dramatically. The misconception that was expressed by over 60% of first- and second-year medical students in a study, and by some medical practitioners, was that heart failure is caused by the heart getting too big, which in turn stretches the cardiac muscle fibres. The force of contraction is determined by mechanical–anatomical factors and activational factors (energetic). The primary cause of congestive heart failure is activational, whereas the misconception emphasized the mechanical overstretching as the cause for heart failure. This study represented the first experiment in a research program designed to characterize students' and

physicians' understanding of significant biomedical concepts and their utilization in clinical contexts. More recently we conducted a detailed study (Kaufman *et al.*, 1992, 1996) to characterize students' and physicians' understanding of biomedical concepts in the domain of cardiovascular physiology. In the experiment, subjects were presented with questions and problems pertaining to the concepts of cardiac output, venous return, and the mechanical properties of the cardiovascular and circulatory system. The stimulus material included several areas of questions and problems including basic physiology (e.g. explain the effects of an increase in pre-load on stroke volume), applied physiology (e.g. extreme exercise), pathophysiology (e.g. the haemodynamic effects of hemorrhage), medical disorders (e.g. congestive heart failure) and brief clinical problems. This afforded us an opportunity to investigate subjects' reasoning within and across levels in the hierarchical chain of biomedicine. The first links in the chain are the physical principles related to the dynamics and statics of the storage and flow of fluids through tubes. In particular, a basic understanding of pressure–volume and pressure–flow relationships is essential to understanding this subject matter.

Our findings indicated a wide range of conceptual errors and errors of analysis, in subjects at different levels of expertise. These errors were prominent in different sections of the study but tended to carry over into other sections. Overall, there was an evident increase in conceptual understanding with levels of training. Students who were tested at the very beginning of medical school began their learning with preconceptions that were not commensurate with the assimilation of new knowledge. For instance, one subject was lacking in basic physical science knowledge and had difficulties reasoning about pressure gradients.

There were particular misconceptions that would appear to be a function of formal learning. For example, a misconception was manifested in the responses of six subjects, including two fourth-year students and two cardiology residents. It was related to a confounding of venous resistance and venous compliance. The notion is that since an increase in venous resistance is associated with a decrease in compliance, then the net effect of resistance would be to increase venous return. If one considers the meaning of resistance, which all of these subjects clearly understood, then it appears quite counterintuitive that resistance can facilitate (as opposed to impede) blood flow. This would suggest that this misconception is a function of formal learning rather than acquired through experience.

The more advanced subjects in our study, including the senior students and physicians, experienced more difficulty in responding to the basic physiology than they did applying the same concepts in more clinically oriented problems. On several occasions, the physicians would use clinical analogies to explain physiological processes (e.g. using aortic stenosis to account for the effects of after-load on end-systolic pressure). More often than not, the analogies did not successfully result in correct explanations. However, when provided with pathophysiological conditions or medical disorders requiring pathophysiological explanations (e.g. congestive heart failure), the physicians drew on their clinical knowledge to great effect. The distance in the hierarchy (e.g. from physical science to pathophysiology) had a considerable effect on the likelihood of successful transfer of knowledge.

Most subjects at each level of training exhibited a strong cardiocentric bias. That is, they tended to construct explanations using concepts related to cardiac function, without any due consideration of the factors that affect venous return. This bias was evident even in response to clinical problems. Understanding of these basic science concepts could have implications for particular therapeutic practices, such as fluid management, where decisions have to be made that take into account factors that affect both the peripheral circuit (vessels of the cardiovascular system) and cardiac function.

Biomedical knowledge and clinical science: two different worlds?

We have considered epistemological and curricular issues related to the role of basic science knowledge in clinical medicine, discussed empirical studies related to the use of biomedical knowledge in clinical reasoning contexts, and considered studies that examined students and physicians understanding of biomedical concepts. What inferences can we make concerning the role of basic science knowledge in clinical practice? We will consider two theoretical hypotheses.

Schmidt and Boshuizen (1992) proposed a learning mechanism, knowledge encapsulation, for explaining how biomedical knowledge becomes subsumed under clinical knowledge as a function of training. Knowledge encapsulation is a learning process which involves the subsumption of biomedical propositions, concepts and their inter-relations in an associative net, under a small number of higher level clinical propositions with the same explanatory power. These authors suggest that through the exposure to clinical training, biomedical knowledge becomes encapsulated and integrated into clinical knowledge. They cite a wide range of clinical reasoning and recall studies which purportedly support this kind of learning process. Of particular importance is the well-documented finding that with increasing levels of expertise, physicians produce explanations at higher levels of generality, using fewer and fewer biomedical concepts while producing consistently accurate responses (Patel *et al.*, 1989).

In our view, the notion of knowledge encapsulation represents an idealized perspective on the integration of basic science in clinical knowledge. The reasons for our scepticism are rooted in several sources. Basic science knowledge plays a different role in different clinical domains. For example, clinical expertise in perceptual domains such as dermatology and radiology necessitates a relatively robust model of anatomical structures, which is the primary source of knowledge for diagnostic classification. In other domains, such as cardiology and endocrinology, basic science knowledge has a more distant relationship with clinical knowledge. Furthermore, the misconceptions evident in physicians' biomedical explanations would argue against well-developed encapsulated knowledge structures where basic science knowledge could easily be retrieved and applied when necessary.

As discussed previously, biomedical knowledge represents a complex multi-levelled hierarchical structure. Given what we know about epistemology of basic science knowledge and what we know about the nature of basic science curricula, then it is not tenable to develop such 'neatly packaged' knowledge structures. Our contention is that neither conventional nor problem-based curricula could foster this kind of learning process. There is a successful integration of basic science knowledge into clinical structure with PBL curriculum. However, it has also created the problem of students' inability to decontextualize it once it is integrated (Patel *et al.*, 1993). This problem should be attended to if one assumes that relevant basic science knowledge is naturally embedded into clinical knowledge. Indeed, that appears to be a basic assumption of the clinical rationale for medical education. On the other hand, the bio-medical sciences have a structure that is quite different from the clinical sciences. If that is the case, then one would expect clinicians to exhibit an inability to decontextualize basic science knowledge learned in a clinical context.

It is our view that the results of research into medical clinical reasoning are consistent with the idea that clinical medicine and the biomedical sciences constitute two distinct and not completely compatible worlds, with distinct modes of reasoning and quite different ways of structuring knowledge (Patel *et al.*, 1989). Clinical knowledge is based on a complex taxonomy which relates disease symptoms to underlying pathology. In contrast, the biomedical sciences are based on general principles defining chains of causal mechanisms. Thus, learning to explain how a set of symptoms is consistent with a diagnosis may be very different from learning how to explain what causes a disease.

Perhaps the key role played by basic science may not be in facilitating clinical reasoning *per se*, but in facilitating explanation and coherent communication (Patel *et al.*, 1989). Physicians do not commonly offer basic science explanations when they are reasonably sure of their diagnoses. However, in times of uncertainty, physicians do resort to scientific explanations which are coherent, even if inaccurate. We also see this in medical students when they attempt to integrate knowledge across domains. Basic science provides a powerful means of connecting disparate phenomena and of generating explanations that, if still inaccurate, are much more coherent. The critical observation, then, is that well-organized, coherent information is easier to remember than disjointed collections of facts. Thus, the ability to explain something, even idiosyncratically to oneself, is necessary if information is to be communicated effectively and retained in memory for further analysis and, more importantly, for learning. It is argued, then, that the role of basic science, besides providing the concepts and vocabulary required to formulate clinical problems, is to create a basis for establishing and assessing coherence in the explanation of biomedical phenomena. Basic science does not provide the axioms, the analogies or the abstractions required to support clinical problem solving. Rather, it provides the principles that make it possible to organize observations that defy ready clinical classification and analysis. We also contend that, because clinical reasoning demands the coordination of multiple tasks and goals, the ability to organize and communicate observations is an absolute prerequisite for medical expertise.

We have proposed that basic science knowledge is a valuable tool in the development of coherence in the explanation of clinical phenomena. This role of basic science is under-appreciated by the general medical and educational communities. In response to the proposal that the teaching of basic science and clinical knowledge should be completely merged, Trelstad (1991) argues that 'basic science is a unique and special activity that when melded into a clinical environment, will only be diluted in focus and quality' (p. 1186). This suggestion echoes the concerns and issues raised in this chapter. While we believe that teaching of basic science in context is important, it is not sufficient for promoting the robust transfer of usable knowledge. The 'two world' hypothesis implies that each body of knowledge be given special status in the medical curriculum and that the correspondences between the two worlds need to be developed.

Common findings in research into scientific domains are that students have inherent difficulty in transferring knowledge across contexts and that instruction fails to promote robust transferable knowledge. This is readily apparent in the lack of utility within clinical contexts of basic science knowledge as it is commonly taught. Salomon and Perkins (1989, 1998) propose a useful distinction for characterizing different kinds of transfer and the relative time points at which transfer occurs.

Forward-reaching transfer occurs when one abstracts basic elements in anticipation of later application. This type of transfer would be expected when one is acquiring basic science knowledge in a classroom setting. Backward-reaching transfer is required when one faces a new situation and deliberately searches for relevant knowledge already acquired. This kind of transfer is exemplified in situations when one is engaged in a clinical reasoning task and needs to abstract particular principles to explain a complex problem. The challenge for medical schools is to present concepts in diverse contexts and make the relationships between the specific and general aspects explicit. This entails striking the right balance between presenting information in applied contexts (e.g. as illustrated by a clinical problem) and allowing students to derive the appropriate abstractions and generalizations to further develop their models of conceptual understanding. This would enhance the opportunities for promoting forward-reaching and backward-reaching transfer, enhancing the role of basic science knowledge as a valuable resource for developing coherent explanations in a clinical reasoning context.

Acknowledgements

The work for updating this chapter was supported by grants from the Social Sciences and Humanities Research Council of Canada (nos 410951206 and 410981356).

References

Arocha, J. F., Patel, V. L. and Patel, Y. C. (1993) Hypothesis generation and the coordination of theory and evidence in novice diagnostic reasoning. *Medical Decision Making*, **13**, 198–211.

Blois, M. S. (1988) Medicine and the nature of vertical reasoning. *New England Journal of Medicine*, **318**, 847–851.

Boshuizen, H. P. A., Schmidt, H. G. and Coughlin, L. D. (1988) On the application of medical basic science in clinical reasoning: Implications for structural knowledge differences between experts and novices. In *Proceedings of the Tenth Annual Conference of the Cognitive Science Society* (V. L. Patel and G. J. Groen, eds), pp. 517–523. Hillsdale, NJ: Lawrence Erlbaum.

Cavazos, L. F. (1984) Basic science studies: Their purpose in medical education. *Journal of Medical Education*, **59**, 763.

Charness, N. (1991) Expertise in chess: The balance between knowledge and search. In *Toward a General Theory of Expertise: Prospects and Limits* (A. Ericsson and J. Smith, eds), pp. 39–63. New York: Cambridge University Press.

Chi, M. T. H., Feltovich, P. J. and Glaser, R. (1981) Categorization and representation of physics problems by experts and novices. *Cognitive Science*, **5**, 121–152.

Clancey, W. J. (1988) Acquiring, representing and evaluating a competence model of diagnostic strategy. In *The Nature of Expertise* (M. T. H. Chi, R. Glaser and M. Farr, eds), pp. 343–418, Hillsdale, NJ: Lawrence Erlbaum.

Cruess, R. L., Patel, V .L. and Groen, G. J. (1985) Basic science studies (Response to the Editorial Comments). *Journal of Medical Education*, **60**, 208.

Dawson-Saunders, B., Feltovich, P. J., Coulson, R. L. and Steward, D. (1990) A survey of medical school teachers to identify basic biomedical concepts medical students should understand. *Academic Medicine*, **7**, 448–454.

Ericsson, A. and Smith, J. (eds) (1991) *Toward a General Theory of Expertise: Prospects and Limits*. New York: Cambridge University Press.

Feinstein, A. R. (1973) An analysis of diagnostic reasoning: The domain and disorders of clinical macrobiology. *Yale Journal of Biology and Medicine*, **46**, 264–283.

Feltovich, P. J. and Barrows, H. A. (1984) Issues of generality in medical problem solving. In *Tutorials in Problem Based Learning* (H. G. Schmidt and M. L. De Volder, eds), pp. 128–142. Assen: van Gorcum.

Feltovich, P. J., Spiro, R. and Coulson, R. L. (1989) The nature of conceptual understanding in biomedicine: The deep structure of complex ideas and the development of misconceptions. In *Cognitive Science in Medicine: Biomedical Modeling* (D. A. Evans and V. L. Patel, eds), pp. 113–172. Cambridge, MA: MIT Press.

Flexner, A. (1910) *Medical Education in the United States and Canada*. Bulletin 4. New York: Carnegie Foundation for the Advancement of Teaching.

Friedman, C. F. and Purcell, E. F. (1983) *The New Biology and Medical Education: Merging the Biological Information, and Cognitive Sciences*. New York: Josiah Macy Jr Foundation.

Joseph, G.-M. and Patel, V. L. (1990) Domain knowledge and hypothesis generation in diagnostic reasoning. *Medical Decision Making*, **10**, 31–46.

Kaufman, D. R., Patel, V. L. and Magder, S. A. (1992) *Development of Conceptual Understanding of Biomedical Concepts*. Technical Report CME92-CS4. Montreal, Quebec: Centre for Medical Education, McGill University.

Kaufman, D. R., Patel, V. L. and Magder, S. A. (1996) The explanatory role of spontaneously generated analogies in a reasoning about physiological concepts. *International Journal of Science Education*, **18**, 369–386.

Lesgold, A. M., Rubinson, H., Feltovich, P. J., Glaser, R., Klopfer, D. and Wang, Y. (1988) Expertise in a complex skill: Diagnosing X-ray pictures. In *The Nature of Expertise* (M. T. H. Chi, R. Glaser and M. J. Farr, eds), pp. 311–342. Hillsdale, NJ: Lawrence Erlbaum.

Neame, R. L. B. (1984) The preclinical course of study: Help or hindrance. *Journal of Medical Education*, **59**, 699–707.

Norman, G., Brooks, L. R., Rosenthal, D., Allen, S. W. and Muzzin, L. J. (1989) The development of expertise in dermatology. *Archives of Dermatology*, **125**, 1063–1068.

Patel, V. L. and Groen, G. J. (1986) Knowledge-based solution strategies in medical reasoning. *Cognitive Science*, **10**, 91–116.

Patel, V. L. and Kaufman, D. R. (1998a) Bridging theory to practice: Medical informatics as a local science of design. *Journal of the American Medical Informatics Association*, **5**, 489–492.

Patel, V. L. and Kaufman, D. R. (1998b) Medical informatics and the science of cognition. *Journal of the American Medical Informatics Association*, **6**, 493–502.

Patel, V. L., Evans, D. A. and Groen, G. J. (1989) Biomedical knowledge and clinical reasoning. In *Cognitive Science in Medicine: Biomedical Modeling* (D. A. Evans and V. L. Patel, eds), pp. 49–108. Cambridge, MA: MIT Press.

Patel, V. L., Evans, D. A. and Kaufman, D. R. (1990a) Reasoning strategies and use of biomedical knowledge by students. *Medical Education*, **24**, 129–136.

Patel, V. L., Groen, G. J. and Arocha J. F. (1990b) Medical expertise as a function of task difficulty. *Memory and Cognition*, **18**, 394–406.

Patel, V. L., Groen, G. J. and Norman, G. R. (1991a) Effects of conventional and problem- based medical curricula on problem solving. *Academic Medicine*, **66**, 380–389.

Patel, V. L., Groen, G. J. and Norman, G. R. (1993) Reasoning and instruction in medical curricula. *Cognition and Instruction*, **10**, 335–378.

Patel, V. L., Groen, G. J. and Scott, H. S. (1988) Biomedical knowledge in explanations of clinical problems by medical students. *Medical Education*, **22**, 398–406.

Patel, V. L., Kaufman, D. R. and Magder, S. (1991b) Causal reasoning about complex physiological concepts by medical students. *International Journal of Science Education*, **13**, 171–185.

Patel, V. L., Kaufman, D. R. and Arocha, J. F. (1999) Conceptual change in the biomedical and health sciences. In: *Advances in Instructional Psychology* (R. Glaser, ed.), Vol. 5, Hillsdale, NJ: Lawrence Erlbaum, in press.

Pople, H. E. (1982) Heuristic methods for imposing structure on ill-structured problems: The structuring of medical diagnostics. In *Artificial Intelligence in Medicine* (P. Szolovitz, ed.), pp. 119–190. Boulder, CO: Western Press.

Prokop, D. J. (1992) Basic science and clinical practice: How much will a physician need to know? In *Medical Education in Transition* (R. Q. Marston and R. M. Jones, eds), pp. 51–57. Princeton, NJ: The Robert Wood Johnson Foundation.

Salomon, G. and Perkins, D. N. (1989) Rocky roads to transfer: Rethinking mechanism of a neglected phenomenon. *Educational Psychologist*, **24**, 113–143.

Salomon, G. and Perkins, D. (1998) Individual and social aspects of learning. In *Review of Research in Education* (P. D. Pearson and A. Iran-Nejad, eds), Vol. 23, pp. 1–24.

Washington, DC: American Educational Research Association.

Schaffner, K. F. (1986) Exemplar reasoning about biological models and diseases: A relation between the philosophy of medicine and philosophy of science. *Journal of Medicine and Philosophy*, **11**, 63–80.

Schmidt, H. G. and Boshuizen, H. P. A. (1992) Encapsulation of biomedical knowledge. In *Advanced Models of Cognition for Medical Training and Practice* (D. A. Evans and V. L. Patel, eds), pp. 265–282. NATO ASI. Series F: Computer and Systems Sciences, Vol. 97. Heidelberg: Springer.

Stead, W. W. (1998) It is the information that's important, not the technology. *Journal of the American Medical Informatics Association*, **5**, 131.

Stritter, F. T. and Mattern, W. D. (1983) Thoughts about the medical school curriculum. In *The New Biology and Medical Education: Merging the Biological Information, and Cognitive Sciences* (C. P. Friedman and E. F. Purcell, eds), pp. 228–235. New York: Josiah Macy Jr Foundation.

Trelstad, R. L. (1991) The nation's medical curriculum in transition: Progression or retrogression? Reactions to the Robert Wood Johnson Foundation Commission on Medical Education. *Human Pathology*, **22**, 1183–1186.

5

Parallels between clinical reasoning and categorization

Brett Hayes and Roger Adams

For some time it has been recognized that the application of concepts and methods from cognitive psychology provides a useful framework for the study of clinical decision making.[1] This chapter continues this theme by exploring the relevance to clinical decision making of theory and research from what has to date been a somewhat neglected area of study, i.e. human categorization. Initially, we consider the applicability of categorization as a descriptor for many of the cognitive processes involved in clinical diagnosis and treatment planning. We then briefly review three competing models of categorization, and discuss their implications for the understanding of clinical reasoning and the teaching of clinical-reasoning skills. Finally, the way in which categorization processes evolve with clinical experience is explored.

What is categorization and why is it important?

Categorization occurs whenever we treat two or more distinguishable cases, objects or events equivalently (Mervis and Rosch, 1981). Categorization processes can be seen to operate routinely in everyday life when we decide that some object is a member of a familiar category such as dog, cat or bird, or when, in the practice of a health profession, a clinically relevant decision is made. For example, in radiology, a clinician might view an X-ray of a lung and on the basis of the observed visual features make a preliminary diagnosis such

as atelectasis (collapsed lung), multiple tumour or pathology free. Similarly, in sports physiotherapy, the clinician will take a history, watch an injured athlete's gait, manually examine the injured limb and subsequently may make a diagnosis of hamstring tear, ACL rupture or no structural damage. Whenever a clinician uses salient features of the patient's condition to assign a diagnostic label to that problem, categorization can be said to have taken place.

In general terms, the ability of human beings to categorize is extremely useful because it allows us to make sense of the almost infinite variety of stimuli in the world and to go beyond the information contained in a particular case or instance. In the context of clinical assessment, diagnostic categorization serves several important functions. It permits the clinician to make concurrent predictions about clinical signs or symptoms that are usually associated with the diagnosed condition but which have not yet been observed in a given patient (Mumma, 1993). It also allows the clinician to make prospective predictions about the likely course of the condition and hence guides the selection of appropriate treatment strategies (Blashfeld et al., 1989). Moreover, diagnosis helps the clinician to see the commonalities between cases that may seem, on first presentation, to be quite diverse. In this way diagnosis facilitates the development of deeper theories of the aetiology and maintenance of the clinical disorder.

Recent research in cognitive psychology has taught us much about how people learn and use categories in everyday life (for reviews, see Heit, 1997; Komatsu, 1992; Medin, 1989) and there is a

[1] See chapters 2, 4 and 9.

growing awareness that many of the issues examined in such research have considerable relevance
to the understanding of clinical reasoning (*cf.*
Mumma, 1993; Norman *et al.*, 1992a; Papa *et al.*,
1990; Schmidt *et al.*, 1990). Our aim is to identify
and review some of this evidence, and to explore
ways in which it can guide approaches to the
teaching of clinical reasoning. Before we proceed,
however, we need to deal with two issues relating
to the scope of application of categorization theory
to clinical domains.

The first issue concerns the nature of the clinical
disciplines which can benefit from a better understanding of categorization processes. Some authors
in the clinical literature (e.g. Norman *et al.*, 1992b)
have suggested that the parallels between categorization processes and the processes involved in
diagnosis may be limited to fields such as radiology, dermatology and pathology, where the rapid
and simultaneous processing of perceptual cues is
important in clinical judgements. Basic categorization processes are considered less important in
primary care or internal medicine, in which self-
reported data about a patient's history, physical
condition and the results of laboratory tests must
be gathered over an extended period of time,
analysed and integrated before a diagnosis can be
made. However, we believe that this emphasis on
the 'pattern recognition' component of categorization is unwarranted and overly conservative in its
estimation of the relevance of categorization
theory. Categorization, while often involving the
recognition of perceptual patterns, should be
regarded as a type of schema abstraction
(Komatsu, 1992) in which we decide the meaning
of objects, events or cases and how we should
behave towards them. Hence categorization theory
has proved useful in the analysis of how people
come to apply categorical labels to complex
stimuli such as personality profiles and biographical descriptions (e.g. Lingle *et al.*, 1983), elaborate semantic concepts (e.g. Lakoff, 1986), and
psychiatric diagnoses (Genero and Cantor, 1987;
Horowitz *et al.*, 1981). There seems no good
reason, therefore, why categorization research
cannot provide useful insights into the complex
clinical decisions associated with fields such as
internal medicine, nursing, occupational therapy
and physiotherapy, where social, emotional and
environmental cues, as well as physical cues, are
important parts of a patient's presentation.

The second important issue concerns the components of the therapeutic process in which categorization might operate. The clearest parallel with
everyday object categorization is in the assignment
of a diagnostic label to a presenting patient and
indeed the main focus of this chapter is on the role
that categorization plays in diagnosis. One should
not assume, however, that this is the only way that
categorization affects clinical reasoning. Categorization also operates whenever we decide on a
particular treatment regimen for an individual or
when we judge a case to have a poor, fair or good
prognosis. To illustrate, let us say that we have two
treatments available, treatment A and treatment B.
Even if we eschew the use of diagnostic labels we
are unlikely to treat every individual case as
completely unique. In choosing a treatment for a
given patient we will be guided by the degree to
which that person is similar to previous patients
who had responded well to treatment A rather than
treatment B or vice versa. Of course, when we draw
on our experience in this way we are categorizing.
Categorization can thus be seen to exert a pervasive
influence on a variety of aspects of the processes of
assessment and treatment of health problems.

Models of category acquisition and representation

One aspect of the usefulness of the categorization
literature to those interested in clinical reasoning is
that much of the research has been concerned with
the way in which novel categories are learned as a
result of experience with individual instances or
case examples. Interest has been centred on the
parameters that affect category acquisition, the way
in which categories are stored in memory, and the
way acquired category knowledge guides the
classification of both familiar and novel instances.
Clearly, a better understanding of such processes
may inform approaches to the teaching of diagnostic
and other pattern recognition skills, and may provide
insights into the ways perception of a case may
change with increasing case experience or expertise.
Moreover, knowing more about the processes by
which individuals learn new diagnostic categories
will provide valuable information for those responsible for teaching diagnostic skills. To this end we
begin with a brief review of the major models and
findings in the area of category learning.

Classical and prototype models of category learning

Until relatively recently, most models of human
category learning assumed that natural categories

were represented in memory as sets of 'defining' features which were both necessary and sufficient for category membership (e.g. Bruner *et al.*, 1956). That is, it was believed that all members of the category shared some common feature or properties, that all instances were equally good members of a category and that the boundaries between categories were distinct. To illustrate the clinical implications of this approach, consider a common diagnostic category such as influenza which might be defined formally as 'an acute infectious disease due to influenza virus. Infection is of the upper respiratory tract with general constitutional symptoms of fever, malaise and muscular aches' (Critchley, 1978, p. 886). The classical categorization view would lead to the highly questionable predictions that all the definitional features should be present in each and every case of influenza and that this symptom set did not overlap with other diagnostic categories.

Both clinical intuition and a wealth of research into everyday human categorization (e.g. Rosch, 1975; Smith and Medin, 1981) suggest that this 'classical' theory of category structure is incorrect. Most researchers studying clinical diagnosis (e.g. Bursztajn *et al.*, 1981; Genero and Cantor, 1987) now assume that the clinical features that a person observes are related only in a probabilistic way to categorical labels. Although certain clinical features may be correlated strongly with the presence of a particular condition, in most cases no single clinical sign or symptom is thought to be both necessary and sufficient for the diagnosis of a particular disease. Like the object categories examined by Rosch (1975), diagnostic categories can be said to have an 'internal structure', with some individual cases or instances judged to be more typical of the disease category as a whole than others. Hence, medical students and doctors judge conditions such as ulcerative colitis and duodenal ulcers as better examples of the general diagnostic category gastrointestinal disorders than problems such as oesophageal spasm (Bordage and Zacks, 1984). Clinicians also diagnose cases that show such typical symptoms more quickly and confidently than less typical cases (Blashfeld *et al.*, 1989; Horowitz *et al.*, 1981).

The rejection of the classical model has led to the search for alternative ways of explaining the process of human categorization. One of the most influential of such approaches is the view that through exposure to category members one comes to abstract the central tendency of these exemplars (e.g. Posner and Keele, 1968). This 'prototype' representation would contain the features that are most frequently associated with category members, and is thought to be used as a basis for categorization decisions. A novel instance is classified as a member of that category whose prototype it most closely resembles. In a diagnostic context it would be argued that as a result of exposure to a variety of cases which share a common underlying pathology, a clinician abstracts and stores a summary of the characteristic symptoms, signs or 'features' of that condition. Future diagnoses involving this condition would involve a comparison between the features of the presenting case and those of the stored diagnostic prototype or schema.

Early evidence that people abstract prototypes during the course of category learning came from studies such as that of Posner and Keele (1968), who trained adult subjects to classify small sets of random dot patterns into a number of alternative categories. Each item was presented individually, the subject made a classification judgement and was given corrective feedback. Importantly, the prototype of each category, which was formed from the statistical average of the category members, was not presented during this training period. Upon learning to classify correctly each of the training items, subjects proceeded to a test phase in which they were presented with training instances, novel category items and the prototypes of each of the training categories. The prototypes, which had not been encountered previously, were classified more accurately and quickly than any other new pattern and as accurately as the training instances. This result, which has been replicated across a wide range of stimuli (Komatsu, 1992), suggests that people routinely form prototypes when they are learning a novel category and that these prototypes play an important part in subsequent classification decisions.

Bordage and Zacks (1984) investigated the use of prototype representations in medical students' and general practitioners' knowledge of physical diseases. They first obtained ratings of how typical a set of individual diseases were of a number of general categories of medical disorder (e.g. respiratory disorders, endocrine disorders, infections, neoplasms, dyspnoea) asking their subjects to list diseases that belonged to each category. Highly typical and atypical diseases were then presented in a semantic verification procedure in which subjects had to make speeded decisions about the truth (e.g. 'diabetes mellitus is a kind of endocrine disorder') or falsity (e.g. 'otitis media is a kind of gastrointestinal disorder') of a number of statements. Both doctors and students responded more quickly and with fewer errors to the statements involving 'typical' disorders than they did for the 'atypical' disorders.

It would of course be wrong to think that prototype abstraction was the only categorization process involved in clinical decision making. Information about the central tendency of previously experienced cases is just one of the many factors that contribute to the assignment of a diagnosis to a patient. Just as important in many ways is knowledge of the degree to which individual cases vary around the central tendency or prototype. Some diseases (e.g. inguinal hernia) might be said to have 'low variability' because their clinical presentation tends to be quite similar across cases. Other disorders (e.g. bowel cancer) manifest themselves in very different ways in different individuals. A skilled clinician relies on his or her knowledge of such clinical variability in arriving at a diagnosis (Regehr and Norman, 1996).

To find solid empirical evidence regarding the learning and use of information about category variability, we need only return to Posner and Keele's (1968) seminal work. In the training phase of their category learning study they systematically manipulated the within-category variability of the sets of visual patterns presented to subjects. The low variability sets contained items that were very similar to one another and to the category prototype, the high variability condition contained both highly typical and atypical items, and the moderate condition was made up of items with an intermediate level of variability. The level of variation in the training items was found to have a significant effect on the subsequent transfer test, with subjects trained on moderately variable items classifying more test patterns correctly than either of the other two groups. This result has since been replicated and extended, with demonstrations that knowledge of property variability within a category may in some cases be the primary basis for categorization decisions (e.g. Rips, 1989) and that training with instances that vary in their typicality leads to better retention of category properties over extended periods of time (Homa and Vosburgh, 1976).

In the disease or injury diagnosis context these findings are significant in two ways. First, they confirm our earlier assertion that object categorization, like clinical diagnosis, involves consideration of both the central tendency (i.e. most typical) of category features as well as the range of feature variability which exists in the category. More importantly, these findings point to a principle that may guide future studies of diagnostic training. Such research indicates that if we wish to equip clinicians to diagnose accurately a range of cases that share the same underlying pathology, we need to train them with cases that vary considerably in the typicality of their clinical signs and symptoms. The presentation of only 'typical' cases of a particular condition will result in a rather narrow and error-prone diagnostic schema.

Although we suspect that many clinical training programs already incorporate this advice, to our knowledge no controlled training study has yet tested the hypothesis. The category learning procedure used by Posner and Keele (1968) and many others subsequently (e.g. Medin, 1989) could, however, be easily adapted for the purpose. One would begin by presenting trainee clinicians with cases belonging to a number of illness or injury categories. By obtaining normative ratings of the typicality of each case relative to the category as a whole, one would also be able to manipulate the degree of within-category variability in the training sets. When the trainees had learned to classify the training items they could be presented with old, novel and prototypical cases, and their accuracy in diagnosis of each of these case types compared.

Exemplar approaches to categorization

Even if we assume that people learning categories routinely store information about both prototypes and category variability, many would argue that we still underestimate the complexity of human categorization processes. Many influential models of categorization assume that category learning is actually a process of storage of the memory traces of individual category members or exemplars. Categorization is thus seen to involve a comparison of a novel instance to some or all of the known exemplars of the category (for a detailed discussion of such models, see Brooks, 1987; Komatsu, 1992). In a diagnostic context, this model would predict that disease and injury categories are represented by the individual cases that a clinician has encountered in the past, and the diagnosis of a new case will be determined by its similarity to past cases of particular illness or injury states.

Exemplar models have little difficulty explaining people's sensitivity to variability within a category (Kruschke, 1996). In direct comparisons of prototype and exemplar models in laboratory-based category learning experiments, the latter have often been found to be more successful (e.g. Brooks, 1987; Komatsu, 1992 for a review).

Brooks *et al.* (1991) provided a clear demonstration of the influence of knowledge of prior instances in the diagnosis of skin disorders. Medical residents and experienced physicians first rated how typical a number of photographs of dermatological lesions were of their respective diagnostic categories. This exposure to concrete examples was found to facilitate the accuracy of the subsequent diagnosis of cases involving perceptually similar lesions, but not of dissimilar cases belonging to the same diagnostic category or cases belonging to an alternative category. This effect was found to persist even when a 2 week delay between the initial and test cases was introduced, and was not affected by instructions to diagnose on the basis of 'first impressions' or to give careful consideration to alternative diagnoses.

Hence, exposure to concrete prior examples of diagnostic categories can and does influence diagnostic classification, even in clinicians with ample experience of the clinical features of the conditions under consideration. It remains to be shown whether such facilitative effects can be found in less 'perceptual' diagnostic domains. Nevertheless, this effect, which was of the order of 10–20% improvement in diagnostic accuracy over cases that did not resemble the old instances, is a compelling argument in favour of greater consideration of the role of exemplar effects in clinical diagnosis.

A further reason for the serious examination of exemplar-based categorization models in the analysis of diagnosis is the fact that such models are better than prototype models at explaining the learning of feature correlations. Although at some early stage of training clinicians learn about each of the individual signs and symptoms of a disorder, many would argue that diagnosis and other important clinical judgements are strongly influenced by the detection of significant clusters of clinical features that tend to co-occur across cases (Schwartz and Griffin, 1986). An analogous process can be seen to occur in everyday categorization, where with sufficient experience we develop a sensitivity to covariation between features. Thus, for example, in the course of learning about members of the category bird one comes to expect that if a particular member of this category is large it will not sing or if it is small it would make its nest in trees.

Exemplar models of categorization have in general been shown to give better accounts of

feature correlation learning than models which assume that only prototype information is stored (Smith and Medin, 1981). The applied implication of this finding is that an exemplar- or case-based approach to training should be the preferred method for teaching students about significant correlations between clinical features. Indirect support for this thesis was found in a recent study by Wattenmaker (1991), who examined ways of facilitating people's sensitivity to feature correlations in artificial categories composed of sets of fictitious biographical descriptions. Each of these categories contained some feature pairs which always appeared together. Subjects were first trained with instructions that either emphasized the memorization of each individual instance (exemplar-based processing) or encouraged them to look for the features that were shared between category members (prototype abstraction). Those given the exemplar-based training performed far better in a subsequent task in which the same subjects were presented with pairs of correlated features and asked to choose the category to which these feature pairs belonged.

The implication of this finding for the teaching of clinical-reasoning skills seems clear. If we wish trainee clinicians to become sensitive to relationships between the clinical features of a disorder then a system that emphasizes the careful analysis of individual cases is to be preferred to one that focuses simply on the common typical features of the diagnostic class.

Which categorization model best fits the clinical context?

We have seen that exemplar approaches to clinical reasoning have some advantages over models which assume that most decisions are based on a consideration of only the prototypical features of a disorder. But surely an extreme exemplar-based account of clinical categorization, in which only individual case examples are stored, is equally misleading. After all, most clinical training courses begin the teaching of diagnosis with a description of the typical clinical features of a problem. Moreover, the implication that skilled diagnosis involves greater reliance on analogy to previously experienced cases seems to run contrary to findings that medical experts are distinguished by their 'chunking' of diagnostic features into abstract, higher order units (e.g. Lesgold *et al.*, 1988; Norman *et al.*, 1979).

A growing number of researchers are now coming to emphasize the flexibility of human categorization, acknowledging that for most categories, people have access to category-wide generalizations as well as the specific details of previous exemplars (cf. Brooks, 1987; Hayes and Taplin, 1993; Kruschke, 1996). Which of these various sources of information has the greatest influence on categorization decisions seems to depend upon the specific structure of the category learning situation. One factor that influences the use of prototype knowledge, namely within-category variation, has already been discussed. A second factor, the size of the category being learned, has also been established as an important determinant of the use of prototype and exemplar information. When a person's experience is limited to only a few category instances, as is the case for the novice clinician, their classification decisions are likely to be strongly influenced by the idiosyncratic features of these cases (Homa *et al.*, 1981). As the number of exemplars to be learned increases, people come to rely more on knowledge of prototypical features in assigning category membership. Other factors that have been shown to modulate the use of exemplar- or prototype-based strategies of categorization are the number of times that a particular case is repeated during training, the number of categories to be learned (Homa *et al.*, 1991), the delay between initial exposure to category members and subsequent classification tasks (Smith and Medin, 1981), and the level of corrective feedback given to subjects about category membership decisions (Klahr and Dunbar, 1988).

In drawing out the implications of these findings for medical diagnosis we are reminded of the comments made by Norman *et al.* (1992b) in their review of research concerning expertise in radiology and dermatology. These authors noted that one of the failings of studies in this area was the absence of detailed studies examining task factors that may influence the use of perceptual and reasoning strategies in the diagnostic process. The literature reviewed above indicates that such task factors are indeed important in determining the approach to, and effectiveness of, diagnosis and identifies a number of specific factors that are well worth investigating in a clinical setting.

A further important factor that impacts on the way in which clinicians might mentally represent diagnostic categories is their level of expertise. Genero and Cantor (1987), when training students to recognize psychiatric conditions, found that pre-novices (undergraduate students) benefited most from information presented in summary, prototype form, while more experienced practitioners (graduate students) appeared to show the greatest benefit from information presented as multiple exemplars. Hence, the model of categorization that best fits the learning process for clinicians may depend critically on levels of training and experience. This point is examined in greater depth in the next section.

The effects of expertise

As well as producing a better grasp of the features of a variety of clinical conditions, increasing clinical experience may result in more subtle and complex changes in the conceptual structure of clinicians. Comparisons of expert and novice clinicians have shown that experts possess more differentiated and flexible diagnostic categories than novices (e.g. Feltovich *et al.*, 1984), as well as a better ability to perceive the abstract similarities between conditions that have very different clinical features (Murphy and Wright, 1984). The importance of such knowledge of the complex relationships between different disorders was further illustrated in a study by Pauker *et al.* (1976). They observed that in taking patient histories, expert doctors not only generated a hypothetical diagnosis more quickly than students but also were able to call to mind more alternative diagnostic categories that plausibly explained the clinical features of a presenting case (e.g. they noted that a case of multiple pulmonary emboli could be mistaken for cardiomyopathy). This rather complex pattern of results is consistent with a growing recognition in the wider categorization literature that, with experience, category knowledge moves beyond a consideration of prototypical features or the details of particular instances. Expert categorizers also develop heuristics, rules of plausible reasoning, and theories about the links between different categories that guide their inferences (Murphy and Medin, 1985).

The effects that such complex knowledge frameworks can have on category learning have been demonstrated by Medin *et al* (1987) using a category-sorting procedure. University undergraduates were asked to sort eight instances of fictitious diseases into two 'sensible' groups of equal size. The set was structured so that it could be divided by attending to either of two pairs of correlated category features. Although in terms of the objective category structure either feature pair was an equally valid way of sorting the categories, subjects showed a strong tendency to sort on the basis of feature pairs for which they could see a plausible causal link (e.g. earache and dizziness) rather than feature pairs that were perceived as less closely connected (e.g. itchiness and weight gain). Hence, the subjects' prior knowledge of the causal relationships between certain symptoms had a profound effect on their learning of feature relationships in a novel category.

The influence that such complex cognitive strategies have on the encoding of clinical features during radiological diagnosis has been investigated by Norman and his colleagues (Norman *et al.*, 1992a). These researchers first provided expert and resident radiologists with X-ray films accompanied by a clinical history that led them to expect that the cases either were normal or showed signs of bronchiolitis. After reading the history the clinicians were asked to list all symptomatic features present in the X-ray and to estimate the probability of disease. When they were biased to expect a positive result from the patient history, the expert and novice radiologists gave higher disease probability ratings and found significantly more symptomatic features in both abnormal and normal films than when the case history was normal. This result is startling in many ways, since it shows that the bias created by the patient histories was strong enough to lead even experienced radiologists to report clinical signs which were not actually present in the normal slides.

Norman *et al.* (1992a) concluded that hypotheses and expectations formed very early in the diagnostic process can directly affect the search for, and encoding of, clinical features and subsequent diagnosis. While this is almost certainly true in some cases, the evidence from the object categorization literature suggests that the relationship between one's expectations about a patient based on background history and the search for clinical features may actually be far more complex (*cf.* Murphy and Medin, 1985; Mumma, 1993). Wisniewski and Medin (1994) examined the interaction between 'top-down' information such as a person's prior expectations or hypotheses about category assignment and 'bottom-up' information such as the presence or absence of particular features in a visual category-learning task. They found evidence for a bidirectional

interaction between these two types of information. As in the Norman *et al.* (1992a) study, people's different expectations led them to attend selectively to different features in generating category membership rules, to treat the same visual features in different ways and to encode particular combinations of features into higher-order chunks. Significantly, however, when subjects were given further information about the accuracy of their category assignments, particularly when they were given negative feedback, they changed their categorization strategies. Some subjects shifted their interpretation of specific visual features, while others changed their criteria for category membership or shifted their focus to consider features that they had previously ignored.

Such results indicate that while top-down expectations may guide the initial feature search in diagnosis, there is an ongoing interaction between expectations and data such that clinical information which strongly contradicts the initial hypotheses may change one's expectations and diagnostic strategies for future cases. This process is illustrated in Figure 5.1. The figure highlights a number of aspects of the process of clinical diagnosis that warrant further investigation. Following Norman *et al.* (1992a), further research is needed to understand exactly how a clinician's initial hypotheses, or any other information which biases his or her expectations about a particular case, affect the search for clinical signs and symptoms. Similarly, we need a better grasp of the ways in which clinicians shift their diagnostic strategies when they receive information which disconfirms their original hypotheses about a case, and the best way to present this negative feedback to them (see Heit, 1997, and Schwartz and Griffin, 1986, for some suggestions regarding how such research should proceed). Finally, the ways in which clinical expertise alters and tunes both the top-down expectations about a patient's condition as well as the actual clinical information which is deemed significant for diagnosis need to be investigated more thoroughly.

Conclusions

The pioneering work of Bordage and Zacks (1984), and of Norman, Brooks and their colleagues has demonstrated the usefulness of theoretical models and methods from the human

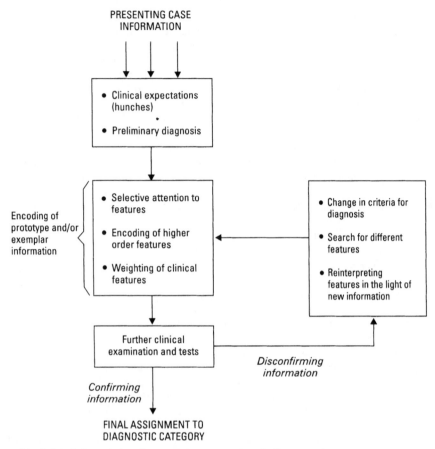

Figure 5.1 A model of clinical diagnosis based upon contemporary categorization research

categorization literature in the exploration of the clinical reasoning process. Our purpose here was to clarify and extend this theoretical framework and to highlight the many areas of clinical decision making that could benefit from an approach that views such decisions as complex categorization tasks. In particular, categorization theory informs the debate about the way in which diagnostic categories might be represented in memory, indicates the significant task variables that may mediate the use of different diagnostic strategies, and provides guidelines for the structure of clinical training to enhance sensitivity to the co-occurrence of significant clinical features. Categorization research concerning the effects of top-down knowledge on feature encoding is also a fertile source of hypotheses about the way in which prior knowledge of a patient or diagnostic expectations influence feature search and how this process might change with clinical expertise.

References

Blashfeld, R. K., Sprock, J., Haymaker, M. A. and Hodgin, J. (1989) The family resemblance hypothesis applied to psychiatric classification. *The Journal of Nervous and Mental Disease*, **177**, 492–497.

Bordage, G. and Zacks, R. (1984) The structure of medical knowledge in the memories of medical students and general practitioners: Categories and prototypes. *Medical Education*, **18**, 406–416.

Brooks, L. R. (1987) Decentralised control of categorization: The role of prior processing episodes. In *Concepts and Conceptual Development: Ecological and Intellectual Factors in Categorization* (U. Neisser, ed.), pp. 141–174. Cambridge: Cambridge University Press.

Brooks, L. R., Norman, G. R. and Allen, S. W. (1991) Role of specific similarity in a medical diagnosis task. *Journal of Experimental Psychology: General*, **120**, 278–287.

Bruner, J. S., Goodnow, J. and Austin, G. (1956) *A Study of Thinking*. New York: Wiley.

Bursztajn, H., Feinbloom, R. I., Hamm, R. M. and Brodsky, A. (1981) *Medical Choices, Medical Chances*. New York: Delacorte Press.

Critchley, M. (ed.) (1978) *Butterworth's Medical Dictionary*, 2nd edn. Oxford: Butterworth-Heinemann.

Feltovich, P. J., Johnson, P. E., Moller, J. H. and Swanson, D. B. (1984) LCS: The role and development of medical knowledge in diagnostic expertise. In *Readings in Medical Artificial Intelligence: The First Decade* (W. J. Clancey and E. H. Shortliffe, eds), pp. 275–319. Reading, MA: Addison-Wesley.

Genero, N. and Cantor, N. (1987) Exemplar prototypes and clinical diagnosis: Toward a cognitive economy. *Journal of Social and Clinical Psychology*, **5**, 59–78.

Hayes, B. K. and Taplin, J. E. (1993) Developmental differences in the use of prototype and exemplar-specific information. *Journal of Experimental Child Psychology*, **55**, 329–352.

Heit, E. (1997) Knowledge and concept learning. In *Knowledge, Concepts, and Categories* (K. Lamberts and D. Shanks, eds.), pp. 7–41. London: Psychology Press.

Homa, D., Dunbar, S. and Nohre, L. (1991) Instance frequency, categorization, and the modulating effect of experience. *Journal of Experimental Psychology: Learning, Memory, and Cognition*, **17**, 444–458.

Homa, D., Sterling, S. and Trepel, L. (1981) Limitations of exemplar-based generalization and the abstraction of categorical information. *Journal of Experimental Psychology: Human Learning and Memory*, **7**, 418–439.

Homa, D. and Vosburgh, R. (1976) Category breadth and the abstraction of prototypical information. *Journal of Experimental Psychology: Human Learning and Memory*, **2**, 322–330.

Horowitz, L., Wright, J. C., Lowenstein, E. and Parad, H. (1981) The prototype as a construct in abnormal psychology: 1. A method for deriving prototypes. *Journal of Abnormal Psychology*, **90**, 568–574.

Klahr, D. and Dunbar, K. (1988) Dual space search during scientific reasoning. *Cognitive Science*, **12**, 139–175.

Komatsu, L. K. (1992) Recent views of conceptual structure. *Psychological Bulletin*, **112**, 500–526.

Kruschke, J. K. (1996) Dimensional relevance shifts in category learning. *Connection Science: Journal of Neural Computing, Artificial Intelligence and Cognitive Research*, **8**, 225–247.

Lakoff, G. (1986) *Women, Fire and Dangerous Things: What Categories Tell us About the Nature of Thought*. Chicago: Chicago University Press.

Lesgold, A. M., Rubinson, H., Feltovich, P., Glaser, R., Klopfer, D. and Wang, Y. (1988) Expertise in a complex skill: Diagnosing X-ray pictures. In *The Nature of Expertise* (M. T. H. Chi, R. Glaser and M. Farr, eds), pp. 322–351. Hillsdale, NJ: Lawrence Erlbaum.

Lingle, J. H., Altom, M. W. and Medin, D. L. (1983) Of cabbages and kings: Assessing the extensibility of natural object concept models to social things. In *Handbook of Social Cognition* (R. Wyer, T. Srull and J. Hartwick, eds), pp. 71–116. Hillsdale, NJ: Lawrence Erlbaum.

Medin, D. L. (1989) Concepts and conceptual structure. *American Psychologist*, **44**, 1469–1481.

Medin, D. L., Wattenmaker, W. D. and Hampson, S. E. (1987) Family resemblance, conceptual cohesiveness and category construction. *Cognitive Psychology*, **18**, 158–194

Mervis, C. B. and Rosch, E. (1981) Categorization of natural objects. *Annual Review of Psychology*, **32**, 89–115.

Mumma, G. H. (1993) Categorization and rule induction in clinical diagnosis and assessment. In *The Psychology of Learning and Motivation*, Vol. 29 (G. V. Nakamura, D. L. Medin and R. Taraban, eds), pp. 283–326. New York: Academic Press.

Murphy, G. L. and Medin, D. L. (1985) The role of theories in conceptual coherence. *Psychological Review*, **92**, 289–316.

Murphy, G. L. and Wright, J. C. (1984) Changes in conceptual structure with expertise: Differences between real-world experts and novices. *Journal of Experimental Psychology: Learning, Memory and Cognition*, **10**, 144–155.

Norman, G. R., Brooks, L. R., Coblentz, C. L. and Babcock, C. J. (1992a) The correlation of feature identification and category judgements in diagnostic radiology. *Memory and Cognition*, **20**, 344–355.

Norman, G. R., Coblentz, C. L., Brooks, L. R. and Babcock, C. J. (1992b) Expertise in visual diagnosis: A review of the literature. *Academic Medicine*, **67**, S78–S83.

Norman, G. R., Jacoby, L. L., Feightner, J. W. and Campbell, E. J. M. (1979) Clinical experience and the structure of memory. *Proceedings of the 18th Annual Conference on Research in Medical Education*, **18**, 163–168.

Papa, F. J., Shores, J. H. and Meyer, S. (1990) Effects of pattern matching, pattern discrimination, and experience in the development of diagnostic expertise. *Academic Medicine*, **65**, S21–S22.

Pauker, S. G., Gorry, G. A., Kassirer, J. P. and Schwartz, W. B. (1976) Towards the simulation of clinical cognition: Taking the present illness by computer. *The American Journal of Medicine*, **60**, 981–996.

Posner, M. I. and Keele, S. W. (1968) On the genesis of abstract ideas. *Journal of Experimental Psychology*, **77**, 353–363.

Regehr, G. and Norman, G. R. (1996) Issues in cognitive psychology: Implications for professional education. *Academic Medicine*, **71**, 988–1001.

Rips, L. J. (1989) Similarity, typicality, and categorization. In *Similarity, Analogy, and Thought* (S. Vosniadou and A. Ortony, eds), pp. 21–60. New York: Cambridge University Press.

Rosch, E. (1975) Cognitive representations of semantic categories. *Journal of Experimental Psychology: General*, **104**, 192–233.

Schmidt, H. G., Norman, G. R. and Boshuizen, H. P. A. (1990) A cognitive perspective on medical expertise: Theory and implications. *Academic Medicine*, **65**, 611–621.

Schwartz, S. and Griffin, T. (1986) *Medical Thinking: The Psychology of Medical Judgment and Decision Making*. New York: Springer.

Smith, E. E. and Medin, D. L. (1981) *Categories and Concepts*. Cambridge, MA: Harvard University Press.

Wattenmaker, W. D. (1991) Learning modes, feature correlations, and memory-based categorization. *Journal of Experimental Psychology: Learning, Memory and Cognition*, **17**, 908–923.

Wisniewski, E. J. and Medin, D. L. (1994) On the interaction of theory and data in concept learning. *Cognitive Science*, **18**, 221–281.

6

Action and narrative: Two dynamics of clinical reasoning

Maureen Hayes Fleming and Cheryl Mattingly

Research in clinical reasoning emerged from the medical problem-solving tradition which emphasized the hypothetical deductive method. Recently many theorists have argued that this strictly cognitive view is too narrow to encompass the myriad ways in which health professionals devise solutions for clients' needs. We have found that the desire to conduct effective treatment, especially in the rehabilitation professions, directs the clinician to understand the client as a person who makes meaning of the illness or injury in the context of a life. By emphasizing the social dimension of clinical reasoning we are highlighting a quality of expert judgement which is by nature improvisational, flexible, and highly attuned to the specifics of the person, the condition and the context.

We discuss two streams of reasoning, active judgement and narrative. Working out narrative possibilities and making active judgements are two dynamic processes which intertwine while the clinician carries out the best treatment with and for the individual patient. We further submit that through making and reflecting on these active judgements and narrative possibilities clinicians develop their own stock of tacit knowledge and enhance their expertise.

We draw upon ethnographic research projects we have conducted over the past decade, primarily (but by no means exclusively) among occupational therapists. This chapter is not a report of findings. We refer to these studies in a general way to illustrate and support a conception of clinical reasoning and expertise grounded in the complexities and nuances of everyday practice in the world of rehabilitation.

Action and judgement

Action is the essence of clinical practice. In occupational, physical and speech therapy the patient *must* act. Without the patient's participation there is no therapy. One common view of action is that action takes place after one has carefully thought about the problem and its possible resolution. The assumption is that one thinks carefully about the problem, decides what the central issue is, determines the best solution and takes action. This sequence may often be the case, but not always. Some philosophers, particularly the phenomenologists, claim that thought and action occur in a rapid dynamic relation to one another, not in a fixed sequence. The word 'judgement' is often used to express this dynamic relationship. Buchler (1955), following on the work of John Dewey, C. S. Pierce and others, points out that action not only expresses the results of a judgement, it can be a judgement itself. Buchler (1955, p.11) comments 'every action is itself a judgement'. Schön (1983) submits that reflective practitioners act first and judge the results afterward. Architecture students develop their expertise by looking at an area of land and sketching out versions of the structure they envision on that space. Action (sketching) is a way of seeing and a way of thinking. It is an act of both imagination and production in which an image becomes visible and can be judged. The imagined building comes briefly to life in the form of a drawing. The structure is 'built' in imagination, action and judgement long before the backhoe arrives. Between the imaginative eye and the artful hand, the practitioner negotiates the route between the creative image and the concrete restrictions of the size, slope and orientation of the site using a dynamic process of active judgement.

Health care practitioners also use imagination and action to make professional judgements about client's problems and potential solutions. The patient is a 'site' where the best structure must be, not constructed, but reconstructed. Health care practitioners work with persons in crisis with whom action must be taken immediately. Many judgements are made before, during and after action. In professional work action and judgement merge. The practitioner often has the advantage of having the patient – the person – as a partner or at least informant in the endeavour. Usually the patient trusts the clinician and is willing to respond to requests for action. The actions that the patient executes give the practitioner a great deal of information. Conversely, the clinician might take action on the patient and this gives the therapist another source of information. The clinician and patient become involved in a coordinated set of actions and interactions which many observers have characterized as a therapeutic dance.

Many professional judgements are based on observations and interpretations of patients' actions. Clinicians want to see if and how a patient can perform an action. The practitioner judges the quality of the motion in order to make clinical judgements regarding the current level of strength or range of motion and estimates the possible functional gains the patient may make during treatment. By judging today's action the clinician can gauge the potential for future functional performance. The patient is asked to perform specific motions or sets of movements, often and with frequent numbers of repetitions. Isolated motions, such as elbow flexion or thumb–finger prehension are requested. Every day the therapist asks for more repetitions, more weight, more concentration, etc. Therapists remind a person that they could not do this last week or yesterday, and point out what they can do today and where they could be tomorrow or next week. The story of progress toward reconstruction is played out in increasingly better and more functional actions. Clinicians want the patient's movements to match the image in the therapist's mind – to meet the perceived potential. Eventually the motions are combined into actions or sets of motions with a motive such as shoulder rotation, elbow extension, wrist stabilization, finger extension and flexion, etc., to reach for an object. Later these and other motions and actions are combined so that desired

functional activities, such as eating, may be performed. In a sense it is not the professional who is the therapist, but rather the patient and his/her ability to invest in meaningful action. Through this investment the person rebuilds the body and reconstructs a sense of self as a person who can function in the world – an actor.

Practitioners take many actions while treating their patients. They also gain information from their interpretations of the sensations they receive from the patient and they learn from their own actions. The therapist tests muscle tone, adjusts the position of finger and thumb in a tenodesis grasp or balances a child in her lap while he works with a toy. In the interest of improving the patient's potential for future action experts evaluate the patient's action, guide their own action, make interpretations simultaneously, make rapid judgements, and change action smoothly and rapidly. Action is both a concrete event and a reasoning strategy that mediates the flow of therapy from image to result. Simultaneously, clinicians learn if and how their own actions worked as effective treatment strategies. In this way a wealth of personal/professional expertise is developed. Much of this expertise knowledge is what Polanyi (1966) referred to as 'tacit knowledge'.

Tacit knowledge and professional judgement

When we conducted our first study we were confident that we would discover that therapists had a great deal of professional knowledge and skill, and had a great stock of tacit knowledge. We did not anticipate the great extent of the knowledge the therapists possessed and the degree to which they were unaware of it. Polanyi coined the term 'tacit knowledge' and described it as the stock of professional knowledge that experts possess, that is not processed in a focused cognitive manner but rather lies at a not quite conscious level where the knowledge is accessible through acting, judging or performing. This level of awareness is what Polanyi calls 'the tacit dimension'. It is a type of knowledge that is acquired through experience. Polanyi (1966, p. 4) called this tacit knowledge because experts were able to act on it but could not always verbalize exactly what they were doing or why. He expressed this concisely in the words 'we know more than we can tell'.

In daily practice the clinician encounters a new situation, takes action, perhaps several variations of a set of actions and reflects on them to evaluate whether this action 'worked'. Was it effective in solving a problem with this particular patient who in some ways was subtly different from the last patient of the same age, gender and diagnosis? Through this action and reflection the therapist builds a stock of tacit knowledge which becomes increasingly nuanced with further experience. Tacit knowledge has some advantages and disadvantages. It contributes to efficiency. The expert can do what is required, quickly and smoothly in much less time than it takes to explain. Since tacit knowledge is developed in action, it remains accessible to immediately guide action. Clinicians often literally act before they think. This is not mindless action, it is an automaticity of expertise which does not have to be processed through the lengthier channels of formal cognition. However, the inability to explain all that one knows causes others to question the credibility of the professional's knowledge. Occupational therapists in our study had a particular problem with this credibility issue because they had a wealth of practical tacit knowledge and confidence in their clinical skills, but did not have a rich language to explain or describe their practice, as do physicians and some other practitioners in the clinical environment. Giving language to some aspects of their practice (Mattingly *et al.*, 1997) gave the therapists a clearer perspective on their practice and a vehicle to examine and advance it.

Tacit knowledge serves in the immediate situation due to its development in the past. It can also work to help a clinician formulate an image of the potential future situation, both as an image and a guide to plan treatment. Following is an example of a clinician whose tacit knowledge was copious, and who could also articulate that knowledge given very little prompting.

A Norwegian therapist we know read a transcript of an American therapist's report on her work with a man with a crush injury to his hand. The report was basically a long list of abbreviations about DIP, PIP and other joints and various soft tissue injuries. This therapist looked up from the notes and sighed. We asked, 'What is the matter?' and she said, 'I can just see it all now. This man is going to get very depressed, lose his job, probably become an alcoholic and his wife will divorce him. He will probably have bad contractures, more surgery, be committed to therapy for a while, and cycle back and forth between depression and attempts to get his life and therapy back on track'. We looked at her in astonishment.

That was exactly what happened to him. 'How did you know?' we asked. She said, 'I've seen it all before. I have been a hand therapist for several years. As soon as I read the description of his injuries, his hand just lit up in my mind. I could just see it. Then his life just rolled along in my mind as well. I knew just how it was going to be. This is a very difficult injury and very devastating to the person'.

This experienced therapist knew similar people in the past and was able to envision this person's situation. The strong imagistic quality, to say nothing of the accuracy, of her comments demonstrate more than simple memory. Her capacity to suddenly see this patient in her mind's eye is part of her expertise. The image is a vivid and powerful portrayal of the person's future life. This therapist's ability to create vivid images of a patient's life, to take a minimal description of a hand injury and envision a host of life consequences, including how these might affect the emotions and motives of the patient, also reveals well developed skills in narrative reasoning.

Narrative reasoning

One might assume that narrative reasoning is related strictly to telling and interpreting stories. However, it has come to be associated with a much broader human capacity. It constitutes a form of meaning-making which is pervasive in human activity (*cf.* Bruner, 1986, 1990, 1996; Carr, 1986; MacIntyre, 1981; Nussbaum, 1990; Ricoeur, 1984). In recent years, narrative thinking has been recognized as important in clinical judgement (Frankenberg, 1993; Good, 1994; Hunt, 1994; Hunter, 1991; Mattingly and Fleming, 1994; Mattingly, 1991, 1998a,b). Narrative reasoning is necessary to interpret the actions of others and respond appropriately to the social context. Bruner (1986, 1996) refers to it as a capacity to 'read other minds', i.e. to make accurate inferences about the motives and intentions of others based on their observable behaviour and the social situation in which they act. When we try to make sense of what another person is up to, we ask, in effect, what story is that person living out? Narrative thinking, as the anthropologist Michael Carrithers (1992, p. 77–78) remarks, 'allows people to comprehend a complex flow of action and to act appropriately within it . . . narrative thinking is the very process we use to understand the social life around us'.

When occupational therapists reason narratively, clinical problems and treatment activities are organized in their minds as an unfolding drama (Mattingly, 1998b). A cast of characters emerges. Motives are inferred or examined. Narrative reasoning is needed when clinicians want to understand concrete events that cannot be comprehended without relating an inner world of desire and motive to an outer world of observable actions and states of affairs. Narrative reasoning concerns the relationship among motives, actions, and consequences as these play out in some specific situation (Bruner, 1986; Dray, 1954; Ricoeur, 1980, 1984). Attention to the specifics of context is not sufficient to distinguish narrative reasoning from other modes of clinical thinking, however. As one scholar notes, 'The individual case is the touchstone of knowledge in medicine' (Hunter, 1991, p. 28). The hallmark of narrative reasoning is that it utilizes specifics of a very special sort: it involves a search for the precise motives that led to certain key actions and for how those critical actions produced some further set of consequences. While narrative reasoning is evidently a generic human capacity, it is prone to tremendous misjudgement. As we all know, it is quite easy to misinterpret the motives and intentions of others, especially if they are strangers and come from unfamiliar social or cultural backgrounds. In some cases, and for some practices, interpretive errors are not especially important. One can make a splint, for example, without needing to have tremendous skills in interpreting the meaning of splint wearing for one's client. However, one cannot make a good decision about when to give a client a splint, or figure out how to get that client to wear it, without developing a capacity to assess the beliefs, values and concerns of the client.

There are practical reasons why expert rehabilitation professionals, in particular, hone their narrative reasoning skills. The most obvious one is that effective treatment depends upon highly motivated patients. As occupational therapists often say, in therapy, patients are not 'done to' but are asked to 'do for themselves'. This 'active healing' process means that patients cannot passively yield their bodies to the expert to receive a cure; rather they need to become highly committed participants in the rehabilitation process. This presents a special challenge to the professional: How do I foster a high level of commitment in my patients? This task calls upon narrative reasoning as the practitioner tries to design a treatment approach which will appeal to a particular patient. Occupational therapists refer to

this as 'individualizing treatment.' Narrative reasoning figures centrally in those health professions, such as rehabilitation therapies, where efficacious practice requires developing a strong collaboration with clients. When motives matter, narrative reasoning is inevitable and poor skills in such reasoning will mean that therapy is likely to fail.

Prospective stories: therapy stories and life stories

However, in occupational therapy at least, narrative reasoning is not merely directed at the problem of attaining the co-operation of a patient during a particular clinical encounter. The therapist's ability to employ narrative reasoning sensitively is essential to another clinical task – helping patients link their past (often a time before illness or disability) to a present and to a future worth pursuing. When therapists ask themselves 'Who is this patient?' they are asking a fundamentally narrative question. They are wondering what might motivate this particular patient in treatment, and, beyond that, which treatment activities and goals would be most appealing and useful, given the life this person will likely be living once therapy is completed. Therapists routinely struggle to develop images of their patients as individuals with unique needs and commitments, with singular life stories. 'Curing' is rare in the world of rehabilitation, and, in any case, it is not possible to transport a patient back in time to younger and healthier years. Instead, occupational therapists work to connect with patients in order to judge which treatment goals are most fitting and which treatment activities make most sense given the patient's conceptions of what is important in life. In fact, collaboration with patients is so central, it is probably more accurate to speak of the co-construction of treatment goals and activities.

The power of narrative as an on-going, largely tacit, reasoning process which guides action and becomes most evident in clinical situations when things break down – when it is difficult for the practitioner to make narrative sense of the clinical encounter or one's patient. When practitioners confront patients who are incomprehensible in some significant way, the whole direction of treatment may falter. The tacit narrative reasoning which practitioners carry into clinical encounters is likely to turn into explicit storytelling as they try to discern what is going on and what 'story they are in' with a particular client. For instance, a patient may insist that he wants to return to his job, show up to all his clinical appointments faithfully, comply with all the tasks set before him during his therapy hour, but never manage to 'get around' to doing the exercises he is supposed to be carrying out at home. Without these home exercises, the therapist may explain several times, treatment will not be successful. He will not be able to use his hand. He will not be able to return to work. Yet, nothing helps. Things continue just as before. Perhaps he has been lying or deceiving himself. Perhaps he does not want his job back after all. But if he were merely non-compliant, uninterested in returning to work, why does he show up to every appointment so faithfully, even arriving early? Why does he try so hard during therapy time? Such mysteries are common. Therapists become increasingly unclear about how to proceed in their treatment interventions, even when 'the good' (outcome) for a patient (say, maximal return of hand function) remains fixed in an abstract sense.

Narrative reasoning is a guide to a therapist's future actions because it provides images of a possible future for the client. When reasoning narratively, practitioners are trying to assess how to act in particular clinical situations, taking into consideration the motives and desires of themselves, their clients and other relevant actors. The on-going construction of a narrative framework provides clinicians with historical contexts in which certain actions emerge as the inevitable next steps leading to the most promising future. Although the question of what 'the good' future is for any particular patient may never be explicitly asked, the process of treatment itself is very often a process of exploring and negotiating a vision of the future good. When clinicians assess how they can help a patient reshape his or her situation for the better, this assessment is often informed by a 'prospective story', an imagined future life story for that patient. Thus, clinicians contemplate how to situate their therapeutic interventions (a kind of 'therapeutic present') in light of a patient's past and some hoped-for vision of what will follow in the future when the patient is discharged.

Narrative reasoning is directed to the future in the sense that it involves judgements about how to act in order to 'further the plot' in desirable directions and to subvert, as far as possible, undesirable ones. While our traditional concept is that stories recount past events, stories in the clinical world are often directed to future possibilities. How are such 'prospective stories' communicated to patients or negotiated with them? Generally, this does not occur by telling the stories in detail. Rather, the stories are sketched through subtle hints or cues, or enacted in clinical dramas that prefigure life after therapy. The prospective story is offered, like the architect's sketch, as a possibility, something to be 'looked at', viewed from different angles, something to make a judgement about. When therapists offer short stories to their patients about what their life will be like 'in a few weeks' or 'when the halo comes off' or when 'you are home with the kids', they are offering images and possibilities of a meaningful future. Therapists hope that a commitment to these narrative images, images that point toward a future life story, will carry the patients through the long, tedious, often painful routines of treatment.

Active judgements, tacit knowledge and narrative images: A case story

The interplay of actions, judgements, tacit knowledge and narrative image making is dauntingly intricate to describe in the abstract but becomes easily visible when examining concrete instances of practice. The following case story, written by an experienced occupational therapist, illustrates how image, action and narrative come together in expert therapeutic practice.

The story of Ann[1]

Ann was a 26-year-old woman who had given birth and subsequently had a stroke. She was admitted to a rehabilitation hospital with right hemiparesis. When I first met Ann, she was very depressed about being separated from her new baby and her main fear was that she would not be able to adequately care for the baby on her own. Adding to this fear was the knowledge that her insurance would not cover any in-home services. Her husband was her only family, he worked construction every day and they lived in a trailer park. In order to go home with the baby, she would need to be very independent.

The initial therapy sessions were centered around tone normalization, with an emphasis on mat activities, along with traditional ADL (activities of daily living) training in the mornings. Ann's husband visited daily and

[1] by Maureen Freda, MA, OTR.

usually brought the baby with him. At first this was extremely frustrating to Ann, since she could not hold the baby unless she was sitting down with pillows supporting her right arm. She continued to voice anxiety around the issue of going home and being able to care for the baby. Her husband was also very worried about how this transformation would take place – from Ann as a patient to Ann as wife and mother. I spent a lot of time talking to both Ann and her husband about the necessity of normalizing the tone and improving the movement of the upper extremity as a sort of foundation to the more complex functional skills Ann was so anxious to relearn.

Eventually it was time to spend the majority of the treatment time on functional skills. The two areas we focused on were homemaking and child-care. The homemaking sessions were fairly routine and traditional in nature. However, it proved to be a bit more difficult to simulate some of the child-care activities.

Our first obstacle was to find something that would be like a baby. We settled on borrowing a 'recus-a-baby' from the nursing education department. We used this 'baby' for the beginning skills such as feeding and diaper changing. Ann had progressed to a point where she had slight weakness and in-co-ordination in the right arm, and she was walking with a straight cane. The next step was to tackle walking with the baby. We of course practised with a baby carrier. We also had to prepare for the event of carrying the baby without the 'carrier'. I wrapped weights about the 'baby' to equal the weight of the now 3-month-old infant at home. Ann walked down the hall carrying the 'baby' and I would be following behind jostling the 'baby' to simulate squirming (we became the talk of the hospital with our daily walks!!). Ann was becoming more and more comfortable and confident with these activities, so it was time to make arrangements to have the real baby spend his days in the rehab with his mother. This was not as easy as it might seem. The administration of the hospital was not used to such requests. But with the right cajoling in the right places this was eventually approved. The real baby now replaced 'recus-a-baby' on our daily walks and in the clinic. While these successes were comforting to Ann and

her husband, the fact remained that we were still in a very protective environment. The big question was yet unanswered – would these skills hold up under the stresses of everyday life – alone – in a trailer for 8 hours daily?

Never being one to hold to tradition, I decided to go to administration another time with one more request. I wanted to do a full day 'home visit' with Ann and her baby. This too was approved and a week before Ann's scheduled discharge, she and I set out for a rigorous day at the home front. Once there all did not go smoothly; Ann fell once and practically dropped the baby. She was very anxious and stressed, but we managed to get through the day. We talked and problem solved every little real or perceived difficulty. Both Ann and the baby survived the fall and the 'almost' dropping. When we got back to the hospital, Ann, her husband, the social worker and I sat down and realistically discussed and decided what kind of outside help was a necessity and what Ann could really accomplish in a day. Ann's husband adjusted his schedule, a teenage neighbor was brought in for 2–3 hours a day and Ann was able to do the majority of the care for her baby.

Action, judgement, narrative and expertise in the story of Ann

In the above story an experienced clinician orchestrates a therapy program for a somewhat unusual patient. Maureen begins her story with a typical medical case history approach but it quickly becomes evident that the patient's particular life situation shapes Maureen's judgements about how to design treatment. It matters, for instance, that one of the primary consequences of Ann's stroke was that Ann was fearful of her ability to care for her newborn baby. Maureen also immediately takes into account key elements that will be at play in Ann's 'future story'. Maureen notes the particular situation to which Ann will be returning as a mother unable to afford child care, with no family to turn to except her husband, who works all day.

Maureen judges what actions Ann will need to relearn, and selects and invents therapeutic activities based on her perception of the social context and personal goals of Ann and her husband. Maureen is sensitive to the husband's insight about the need for Ann's transformation from patient to wife and mother. She situates her treatment goals within the notion of transformation. Her treatment approach develops as a powerful 'short story' which aids in Ann's transformation from fearful patient to confident mother able to handle even the difficult task of carrying her baby in her arms. Maureen makes continual judgements about how to shift treatment from safer and easier tasks to those more closely approximating Ann's 'real world' life situation.

In creating this unique treatment story, Maureen relies on her accumulated tacit knowledge culled from years of experience. She draws upon a typical treatment sequence, from building individual motions, to actions, to coordinated functional skills. She clearly has a great deal of tacit knowledge regarding how to help patients build their ADL skills. While this occupational therapist can draw upon a wealth of tacit knowledge, in many ways she faces a singular situation which requires her to make judgements specifically tailored to Ann's needs.

The symbolic plays a powerful role in this treatment. Maureen sees the need for a substitute or symbolic baby, not just a pretend baby in the form of a pillow. She borrows a model from another clinical department and this seems to do the trick. Maureen moves on with Ann from sedentary baby care activities to the more challenging, complex and risky activity of walking with the baby. She rises to this challenge by developing novel therapeutic activities, such as adding weights and simulating the baby's squirming. These increasingly active qualities of the 'recus-a-baby' stand in for the real baby who now enters the picture as a more viable image. The more realistic the 'baby's' actions become, the more Ann becomes prepared to make the transition from patient to mother.

Maureen judges when it is time for the real baby to make an appearance on the rehabilitation floor. Maureen's confidence in her own judgements prepares her to make and win the case with administration for the baby – Danny – to participate in his mother's therapy. The therapy worked. It was clear to everyone that this move beyond conventional practice reaped benefits far greater than would have been attained had Maureen stuck to conventional exercise and routine ADL activities.

Finally, the therapist determines that it is time to take what they have learned and see how they work in the real-life situation of Ann's home. Here we see that Maureen's perception of her own judgement and tacit knowledge vary. She is thoroughly confident that the home visit is the right thing to do. However, she is somewhat less confident regarding potential success that Ann will have in some of the specific activities of baby care. Ann and Maureen now have enough trust in each other and in the plan to believe that this practice session is well worth any potential risks. Although she does not say so, we can infer that the clinician is constantly attentive to the small details of the activities that she asks Ann to carry out in the home and has set up subtle safety features, including her heightened attention and undoubted physical closeness to mother and child.

This confluence of image and action is typical of experienced therapists who are able to see opportunities in the midst of action to gradually or dramatically change their treatment plan in response to particular details of a patient's skills and needs. Notably, this capacity for flexible plan development is central because, as Ann illustrates, a patient's needs and concerns will often change over the course of therapy. Maureen, through her sensitivity to 'this patient' and her personal and social context was able to both speed up and 'individualize' treatment in order to maximize her ability to act and return Ann to her desired social roles.

We have described this treatment process as the creation of a 'short story' within the larger life story of the patient, Ann. (Including, of course, the life stories of her husband and baby as well.) Notably, this is a short story which not only connects to Ann's past, a young woman who has recently given birth, but to a future, i.e. to events and experiences which have not yet taken place. With the careful guiding of treatment activities, the therapist is able to steer Ann toward her hoped-for future, the one where she can independently care for her child, and steer her away from a very undesirable future, one where she remains depressed and fearful of her capacities to take on such care.

The power of any therapeutic short story is its capacity to help patients and their families realize some future story which deeply matters to them. The therapist cannot simply impose this desired future upon Ann, even if it is a future Ann dearly wants. She must look for signals that Ann is ready to move toward it. This requires the therapist's continual judgement about what constitutes the 'just right challenge' (Csikszentmihalyi, 1975) for Ann at any moment in therapy. Such judgements involve assessing Ann's physical capabilities but also require narrative reasoning, assessing the state of Ann's inner world of emotions, desires and beliefs, as these are expressed in her outward actions and words.

Narrative reasoning is also utilized when as Maureen helps to create symbolically potent images for Ann, helping her to envision what life will be like with her baby. Maureen creates dramatic situations in which Ann can test her abilities and face her fears. This dramatic play even allows Ann to face one of her worst nightmares, as she nearly drops her child upon returning home for a trial run with Maureen. Notably, these experiences helped Maureen to talk with Ann, her husband and a social worker in order to make a more realistic plan about how Ann might care for her child upon discharge, including changes in the husband's work schedule and bringing in a neighborhood babysitter to help out.

Conclusion

We have found that clinical reasoning is not just one cognitive process and is not limited to the task of making decisions about concrete biological problems. We claim that in order to be truly therapeutic clinicians must understand their patients and the ways in which they make meaning in lives that are changed by illness or injury. Two of the ways practitioners perceive patient's perceptions of their past and future lives and orchestrate treatment programs to achieve that future vision have been briefly discussed. These strategies are narrative reasoning and active judgement. These forms of reasoning serve to enlarge the clinician's stock of tacit knowledge and expand their expertise.

References

Bruner, J. (1986) *Actual Minds, Possible Worlds*. Cambridge, MA: Harvard University Press.

Bruner, J. (1990) *Acts of Meaning*. Cambridge, MA: Harvard University Press.

Bruner, J. (1996) *The Culture of Education*. Cambridge, MA: Harvard University Press.

Buchler, J. (1955) *Nature and Judgement*. New York: Grosset and Dunlap/Columbia University Press.

Carr, D. (1986) *Time, Narrative, and History*. Bloomington, IN: Indiana University Press.

Carrithers, M. B. (1992) *Why Humans Have Cultures*. Oxford: Oxford University Press.

Csikszentmihalyi, M. (1975) *Beyond Boredom and Anxiety: The Experience of Play in Work and Game*. San Francisco: Jossey-Bass.

Dray, W. (1954) Explanatory narrative in history. *Philosophical Quarterly*, **23**, 15–27.

Frankenberg, R. (1993) Risk: Anthropological and epidemiological narratives of prevention. In *Knowledge, Power and Practice: The Anthropology of Everyday Life* (S. Lindenbaum and M. Lock, eds), pp. 219–242. Berkeley, CA: University of California Press.

Good, B. (1994) *Medicine, Rationality, and Experience: An Anthropological Perspective*. New York: Cambridge University Press.

Hunt, L. (1994) Practicing oncology in provincial Mexico: A narrative analysis. *Social Science and Medicine*, **38**, 843–853.

Hunter, K. (1991) *Doctor's Stories*: Princeton, NJ: Princeton University Press.

MacIntyre, A. (1981) *After Virtue: A Study in Moral Theory*. Notre Dame, IN: University of Notre Dame Press.

Mattingly, C. (1991) The narrative nature of clinical reasoning. *American Journal of Occupational Therapy*, **45**, 998–1005.

Mattingly, C. (1998a) *Healing Dramas and Clinical Plots: The Narrative Structure of Experience*. Cambridge: Cambridge University Press.

Mattingly, C. (1998b) In search of the good: Narrative reasoning in clinical practice. *Medical Anthropology Quarterly*, **12**, 273–297.

Mattingly, C. and Fleming, M. H. (1994) *Clinical Reasoning: Forms of Inquiry in a Therapeutic Practice*. Philadelphia, PA: F. A. Davis.

Mattingly, C, Fleming, M. H. and Gillette, N. (1997) Narrative explorations in the tacit dimension: Bringing language to clinical practice. *Nordiske Udkast*, **1**, 65–77.

Nussbaum, M. (1990) *Love's Knowledge*. New York: Oxford University Press.

Polanyi, M. (1966) *The Tacit Dimension*. Garden City, NY: Doubleday.

Ricoeur, P. (1980) Narrative Time. In *On Narrative* (T. J. Mitchell, ed.), pp. 165–186. Chicago: University of Chicago Press.

Ricoeur, P. (1984) *Time and Narrative*, Vol. 1. Chicago: University of Chicago Press.

Schön, D. (1983) *The Reflective Practitioner: How Professionals Think in Action*. New York: Basic Books.

7

Clinical reasoning and generic thinking skills

Stephen Brookfield

The role of thinking in clinical reasoning

Clinical practice, as most clinicians know, is frequently located in a zone of ambiguity. The actuality of clinical experience often stands in marked contrast to the patterns of practice laid out in introductory texts and pre-service education. Indeed, the contrast between the neatness of professional education and the apparent chaos of clinical experience calls into question the usefulness of pre-service education. If the world refuses to conform to models, concepts and research, then what use is it to study theory? If techniques and responses acquired in school are constantly rendered irrelevant, or distorted, by the exigencies of practice, then why should we bother learning them?

In this chapter I want to argue that pre-service education still plays a crucial role in professional development, but only if curricula place the acquisition of the thinking skills of clinical reasoning, particularly that of critical appraisal, at their centre. Such skills might be regarded as the meta-level skills of clinical practice. They shape the way practitioners approach, analyse and respond to the multiple settings and idiosyncrasies of practice. They do not displace the learning of specific skills or protocols, but they do frame how we determine the appropriateness of these protocols for different situations and how we modify the application of these skills in practice.

One can be technically proficient to a high level but if one is unable to apply thinking in the way clinical reasoning demands, then this proficiency is exercised haphazardly. A reliance on protocol and habitual responses works well as long as the world does not trip you up by refusing to conform to the shape you anticipate. Since the one constant of clinical practice is that nothing stays the same, it follows that the best form of education develops generic skills of analysis that can increase the likelihood of practitioners taking informed clinical action.

At the heart of clinical reasoning are three inter-related skills that might be described as apprehension/scanning, gathering and critical appraisal. These skills are thinking skills; they involve thought rather than instrumental competence. *Scanning* is an act of apprehension. It describes the ways we determine what are the central features of a clinical situation. In scanning a situation we decide what its boundaries are, which patterns of the situation are familiar and grounded in past experience (and which are in new or unusual configurations), and which of the cues that we notice should be attended to. Scanning is the initial sweep or experiential trawl in which we diagnose the big picture.

In the *gathering* phase of clinical reasoning we collect the interpretive resources and analytic protocols available to help us understand the situation correctly. These include the general clinical guidelines we have learned as part of our professional preparation or through in-service development. We remember superiors' instructions regarding what to do in such situations and also colleagues' suggestions we have heard or practices we have seen. Finally, we call on our own intuition. We attend to the instinctive analyses and responses that immediately suggest themselves as relevant.

In the *appraisal* phase we sort through the interpretations we have gathered. We decide which of those seem to fit most closely with the situation we are reviewing, and on that basis we take action. Reasoning is central to this phase. Scanning and gathering involve looking for patterns and broad similarities between a new situation and previous experiences; however, in appraisal we judge the accuracy and validity of the assumptions and interpretations we have gathered. This occurs through a number of interconnected processes: by sifting through past experiences and judging the closeness of their fit to the current situation, by intentionally following prescribed clinical protocols and introducing experimental adaptations of these when they suggest themselves, by consulting peers prior to making clinical decisions or in the midst of action, and by attempting to analyse which of our instinctive judgements and readings we should take seriously, and which we should hold in abeyance. As a result of this appraisal we take action regarding those procedures and responses that make the most sense in the current situation.

In this chapter I want to focus on this third phase of appraisal as the phase of clinical reasoning in which thinking is most central. Appraisal entails a detailed critical review of multiple sources during which we decide to attend to some cues, to discard others, and to reframe those which hold promise but do not entirely explain what we are confronting. In the language of formal research this involves us in determining the accuracy and validity of the assumptions and interpretations that we decide are most appropriate to a situation. In more colloquial terms we try to judge the fit between what we think is happening and the responses that seem to make most sense.

The process of appraisal: a deeper analysis

As a process, clinical appraisal involves practitioners in recognizing and researching the assumptions that undergird their clinical practice. Assumptions are the taken for granted beliefs about the world, and our place within it, that seem so obvious to us that they do not need to be stated explicitly. Assumptions give meaning and purpose to who we are and what we do. In many ways we are our assumptions. So much of what we think,

say and do is based on assumptions about how the world should work, and what we think counts as clinically appropriate, ethical action within it. Yet frequently these assumptions are not recognized for the provisional understandings that they really are. Ideas and practices that we regard as commonsense conventional wisdoms are often based on uncritically accepted assumptions. Some person, institution or authority source that we either trust or fear has told us that this is the way things are and we have accepted their judgement unquestioningly. Clinical appraisal requires that we research these assumptions for the evidence and experiences that inform them. In particular, we try to see our assumptions from as many unfamiliar perspectives as we can.

Sometimes we find that assumptions about appropriate clinical responses are justified by our own or others' experiences, in which case we feel a confidence in their accuracy and validity. When we can say why we hold an assumption, and when we can cite the clinical experiences on which it is grounded, we possess an informed commitment to it. At other times, however, we find that our assumptions are flawed, distorted, or accurate only within a much narrower range of clinical situations than we had originally thought. When this happens we realize we need to abandon or reframe these assumptions so that they provide more accurate guides to, and justifications for, our actions.

One of the most salient features of clinical appraisal is that it is irrevocably context-bound. The same person can be highly open to re-examining one set of clinical practices, but completely closed to critically reappraising another situation or idea. Neither is a facility for clinical appraisal learned developmentally. There is plenty of evidence to show that after a breakthrough in clinical reasoning people can quite easily revert to an earlier, more naive way of thinking and being. So clinical reasoning can only be understood, and its development gauged, within a specific context.

Clinical reasoning is also an irreducibly social process. It happens best when we enlist the help of others (clients, patients, supervisors, peers and colleagues) to see our ideas and actions in new ways. Very few of us can get very far probing our assumptions on our own. No matter how much we may think we have an accurate sense of our practice, we are stymied by the fact that we are using our own interpretive filters to become aware of our own interpretive filters! This is the pedagogic equivalent of a dog trying to catch its tail or of trying to see the back of your head while looking in the bathroom mirror. To some extent we are all prisoners trapped within the perceptual frameworks that determine how we view our experiences. A self-confirming cycle often develops whereby our uncritically accepted assumptions shape clinical actions which then serve only to confirm the truth of those assumptions. We find it very difficult to stand outside ourselves and see how some of our most deeply held values and beliefs lead us into distorted and constrained ways of thinking and practising. Our most influential assumptions are too close to us to be seen clearly by an act of self will.

If clinical reasoning, and especially the process of appraisal, is conceived as an irreducibly social process then our peers (and teachers) become important critical mirrors. To become critically reflective we need to find some lenses that reflect back to us a stark and differently highlighted picture of who we are and what we do. When our peers listen to our stories and then reflect back to us what they see and hear in them, we are often presented with a version of ourselves and our actions that comes as a surprise. Hearing their perceptions helps us gain a clearer perspective on the dimensions to our thoughts and actions that need closer critical scrutiny. It also helps us realize the commonality of our individual clinical experiences. Although no-one lives practice in exactly the same way as someone else, there is often much more that unites us than we realize. Talking to colleagues helps us realize how much we take for granted about in our own practice. It also alerts us to our judgemental ways of seeing. Sometimes it confirms the correctness of instincts that we felt privately but doubted because we thought they contradicted conventional wisdom or accepted clinical protocols. Peer conversation can also help break down the isolation many of us feel. Talking to other practitioners can open up unfamiliar avenues for inquiry, and can allow them to give us advice on how they deal with the problems we are facing.

The praxis of clinical appraisal

Appraisal involves a well-documented praxis of action, reflection on action, further action, reflection on the further action and so on, in a continuous cyclical loop. But these alternating phases need not be separated by extensive periods of time. Action can be mindful, thoughtful and informed. At any one point in the phases described we are engaged in a complex series of operations, some of which involve scrutinizing past assumptions, some of which involve exploring new meaning schemes, some of which require us to try on new identities, etc.

In learning clinical appraisal we can posit the following pattern. Initial reflection is usually prompted by some unexpected occurrence. Something is happening which does not feel right, which does not fit. This disorienting dilemma, to use Mezirow's (1991) term, occasions reflection on the discrepancy between the assumptions, rules and criteria informing our practice and our experiences of clinical reality. Triggers to clinical reasoning are usually presented as traumatic or troublesome in some way, as cognitive dissonances, or perceptions of anomalies, disjunctions and contradictions between our expectations of clinical practice and its actuality. Practically every theorist of critical thinking emphasizes how trauma triggers appraisal through such life shaking incidents such as divorce, bereavement, unemployment, disability, conscription, forced job change or geographical mobility.

Following the trigger event, periods of denial and depression alternate with attempts to understand the nature of the contradiction or dilemma in practice. During this period workers seek desperately for others who are confronting similar anomalies. In formal or informal peer reflection groups practitioners make an active effort to come to terms with the tension they feel. They reinterpret their experiences to create new meanings as they try to reduce feelings of discomfort or alienation. They may flirt with new identities or conceptualizations of what it means to be a clinician. They make a deliberate effort to draw on the experiences of others and to see the situation from their point of view so that the situation can be interpreted from multiple perspectives.

Arising out of this process of exploring and testing new assumptions and beliefs about practice is the development of a changed way of thinking and acting which 'makes sense' or 'fits' the clinical situation. This new perspective on practice is liable to be, initially at least, partial, tentative and fragile. Indeed, there is often a series of incremental confirmations of the validity of this new perspective as clinical experience confirms its accuracy. Having decided that new assumptions and practices make sense in the context of our clinical experiences, we seek ways to integrate them permanently into our practice.

Experiential lenses of clinical appraisal

Exploring the discrepancy between what *is* and what *should be* is at the heart of clinical appraisal. When we embark on this process we have three experiential lenses through which we can view our clinical practice: (1) our autobiographies as practitioners, teachers and clients, (2) our patients' eyes, and (3) our colleagues' experiences. Viewing what we do through these different lenses alerts us to distorted or incomplete aspects of our assumptions that need further investigation.

Lens 1: Our autobiographies as practitioners, teachers and clients

Our autobiographies as practitioners, teachers and clients represent some of the most important sources of insight into practice to which we have access. Yet, in much talk and writing about practice, personal experience is dismissed and demeaned as 'merely anecdotal'; in other words, as hopelessly subjective and impressionistic. It is true, of course, that at one level all experience is inherently idiosyncratic. For example, no-one experiences the death of a patient in exactly the same way as anyone else, with the same mix of memories, regrets, affirmations and pain. Yet at the same time, bereavement as a process of recognizing and accepting loss contains a number of patterns and rhythms that could be described as generic.

The fact that people recognize aspects of their own individual experiences in the stories others tell is one reason for the success of peer support groups for those in crisis or transition. As I hear you talk about going through a divorce, struggling with illness or addiction, or dealing with the death of partners, friends and parents, I am likely to hear echoes of, and direct parallels to, my own experience of these events. The same dynamic holds true in practitioner reflection groups. As we talk to each other about critical events in our practice we start to realize that individual clinical crises are usually collectively experienced dilemmas. The details and characters may differ, but the tensions are essentially the same.

Lens 2: Our patients' eyes

Seeing ourselves through patients' eyes constitutes one of the most consistently surprising elements in any clinical practitioner's career. Each time we do this we learn something. Sometimes what we find out is reassuring. We discover that patients are interpreting our actions in the way that we mean them. They are hearing what we wanted them to hear and seeing what we wanted them to see. However, often we are profoundly surprised by the diversity of meanings patients read into our words and actions. Comments we made incidentally that had no particular significance to us are heard as imperatives. Answers we gave 'off the cuff' to what seemed like inconsequential questions return to haunt us. Long after we have forgotten them they are quoted back at us by patients to prove that what we are saying now is contradicting our earlier advice. What we think is reassuring behaviour on our part is sometimes interpreted as over-protective coddling. A joking aside appreciated by some leaves others insulted.

Lens 3: Our colleagues' experiences

Talking to colleagues about what we do unravels the shroud of silence in which our clinical practice is wrapped. Participating in critical conversation with peers opens us to their versions of events we have experienced. Our colleagues serve as critical mirrors, reflecting back to us images of our actions that often take us by surprise. As they describe their own experiences dealing with the same crises and dilemmas that we face, we are able to check, reframe and broaden our own theories of practice. Talking to colleagues about problems we have in common, and gaining their perspectives on them, increases our chances of stumbling across an interpretation that fits what is happening in a particular situation. A colleague's experiences may suggest dynamics and causes that make much more sense than the explanations we have evolved. If this happens we are helped enormously in our effort to work out just what we should be doing to deal with the problem. Without an accurate reading of the causes of a problem (are these embedded in our own actions, in our patients' past histories, in the wider political or professional constraints placed on our clinical practice, or in a particular intersection of all of these?) we are crippled in our attempts to work through it.

Checking our readings of problems, responses, assumptions and justifications against the readings offered by colleagues is crucial if we are to claw a path to critical clarity. Doing this also provides us with a great deal of emotional sustenance. We start to see that what we thought were unique problems and idiosyncratic failings are shared by many others who work in situations like ours. Just knowing that we are not alone in our struggles can be a life-saving realization. Although clinical appraisal often begins alone, it is ultimately a collective endeavour.

Clinical reasoning and the struggle against impostorship

Thinking in the way that clinical reasoning involves is not without risks. Perhaps the chief of these is the risk of admitting one's own *impostorship*. Clinical practitioners often feel like impostors. They have a hidden sense that they do not really deserve to be taken seriously as competent professionals, because in their heart of hearts they know that they do not really know what they are doing. All they are certain of is that unless they are very careful they will be found out to be practising under false pretences. Such feelings are made worse because of the privacy ethic that prevails in many professional settings. There is no safe place to air uncertainties and request help. Clinicians smitten by impostorship have the conviction that they do not really merit any professional recognition or acclaim that comes their way. De Vries (1993, p. 129) summarizes their feelings as follows:

> These people have an abiding feeling that they have fooled everyone and are not as competent and intelligent as others think they are. They attribute their success to hard luck, compensatory hard work, or superficial factors such as physical attractiveness and likeability. Some are incredibly hardworking, always overprepared. However, they are unable to accept that they have intellectual gifts and ability. They live in constant fear that their imposturous existence will be exposed – that they will not be able to measure up to others' expectations and that catastrophe will follow.

The presentation of the false face that impostorship entails is usually done for reasons of survival. We believe that if we do not look as though we know what we're doing then our patients, colleagues and superiors will eat us alive. We think that admitting frailty will be interpreted as a sign of failure. Impostorship also means that many of us go through our professional lives fearing that at some unspecified point in the future we will undergo a humiliating public unveiling. We wear an external mask of control but beneath it we know that really we are frail figures, struggling to make it through to the end of each day. There is the sense that around the corner is an unforeseen but cataclysmic

clinical event that will reveal us as frauds. When this event happens we imagine that our colleagues' jaws will drop in synchronization. With their collective mouths agape they will wonder out loud, 'How could we possibly have been so stupid as to hire this obvious incompetent in the first place?'.

Viewing our practice through any of the experiential lenses of clinical reasoning heightens considerably the chances of our feeling like impostors. For anyone who is desperately trying to avoid being found out, the last thing they want to endure is a systematic scrutiny of their practice by colleagues. There is always the fear that once their impostorship has been discovered they will be punished. So one of the most important aids to clinical appraisal, having one's practice observed by peers, is also one of the most common triggers to impostorship.

Feelings of impostorship also accompany most attempts at clinical experimentation that spring from our reflection. Any time we depart from comfortable ways of acting or thinking to experiment with a new way of practice, we are almost bound to be taken by surprise. The further we travel from our habitual practices the more we run the risk of looking incompetent. The moments of failure that inevitably accompany change and experimentation increase the sense of impostorship by emphasizing how little we can predict and control the consequences of our actions. In the midst of experimentation it is not uncommon for practitioners to resolve never again to put themselves through the experience of looking foolish in front of colleagues and trying desperately to conceal the fact that they do not really know what they are doing.

How can this feeling of impostorship be kept under control? The key, I think, is to make the phenomenon public. Once impostorship is named as an everyday experience it loses much of its power. It becomes commonplace and quotidian rather than a shameful, malevolent secret. To hear colleagues you admire talking graphically and convincingly about their own regular moments of impostorship is enormously reassuring. If they feel exactly the way we do, then perhaps we are not so bad after all. In public forums and private conversations, practitioners who are acclaimed as successful can do a great deal to defuse the worst effects of impostorship by admitting to its reality in their lives.

Being involved in team practice also makes us less prone to being smitten by impostorship. In clinical situations where teaming is required you have built in reflective mirrors available to you. As you walk to the cafeteria after what you think is a bad clinical experience and you start to engage in your usual enthusiastic bout of self-flagellation, your colleagues are likely to point out the things that went well. They will tell you about the situations you handled confidently and how impressed they were with your abilities. They will provide you with immediate multiple perspectives on events that you have seen in only one way and suggest readings of patients' actions that would never have occurred to you.

Clinical conversation groups invariably surface the theme of impostorship. Once one person has revealed these feelings and experiences, a ripple or domino effect occurs. One after the other, the members of the group give their own illustrations of the phenomenon. The tricky part is to get someone to admit to it in the first place. This is where experienced practitioners and preceptors can be particularly helpful. By admitting to their own feelings of impostorship, experienced practitioners can ease the way for junior colleagues to speak. So joining or forming a reflection group is an important strategy to keep impostorship in its proper place.

Conclusion

Clinical appraisal allows us to stand outside situations and see what we do from wider perspectives. It helps us develop a well-grounded rationale for our actions that we call on to help us make difficult decisions in unpredictable situations. This rationale, a set of critically examined core assumptions about why we do what we do in the way that we do it, is a survival necessity. It gives us an organizing vision of what we are trying to accomplish in our practice.

References

Mezirow, J. (1991) *Transformative Dimensions of Adult Learning*. San Francisco: Jossey-Bass.

De Vries, M. F. R. K. (1993) *Leaders, Fools, and Impostors: Essays on the Psychology of Leadership*. San Francisco: Jossey-Bass.

8

Clinical reasoning and patient-centred care

Steven J. Ersser and Sue Atkins

Developing health services depends not only on technological and organizational development but also on improvements in the way health professionals relate to patients and each other, in an effort to make better health care decisions. Clinical reasoning refers to 'the thinking and decision making processes which are integral to clinical practice' (Higgs and Jones, 1995, p. xiv). Fundamental questions may be asked about the part the patient should or can play in these processes and how this may be achieved. This chapter is based on the belief that patient-centred decision making is likely to result in better clinical decisions, both in terms of achieving clinical effectiveness, and ensuring ethical and humane practice.

It may appear self-evident that clinical decision making would always be formulated in the best interests of the patient. However, there are times when organizational or professional objectives can obscure effective decisions that take sufficient account of the patient's interests, both in terms of objective clinical facts, and patient experience and values. Also, practitioners' varying levels of skill when relating to patients may lead to insufficient account being taken of their concerns and preferences. This in turn can have adverse clinical effects, such as not achieving a desirable degree of co-operation with the clinical plan.

This chapter reviews the significance of a patient-centred approach to clinical reasoning. Relevant theoretical frameworks are introduced to orient the reader to the range of different social, psychological and ethical dimensions relevant to patient-centred care. Practical strategies for achieving patient-centred practice and the limitations of this process are examined. Finally, a case is made for the promotion of patient-centred reasoning as a means to help achieve more effective and humane health care.

Patient-centred care

Patient-centred care involves valuing the individual needs and rights of patients, understanding patients' illness and health care experiences, and embracing them within effective relationships which enable patients to participate in clinical reasoning. It is widely assumed that most patients want and benefit from an active role. Concepts of patient choice, participation, empowerment and working in partnership are being widely examined, advocated and challenged within professional literature as a means of enhancing patient-centred care (Brearley, 1990). Patient-centred decision making is being promoted by government policy initiatives, such as the *Patient's Charter* (Department of Health, 1991) and Changing Childbirth (Department of Health, 1993) in the UK.

Patient-centred reasoning may involve patients participating in determining appropriate management plans, as their condition and motivation allow. Clinical decisions require information of a necessary type and quality. Professionals take account of both objective and subjective data during the clinical assessment process to decide on a patient's health care need and care plan. The difficulty lies in professionals understanding how best to reconcile their objective perspective with that of the patient, when formulating clinical judgements.

Evidence suggests that a level of participation in clinical reasoning, appropriate for the individual, contributes to the patient's sense of control. This may positively affect psychological well-being, physical recovery and satisfaction, and lead to patients accepting greater responsibility for their health (Cahill, 1996; Cooke, 1995). It is argued that anticipated health outcomes associated with patient involvement in decision making need to be fully evaluated (Entwistle *et al.*, 1998). However, patient-centredness is fundamentally about the process of care. When enabling patients to make informed choices, views of the professional and patient may be at variance, and a decision taken may not necessarily lead to the best clinical outcomes. The refusal of Jehovah's Witnesses to accept blood transfusions is a clear example of the ethical dilemmas which may arise from these situations.

There are important consequences or risks of clinical reasoning not being patient-centred. Patients may become passive and disempowered at a time when they need to take more responsibility for their health. There may be difficulties in achieving concordance with the care plan which may impact on clinical effectiveness. Further, professionals may lose important sources of information about patients' health, health care experiences and health and illness behaviours.

Theoretical frameworks

Theoretical perspectives drawn from sociology, psychology, ethics and professional literature can contribute to an understanding of the rationale for advocating more patient-centred decision making.

Sociological perspectives

Concepts of health and illness behaviour and professional and patient roles are fundamental to understanding the way in which social factors may shape whether and how professionals adopt a patient-centred approach to decision making. Fulford (1996, p. 2) views patient-centred care as embracing 'a model of care that incorporates both values and facts, the lived experience of illness and scientific knowledge of disease'. Illness and health behaviour play a fundamental part in health care, both in terms of the behaviours that may lead to ill-health, or its prevention, and the part the patient plays in contributing to the therapeutic plan.

Parsons (1978) recognized the cultural character of health and illness. Health and illness behaviour are related to peoples' concepts of health and illness (Scambler, 1997). Illness behaviour is influenced by the phenomenology of the patient's symptoms and how these are interpreted, alongside the perceived costs and benefits of treatment and care. Health behaviour is shaped by lifestyle, which will influence co-operation with treatment and subsequently recovery and rehabilitation. The importance of understanding illness experience and its implications for informing effective clinical action is highlighted in interpretative studies (Morse and Johnson, 1991).

Role theory has traditionally portrayed the patient as a passive recipient of medical expertise. Parsons' (1951) classic structural-functionalist view of the *sick role* considered the patient as exempt from normal social obligations but with the requirement to co-operate with treatment. The sick role is circumscribed by patients who are unable to fulfil the obligations and expectations which it entails, such as the chronically sick. However, there is duty upon the physician to be solely guided by patients' welfare and to apply the highest standards of professional competence and scientific knowledge (Gerhardt, 1989).

Friedson's (1970, p. 132) analysis of the medical profession distinguishes between the 'medical intervention' pattern and the 'therapeutic pattern' of professional performance. The former views the patient as incompetent to judge medical needs. To achieve cure patients are required to put themselves passively into the hands of staff. In contrast the therapeutic pattern, as commonly used in psychotherapy, involves the patient as an active participant in therapy. The patient's motivation is an essential part of the therapeutic pattern. These patterns remain recognizable in today's health service, raising questions about the extent to which the knowledge of patients, their personal history, experience, values and preferences, may contribute to clinical reasoning.

Sociological theory highlights the nature of professions in controlling knowledge and expertise to secure a position of power in society (Friedson, 1970). Whether intentional or not, there is a risk of professionals withholding information from patients about their condition and treatment, thereby limiting their scope for participation in decision making. A more patient-centred approach therefore requires a review of the professional role and the impact of professionalization. Professional action involves responsibility to make independent and accountable clinical decisions. However, the medical profession has been criticized for exerting undue social control on patients, for example by withholding information (Illich, 1976). While Davis (1976) argues that historically, nursing's occupational strategy has not sought greater control over patients, there are risks of this occurring within contemporary nursing reforms (Ersser and Tutton, 1991). Nevertheless, nurses have scope to empower patients by giving them information and helping them to participate in decision making (Gibson, 1991).

Humanistic and social psychology

Patient-centred care requires an understanding of patient–professional relationships. Irrespective of the profession and its technical character, the whole orientation and comportment of the practitioner, in terms of how they view and respond to the patient, may have a fundamental bearing on the therapeutic consequences of that interaction (Ersser, 1997). Patient-centredness must be characterized by the health professional's beliefs, values and attitudes toward patients in the planning and delivery of care. Patient-centredness encompasses beliefs about the rights of people and their potential to help themselves, with support. The psychology literature suggests that the character of all therapeutic or helping relationships requires qualities of self-awareness, authenticity and empathy (Brammer, 1988). These ideas have been influenced by humanistic psychology (Graham, 1986) and human-existential psychotherapy (e.g. Mitchell *et al.*, 1977).

Ethical theory

A process of ethical reasoning and reflection underpins the decision making of health care professionals (Fleming, 1991a; Robertson, 1996). Ethical theory provides a framework to inform, guide and justify clinical reasoning. In particular, the bioethical principles of autonomy, beneficence and justice are widely used (Smith and Bodurtha, 1995).

Patient-centred decisions require professionals to achieve an appropriate balance between respecting the autonomy of 'competent' patients to make their own decisions and meeting their duty of beneficence. Beneficence is the primary obligation of all health professionals to do good and act in the patient's best interests. However, there are examples of professionals adopting a paternalistic approach, relying almost exclusively on their professional knowledge and judgement about patients' needs, without due regard for patients' concerns and knowledge. Beneficence should be reconciled with and not compete with respect for patient autonomy. Professionals are also obligated to be fair to all patients and uphold the principle of justice. The theory of individualism is based on the assumption that all people have inalienable rights. The morality of a situation is partly based on whether an individual's rights are violated or not, such as the patient's autonomy.

Despite the value of ethical theory, clinical reasoning involves more than the application of principles and rules. When conflicts occur between *prima facie* obligations, it rests with the integrity of the professional to make a judgement in a particular situation.

Professional models

Models of professional practice convey different views about the respective roles of professional and patient, the goals of specific types of health care, and the beliefs and values that ought to underpin the practice. They may also provide pointers to the desirability of patient involvement in clinical reasoning. There are differences in how professions have viewed and interpreted the concept of patient-centred care. Traditionally, the medical model has placed scientific knowledge of disease processes as the central concern of doctors, with a consequent belief that the 'doctor knows best'. Recently there have been efforts to examine and develop more patient-centred approaches to medical consultations (Winefield *et al.*, 1996). Fulford (1996) advocates a more balanced professional model where patients' values and experiences are central, but no less important than clinical knowledge and scientific facts, thereby balancing the power relationship between doctors and patients. Quill and Brody (1996, p. 763) argue that the physician's primary duty is 'to support and enhance patients' abilities to make autonomous choices about their health care'.

Occupational therapy, in contrast, was founded on a client-centred philosophy which aims to improve the independence of clients with disability, respecting client autonomy and choice in developing life skills (Hopkins, 1988). This approach has been reflected in theories and models explaining and guiding practice (Hagedorn, 1992). A primary goal of clinical reasoning in occupational therapy has been to identify the meaning of disability from the disabled client's perspective (Fleming, 1991b). This requires knowledge of client motivation, tolerances, environment, abilities and deficits. Occupational therapists also require insight into their relationship with the client and the ability to make a predictive judgement of long-term potential (Fleming, 1991b).

Within nursing, various theoretical models have been developed to explain the nurse's role and guide the education and practice of nurses throughout the Western world, from the time of Nightingale. The concept of patient-centred care is usually implicit within nursing models. However, the work of Hall (1969), King (1981) and Riehl-Sisca (1980) emphasizes the importance of the patient's stance. Hall's theory focuses on the nurse–patient relationship, influenced by Carl Rogers' (1965) philosophy of 'client-centred therapy'. Hall emphasizes the importance of a non-directive method to enable the patient to develop self-awareness, explore feelings and behaviour, and thereby aid adjustment and recovery. Riehl-Sisca's (1980) model, based on symbolic interactionism (Blumer, 1969), views nursing as a guiding activity in which the nurse seeks to understand and interpret patient behaviour and the meanings patients give to situations. King's (1981) systems theory of goal attainment advocates mutual goal setting and negotiating the nursing plan to achieve satisfactory health outcomes.

Theories of clinical reasoning

Clinical reasoning theories, such as the information processing theory (Newell and Simon, 1972), the hypothetico-deductive model (Elstein *et al.*, 1978) and the phenomenological perspective (Dreyfus and Dreyfus, 1986), focus on the reasoning of professionals. However, more recent models of decision making emphasize the importance of patient involvement (Higgs and Jones, 1995). Interpretive studies comparing clinical judgements of novice and expert professionals suggest that patient-centredness may be a feature of professional expertise (Benner *et al.*, 1992; Fleming, 1991b). A study of expertise in critical care nursing indicates that beginning nurses were more task-oriented than experienced nurses, who focused more on understanding patients' perspectives and priorities (Benner at al., 1992). Similarly, a study of physical therapists in orthopaedic settings (Jensen *et al.*, 1992) found that master clinicians were more likely than novices to gather data reflecting patients' perceptions and to design exercise interventions to fit their environment.

Factors influencing patient involvement in clinical reasoning

A number of factors influence the extent to which patients are involved in clinical reasoning. Extensive studies of patients' preferences for involvement identify age, educational background and the level of medical knowledge required as predictors of the patient's wish to participate (Thompson *et al.*, 1993). A review of studies in this field suggests that demographic and situational characteristics explain 20% or less of the variability in patient preferences for involvement in decision making (Benbassat *et al.*, 1998), highlighting the importance of effective professional–patient relationships in the process. People who expressed a desire for greater involvement were more likely to be younger and better educated. Thompson *et al.* (1993) found significantly lower preference amongst patients for participating in those decisions that required medical expertise. However, when medical decisions involve important patient outcomes, such as a choice between treatment options with varying effects on lifestyle, disfigurement, pain or a trade-off between quality of life and length of life, patients considered that involvement was more important. Age and level of education have been demonstrated to be key factors in the understanding of information for effective decision making. Research evidence has identified impaired understanding in older adults and those with less formal education in the giving of informed consent (Sugarman *et al.*, 1988) and among elderly hospitalized patients in making advanced resuscitation decisions (Sayers *et al.*, 1997).

The patient's opportunity, ability and willingness to participate in decision making will be fundamentally affected by the socio-cultural context. Cultural norms will dictate the legitimacy of health professionals seeking and giving information and involving patients in decision making about their care. Sub-cultural factors, such as patients' social class and ethnicity, will also operate here (Blackhall *et al.*, 1995). Knowledge that is perceived to be broadly within the lay sphere, such as that associated with activities of daily living used in nursing and occupational therapy, may be viewed as more accessible for patients compared with biomedical knowledge which is perceived as more specialized.

The patient's clinical condition may affect involvement in decision making. Chronically ill patients may be more knowledgeable about their condition and treatment, and thus more likely to want to participate in care planning. Patient decision making in palliative care has been found to be more difficult because of the complexity, uncertainty and unpredictability of the terminal illness (Bottorff *et al.*, 1998). Surgical patients' wishes and ability to participate in decision making about nursing care may be limited by the degree of physical illness, the amount of technical information required and the organizational constraints of the hospital (Biley, 1992). Where acute events are likely, attempts can be made by clinical staff to ascertain patients' or relatives views in advance. In emergency situations, such as cardio-respiratory resuscitation, decisions may have been made in advance, although they should be informed by the patient's and family's cultural and religious views about dignity and sanctity of life.

Maternity care is a speciality where there is a growing demand for patient choice. Decision making about performing caesarean sections in the UK is becoming increasingly based on maternal choice (Paterson-Brown and Fisk, 1997). However, Cooke's (1995) analysis of women's experiences indicates that while choice is important, in emergency situations personal preferences are modified and superseded by concerns about the baby's safety.

Strategies promoting patient-centred clinical reasoning

Specific strategies to promote patient-centred clinical reasoning can be identified; their contributions are now examined.

Styles of patient–professional relationship

The ways in which professionals relate to patients are likely to directly influence the degree of involvement patients have in their care. Szasz and Hollender's (1956) classic paper examined the way in which different models of the doctor–patient relationship related to patients' degree of participation in care, along a continuum from the passive patient to active participation. For example, at a minimal level of involvement, the patient's consent is sought for help in dressing or for undergoing surgery. However, the professional may enter into a more complex negotiated relationship, with the patient being assisted to take more responsibility and play an active part in clinical reasoning. This is illustrated in the nursing–rehabilitation setting

(Ersser, 1988) and is often appropriate in care of chronically ill patients. The patient's active participation in care has been defined as 'getting involved or being allowed to become involved in a decision-making process or the delivery of a service or the evaluation of a service, or even simply to become one of a number of people consulted on an issue or a matter' (Brownlea, 1987, p. 605).

Doctor–patient relationships based upon a mutual-participation style may have greater therapeutic potential (Hays and Dimatteo, 1986). Similarly, Hames and Stirling's (1987) nursing study highlights that giving patients choice in their care may contribute to their recovery. Some evidence suggests that the patient control gained through participating in care may be beneficial in itself, regardless of outcome (Smith *et al.*, 1984). However, Brearley's review (1990) indicates the problems of generalizing research findings about patient participation, since many studies have been conducted in the outpatient setting and focus on doctor-patient interaction.

Strategies to actively involve patients in their care are not without difficulty, as illustrated in nursing. Ersser (1997) found that if nurses use a non-directive style of care patients may misconstrue their therapeutic intentions. For example, the simple activity of inviting the patient to consider walking to a washroom for rehabilitation was misinterpreted as the nurse not bothering to bring a wash bowl (Ersser, 1997). This example reinforces earlier evidence that patients may be reluctant collaborators in care (Waterworth and Luker, 1990).

Patient teaching and information giving

A key strategy for involving patients in clinical decision making requires them to be given appropriate information about their situation, principally through teaching. Patient teaching is now recognized as one of the most effective strategies for empowering patients, especially for those with chronic illness who have to integrate their illness with their lifestyle and manage their own condition (Miller, 1992). Self-medication approaches for patients in hospital create opportunities for teaching prior to discharge and help to minimize the problems that can arise from poor therapy compliance (Bird and Hassall, 1993). Family education is also important for parents to be able to care for their sick child in both home and hospital settings (Darbyshire, 1994).

Effective patient teaching has significant resource implications. Support is needed for the development and dissemination of appropriate materials, the time taken for patients and professionals to discuss the various options and the cost implications of the preferences expressed (Entwistle *et al.*, 1997).

Patients' need for information may not necessarily lead to involvement in decision making. Research evidence from a study of cancer patients suggests that patients may actively seek information to satisfy an as yet unidentified aspect of psychological autonomy that does not necessarily include participation in decision making (Sutherland *et al.*, 1989).

Decision analysis

Patients can participate in decision analysis, a systematic process of formulating clinical decisions by specifying the preferences or utilities they place on the different outcomes of care that may arise from specific actions, according to known probabilities (Sackett *et al.*, 1997). For example, Corcoran (1985) describes the way in which patients can review the various combinations of therapeutic effect against related side effects of analgesic drugs, when titrated from a low dosage to a higher one, or from a high dosage downwards. The decision tree may be useful when there is lack of clarity about a patient's values and preferences relating to a therapeutic regimen. Decision analysis is confined to those decisions that involve mutually exclusive alternative options; this can sometimes limit their use. Patient utilities may be employed for alternative health outcome states. Computer software is now available to assist in the process of designing decision trees.[1] Pictorial tools, such as a thermometer diagram, may be drawn with one pole labelled 'perfect health' and the other 'death' for which the patient marks one point. Decision trees have been used in various clinical contexts, including oncology (Buchanan, 1983) and screening choices for Down syndrome using amniocentesis (Fletcher *et al.*, 1995).

Patient advocacy and representation

Some health professionals, such as nurses, express aspirations to act as the patient's advocate (UKCC, 1992), although their involvement in delivering care may impede their ability to exercise this role effectively. Nurses have developed

methods of organizing hospital care that help to create the conditions of continuity which may enhance effective exchange and good relations with patients, although there may be limitations of individuals and/or the system of which they are a part (Ersser and Tutton, 1991). Porter (1988) argues that nurses' attempts to act as patient advocates are impractical because of their tendency to exercise social control as they professionalize, as highlighted earlier. Indeed, there is a view that nurses may in fact make patients more passive in their involvement in health care (Fagin and Diers, 1983).

Significant developments have taken place in the USA in the patient advocate movement, by employing patient representatives who do not belong to any specific health care profession. Ravich and Schmolka (1996) track the development of patient representation with reference to pioneering work undertaken at the Mount Sinai Hospital in New York. This strategy has developed in response to concerns about the depersonalization of medical care, the variable provision of comprehensive information being given to patients and the increasing differentiation and technical specialization of health professionals. Patient representatives play a key role in discussing issues of 'advance directives' with patients. For example, at St Vincent's Hospital in New York, patients are issued with a State booklet specifying their rights. A representative discusses with relevant patients advance directives on issues such as 'do not resuscitate' instructions, health care proxies and living wills (New York State, 1998).

Patient representation is underpinned by a supportive legal framework in the USA. Patient literature at St Vincent's refers to the 'Patients' Bill of Rights' which is embodied in law. Emphasis is given to the importance of informing patients and then providing clear written and spoken information to allow them to see their medical records, participate in discharge planning, receive a second opinion and turn to an ethics consultant or committee. Patient representatives may also participate in case conferences. *The Federal Patient Self-Determination Act (PSDA) (Omnibus Reconciliation Act)* of 1990 mandates that patients be informed about and assisted in executing advance directives about the care they wish to receive in the event that they cannot make decisions for themselves, such as in the case of terminal illness. The use of advance directives has received significant support in large population surveys (Eisemann and Richter, 1999). A move towards making patient

---

[1] *Smltree decision analysis software.* J. Hollonberg, 16B Pine North, Roslyn, NY 11576, USA.

rights and universal standards of care explicit to patients in the UK has been made through the creation of a *Patient's Charter* (Department of Health, 1991).

Technological strategies

Technology can also assist patients to play a more active role in clinical decision making. Thomas (1996) provides a research-based analysis of patient controlled analgesia using analgesic pumps. Chronically ill patients can be helped to play a more active part in managing their condition through helping them to monitor their condition and act on the data obtained, where appropriate. Examples include diabetics accurately monitoring their blood glucose levels using a glucometer or mothers taking their asthmatic child's peak flow measurement using a meter. Computer-assisted devices can enable those with disabilities to communicate their views as a basis for involvement in decision making (Thorton, 1993).

Creating a humane patient-centred hospital environment

Hospital environments may be experienced by patients as dehumanizing, due to the attitudes of staff, ward organization, the presence of technology (Ersser and Tutton, 1991) and ward atmosphere (Ersser, 1997). These factors can stifle patient involvement in decision making or simply their willingness to express their needs (Biley, 1992). They can lead to patients experiencing uncertainty and anxiety, and losing their ability to cope effectively (Levanthal, 1975).

Horowitz (1996) illustrates the importance of creating a patient-centred hospital environment using the Planetree Model Hospital Project. The Beth Israel Medical Centre in New York aimed to create a more humanistic, patient-oriented hospital environment responsive to patients' emotional and educational needs. Efforts were made to create a less institutional interior in the ward. Attention was given to the aesthetic quality of the setting, through use of lighting and art. Modifications were made to key features of the ward, such as the accessibility of the nursing desk for patients. These developments took place in an acute setting. The West Dorset Hospital NHS Trust was one of the first 'patient focus' hospitals to be designed in the UK (Martin, 1996). Low-cost initiatives to create a more therapeutic environment for patients within an old hospital setting were undertaken by nurses

working at the Oxford Nursing Development Unit (Ersser, 1988).

Aside from the physical environment, attention needs to be given to the organization of care within hospitals to effectively address patient and staff needs. The 'named nurse' initiative was launched by the UK government and helped to disseminate established good practice (Wright, 1996). One such system is primary nursing which offers the potential to achieve a high level of continuity of care, thereby helping to create improved conditions for effective nurse–patient communication (Ersser and Tutton, 1991). Similarly, attention should be given to the organization of ward rounds and case conferences to reduce undue intrusion for patients and their alienation from decision-making processes.

Limitations and boundaries of patient-centred decision making

The foregoing analysis highlights that effecting patient-centred reasoning is largely dependent upon the attitudes, skills and knowledge of individual patients and professionals, and the context within which they interact. There are limits to the extent that health care professionals can set aside their values and perspectives and achieve the level of empathy necessary to reach a full understanding of the patient's perspectives. They must also develop the ability to recognize and acknowledge the influence of their beliefs and values and their level of interpersonal skill on patients. Furthermore, promoting patient-centred reasoning has resource implications. It is likely to be more time consuming for professionals and therefore may not necessarily be either cost effective in some situations.

The organizational culture, including aspects such as the scope for continuity of care and the prominence of hierarchies, will influence the opportunities for patient and professional to exchange information. Consideration is also needed of the extent to which organizational and professional practices are focused on patient needs and concerns, rather than simply on professional convenience and the following of tradition.

Conclusions

The development of patient-centred care is a complex issue that requires an understanding of the range of factors that come to influence how individuals, professional groups and organizations create or block opportunity for patient involvement. Careful account needs to be taken of the range of factors that impinge on the readiness and ability of the patient to benefit from any opportunity created. Patient-centred decision making is a broader concept than simply encouraging patients to participate in their care. Broader perspectives are needed to understand the complexities of the issues, to develop a collective understanding and vision of what a patient-centred health service might be and to discover how different theoretical positions can provide explanations and pointers to effective action.

Among the strategies to help promote more active patient involvement in decision making, the professional–patient relationship is of fundamental importance. It provides an anchor for the patient to take more responsibility for decision making, for the building of trust, and for discovery of the patient's and family's capacities. Such relationships can be cultivated only within an appropriate environment and an organizational system that values patient involvement and a different style of professional practice, and recognizes the alienating aspects of health care for patients and their families.

Much emphasis has been given to the importance of the process of care delivery being patient-centred and the fact that this may not necessarily lead to effective clinical outcomes. However, it is clearly a research priority to ascertain any demonstrable benefits of patient-centred involvement in decision making.

The key factors influencing patient involvement have major implications for the education of health professionals. Health service development will take place only when health professionals have the necessary level of awareness and preparation to relate effectively to patients and to influence the organizational changes necessary to bring about change in practice. There remains considerable scope to reform health services and to radically shift health care practice from a professional-centred stance to one that is patient-centred, with greater patient involvement in decision making being a central feature.

References

Benbassat, J., Pipel, D. and Tidhar, M. (1998) Patients' preferences for participation in clinical decision making: A review of published surveys. *Behavioural Medicine*, **24**, 81–88.

Benner, P., Tanner, C. and Chesla, C. (1992) From beginner to expert: Gaining a differentiated clinical world in critical care nursing. *Advances in Nursing Science*, **14**, 13–28.

Biley, F. (1992) Some determinants that effect patient participation in decision-making about nursing care. *Journal of Advanced Nursing*, **17**, 414–421.

Bird, C. and Hassall, J. (1993) *Self-Administration of Drugs: A Guide to Implementation*. London: Scutari.

Blackhall, L. J., Murphy S. T., Frank G., Michel, V. and Azen, S. (1995) Ethnicity and attitudes toward patient autonomy. *Journal of the American Medical Association*, **274**, 820–825.

Blumer, H. (1969) *Symbolic Interactionism: Perspective and Method*. Englewood Cliffs, NJ: Prentice-Hall.

Bottorff, J. F., Steele, R., Davies, B., Garossino, C., Porterfield, P. and Shaw, M. (1998) Striving for balance: Palliative care patients' experiences of making everyday choices. *Journal of Palliative Care*, **14**, 7–17.

Brammer, L. M (1988), *The Helping Relationship, Process and Skills*. London: Prentice-Hall International.

Brearley, S. (1990) *Patient Participation: The Literature*. London: Scutari Press.

Brownlea, A. (1987) Participation: Myths, realities and prognosis. *Social Science and Medicine*, **25**, 605–614.

Buchanan, J. G. (1983) An introduction to clinical decision analysis: Bone marrow transplantation for aplastic anaemia. *Australian and New Zealand Journal of Medicine*, **13**, 451–456.

Cahill, J. (1996) Patient participation: A concept analysis. *Journal of Advanced Nursing*, **24**, 561–571.

Cooke, P. (1995) Choice in childbirth. *MSc Dissertation*. School of Health Care, Oxford Brookes University, Oxford.

Corcoran, S. (1985) Decision analysis: A step-by-step guide for making clinical decisions. *Nursing and Health Care*, **7**(3), 149–154.

Darbyshire, P. (1994) *Living with a Sick Child in Hospital: The Experiences of Parents and Nurses*. London: Chapman & Hall.

Davis, C. (1976) Experience of dependency in work. *Journal of Advanced Nursing*, **1**, 273–282.

Department of Health (1991) *The Patient's Charter*. London: HMSO

Department of Health (1993) *Changing Childbirth Part 1: Report of the Expert Maternity Group*. London: HMSO.

Dreyfus, H. L. and Dreyfus S. E. (1986) *Mind over Machine*. New York: McMillan Free Press.

Eisemann, M. and Richter, J. (1999) Relationships between various attitudes towards self-determination in health care with special reference to an advance directive. *Journal of Medical Ethics*, **25**, 37–41.

Elstein, A. S., Shulman, L. S, and Sprafka, S. A. (1978) *Medical Problem Solving: An Analysis of Clinical Reasoning*. Cambridge, MA: Harvard University Press.

Entwistle, V. A., Sowden, A. J. and Watt I. S. (1998) Evaluating interventions to promote patient involvement in decision making: By what criteria should effectiveness be judged? *Journal of Health Service Research Policy*, **3**, 100–107 .

Entwistle, V. A., Watt, I. S. and Sowden, A. J. (1997) Information to facilitate patient involvement in decision making – Some issues. *Journal of Clinical Effectiveness*, **2**(3), 69–72.

Ersser S. J. (1997) *Nursing as a Therapeutic Activity: An Ethnography*. Aldershot: Avebury.

Ersser, S. (1988) Nursing beds and nursing therapy. In *Primary Nursing: Nursing in the Burford and Oxford Nursing Development Units* (A. Pearson, ed.), pp. 60–88. London: Chapman & Hall.

Ersser, S. J. and Tutton, E. (eds) (1991) *Primary Nursing in Perspective*. London: Scutari.

Fagin, C. and Diers, D. (1983) Nursing on a metaphor. *New England Journal of Medicine*, **309**, 116–117.

Fleming, M. H. (1991a) Clinical reasoning in medicine compared with clinical reasoning in occupational therapy. *American Journal of Occupational Therapy*, **45**, 988–996.

Fleming, M. H. (1991b) The therapist with the three track mind. *American Journal of Occupational Therapy*, **45**, 1007–1014.

Fletcher, J., Hicks, N. R, Kay, J. D. S and Boyd P. A. (1995) Using decision analysis to compare policies for ante-natal screening for Down's Syndrome. *British Medical Journal*, **311**, 351–356 .

Friedson, E. (1970) *Profession of Medicine: A Study of the Sociology of Applied Knowledge*. New York: Dodd, Mead.

Fulford, K. W. M. (1996) Concepts of disease and the meaning of patient-centred care. In *Essential Practice in Patient-Centred Care* (K. Fulford, S. Ersser and T. Hope, eds), pp. 1–16. Oxford: Blackwell Science.

Gerhardt, U. (1989) *Ideas About Illness: An Intellectual and Political History of Medical Sociology*. New York: New York University Press.

Gibson, C. H. (1991) A concept analysis of empowerment. *Journal of Advanced Nursing*, **16**, 354–361.

Graham, H. (1986) *The Human Face of Psychology: Humanistic Psychology in Its Historical, Social and Cultural Contexts*. Milton Keynes: Open University Press.

Hagedorn, R. (1992) *Occupational Therapy: Foundations for Practice. Models, Frames of Reference and Core Skills*. London: Churchill Livingstone.

Hall, L. (1969) The Loeb Centre for Nursing and Rehabilitation, Montefiore Hospital and Medical Centre, Bronx, New York. *International Journal of Nursing Studies*, **6**, 81–95.

Hames, A. and Stirling, E. (1987) Choice aids recovery. *Nursing Times*, **23**(8), 49–51.

Hays, R. and Dimatteo, M. R. (1986) Towards a more therapeutic physician–patient relationship. In *Personal Relationships 5: Repairing Personal Relationships* (S. W. Duck, ed.), pp. 1–20, London: Academic Press.

Higgs, J. and Jones, M. (1995) Introduction. In *Clinical Reasoning in the Health Professions* (J. Higgs and M. Jones, eds), pp. xiii–xvi. Oxford: Butterworth Heinemann.

Hopkins, H. L. (1988) An historical perspective on occupational therapy. In *Willard and Spackman's Occupational Therapy*, 7th edn (H. L. Hopkins and H. D. Smith, eds), pp. 16–37, Philadelphia, PA: Lippincott.

Horowitz, S. F. (1996) The Planetree Model Hospital Project. In *Essential Practice in Patient-Centred Care*. (K. Fulford, S. Ersser and T. Hope, eds), pp. 155–161. Oxford: Blackwell Science.

Illich, I. (1976) *Limits to Medicine, Medical Nemesis: The Expropriation of Health*. Harmondsworth: Penguin.

Jensen, G. M., Shepard, K. F. and Hack, L. M. (1992) Attribute dimensions that distinguish master and novice physical therapy clinicians in orthopaedic settings. *Physical Therapy*, **72**, 711–722.

King, I. M. (1981) *A Theory for Nursing: General Concepts of Human Behaviour*. New York: Wiley.

Levanthal, H. (1975) The consequences of depersonalization during illness and treatment. In *Humanizing Health Care* (J. Howard and A. Strauss, eds), pp. 110–119. New York: Wiley.

Martin, T. (1996) Commentary on Chapter 10 (see Horowitz, S.). In *Essential Practice in Patient-Centred Care*. (K. Fulford, S. Ersser and T. Hope, eds), pp. 162–165. Oxford: Blackwell Science.

Miller, J. F. (1992) *Coping With Chronic Illness: Overcoming Powerlessness*. Philadelphia, PA: F. A. Davis.

Mitchell, K., Bozanth, J. and Kauft, C. (1977) A reappraisal of the therapeutic effectiveness of accurate empathy, possessive warmth and genuineness. In *Effective Psychotherapy* (A. Gurucan and A. Raizin, eds), pp. 482–502. Oxford: Pergamon Press.

Morse, J. M. and Johnson, J. L. (eds) (1991) *The Illness Experience: Dimensions of Suffering*. London: Sage.

New York State (1998) *Your Rights as a Hospital Patient in New York State*. New York State.

Newell, A. and Simon, H. A. (1972) *Human Problem Solving*. Englewood Cliffs, NJ: Prentice-Hall.

Parsons, T. (1951) *The Social System*. New York: Free Press.

Parsons, T. (1978) *Action Theory and the Human Condition*. New York: Free Press.

Paterson-Brown, S. and Fisk, N. M. (1997) Caesarian section: Every woman's right to choose? *Current Opinion Obstetrics and Gynaecology*, **9**, 351–355.

Porter, S. (1988) Siding with the system. *Nursing Times*, **84**(41), 30–31.

Quill, T. E. and Brody, H. (1996) Physican recommendations and patient autonomy: Finding a balance between physican power and patient choice. *Annals of Internal Medicine*, **125**, 763–769.

Ravich, R. and Schmolka, L. (1996) Patient representation: A patient-centred approach to the provision of health services. In *Essential Practice in Patient-Centred Care* (K. Fulford, S. Ersser and T. Hope, eds), pp. 64–84. Oxford: Blackwell Science.

Riehl-Sisca, J. (1989) The Riehl interaction model: An update. In *Conceptual Models for Nursing Practice* (J. Riehl-Sisca, ed.), 3rd edn, pp. 383–402. Norwalk, CT: Appleton Century Crofts.

Robertson D. W. (1996) Ethical theory, ethnography and differences between doctors and nurses in approaches to patient care. *Journal of Medical Ethics*, **22**, 292–299.

Rogers, C. R. (1965) The therapeutic relationship: recent theory and research. *Australian Journal of Psychology*, **17**, 95–108.

Sackett, D. L., Richardson, W. S., Rosenberg, W. and Haynes, R. B. (1997) *Evidence-Based Medicine: How to Practice and Teach Evidence-Based Medicine*. New York: Churchill Livingstone.

Sayers, G. M., Schofield, I. and Aziz, M. (1997) An analysis of CPR decision-making by elderly patients. *Journal of Medical Ethics*, **23**, 207–212.

Scambler, G. (ed.) (1997) *Sociology as Applied to Medicine*. London: Saunders.

Smith, R. A., Wallston, B. S., Wallston, K. A., Forsberg, P. R. and King, J E. (1984) Measuring desire of health care processes. *Journal of Personal and Social Psychology*, **46**, 415–426.

Smith, T. J. and Bodurtha, J. N. (1995) Ethical considerations in oncology: Balancing the interests of patients, oncologists and society. *Journal of Clinical Oncology*, **13**, 2464–2470.

Sugarman, J., McCrory, D. C. and Hubal, R. C. (1998) Getting meaningful informed consent from older adults: A structured literature review of empirical research. *Journal of the American Geriatric Society*, **46**, 517–524.

Sutherland, H. J., Llewellyn-Thomas, H. A., Lockwood, G. A., Tritchler, D. L. and Till, J. E. (1989) Cancer patients: Their desire for information and participation in treatment decisions. *Journal of the Royal Society of Medicine*, **82**, 260–263.

Szasz, T. S. and Hollender, M. H. (1956) A contribution to the philosophy of medicine: The basic models of the doctor–patient relationship. *Archives of Internal Medicine*, **97**, 585–592.

Thomas, V. (1996) Patient controlled analgesia and the concept of patient-centred care. In *Essential Practice in Patient-Centred Care* (K. Fulford, S. Ersser and T. Hope, eds), pp. 103–115. Oxford: Blackwell Science.

Thompson, S. C., Pitts, J. S. and Schwankovsky, L. (1993) Preferences for involvement in medical decision making: Situational and demographic influences. *Patient Education and Counselling*, **22**, 133–140.

Thorton, P. (1993) Communications technology – Empowerment or disempowerment? *Disability, Handicap and Society*, **8**, 339–349.

United Kingdom Central Council for Nursing, Midwifery and Health Visiting (1992) *Code of Professional Conduct*. London: UKCC.

Waterworth, S. and Luker, K. (1990) Reluctant collaborators: Do patients want to be involved in decisions concerning care? *Journal of Advanced Nursing*, **15**, 971–976.

Winefield, H., Murrell, T., Clifford, J. and Farmer, E. (1996) The search for reliable and valid measures of patient-centredness. *Psychology and Health Care*, **11**, 811–824.

Wright S. G. (1996) The named nurse. In *Essential Practice in Patient-Centred Care* (K. Fulford, S. Ersser and T. Hope, eds), pp. 89–98. Oxford: Blackwell Science.

9

Methods in the study of clinical reasoning

Vimla L. Patel and José F. Arocha

This chapter presents an overview of some of the methods used in the study of clinical reasoning. It does not constitute an exhaustive overview. Instead, it presents major features of the most common approaches used in the study of clinical reasoning. In addition, we include a range of new and promising research methodologies used in clinical reasoning research and elsewhere.

Historical sketch

The development of the methodologies used in the study of clinical reasoning in the health sciences has followed from developments in other areas of thinking and reasoning. What started mostly as a study within the psychometric tradition has evolved to include a variety of methods. The study of clinical reasoning is pluralistic. The evolution of this pluralism is reflected in this section.

We have found it useful to divide the historical development into two main periods. The first covers the early investigations of clinical reasoning from the 1950s to the 1970s. It was dominated by the psychometric approach and was devoted mainly to assessment of clinical reasoning performance rather than to basic research. The latter two decades saw a paradigm shift in the behavioural sciences: a shift marked by the change from the behaviourist to the cognitive paradigm and later by an increasing emphasis on alternative research perspectives, such as hermeneutics and situated cognition. This shift had a profound impact on the methods used, leading to a broadening of the methodologies to include a multiplicity of new data gathering and analysis

techniques and a change of focus, from an emphasis on describing overt behaviour to an emphasis on describing and modelling cognitive processes.

The precognitive era

The topic of clinical reasoning has always drawn the attention of medical education researchers. The way the research has been carried out has been determined by the particular theoretical and methodological frameworks dominant at the time.

The first studies of medical reasoning had as their goal the assessment of the clinical skills of physicians and medical students, as these skills were viewed as extremely important for achieving mastery. To this end, the research paradigm dominant during the 1950s and 1960s was the psychometric paradigm, in which emphasis was placed on the identification of general skills, defined in terms of observable behaviours, through the use of psychometric tests.

The purpose of most early studies of clinical reasoning was to develop instruments for assessing clinical performance, rather than characterizing clinical reasoning. An overview of methods for studying clinical reasoning by Vu (1979) distinguished between observational, record-based and simulation methods. For the purposes of the present chapter simulation methods are the most interesting, because they deal with the actual reasoning processes used by subjects, whereas the others attempt to re-construct these processes from either observations or past records.

Simulation methods, which consist of simulating the physician–patient encounter, are of various kinds, including written patient descriptions, real patient simulations and computer simulations (Vu, 1979). What is common to them all is that the information about a problem to be solved is presented to the subjects. The problem posed to the subjects can take several forms, from written patient presentations to computerized presentation systems to the use of live patient simulations. Based on the information presented, an inquiry process begins, in which the subjects request new information and make a diagnosis.

Rimoldi's (1961) test of diagnostic skills was among the first to study the diagnostic process from a psychometric perspective. The test consists of a clinical case which describes a preliminary report on a patient. The subject then inquires about the patient by requesting additional information. The information is given to the subject on cue-cards with a question presented on one side and the answer on the other side. By studying the nature and the chronological sequence of questions asked, it is possible to evaluate the subject's level of clinical reasoning skills. The results of Rimoldi's study (1961) served to characterize the behaviour of physicians as more focused (they asked fewer and more appropriate questions) than that of medical students.

A second form of simulation method is used in the assessment of reasoning skills (Barro, 1973; Elstein *et al.*, 1978; McGuire, 1985). These assessments are variations of the Patient Management Problem (PMP), a test to assess the clinical process. The procedure basically consists of presenting an unfolding patient problem that the subject studies and then attempts to solve by making decisions about the course of action to be taken. In some forms of PMP, subjects receive feedback about the results of their decisions. Different reasoning paths, then, could be followed depending on the previous choices made.

It is important to note that these simulation methods were developed for the purposes of assessment. Because of this, one of the criteria in their creation has been ease of administration. This may have limited their utility as research tools, since the practical goals of assessment had to be reconciled with the conceptual goals of research. Furthermore, most of the literature on these methods concerns psychometric issues such as reliability and various forms of validity.

The cognitive era

The study of clinical reasoning and problem solving in its current form had, as a background, a series of theoretical and methodological developments that took place in other areas of research, notably the development of computer science and, with it, the first simulations of thought processes (Hovland, 1960; Newell *et al.*, 1958). This background suggested that a different approach to research in clinical reasoning was needed. The emphasis was not on testing isolated quantitative hypotheses, but on testing models of reasoning (Newell and Simon, 1972). This requires a more qualitative approach to research than is traditionally accepted. A second line of research was inaugurated with the publication in 1956 of the book *A Study of Thinking* by Bruner *et al.* (1956). The emphasis of this research was on concept formation. As with Newell and Simon's research, this work marked a departure from the behaviouristic framework that had dominated behavioural science at the time. In medicine, these new lines of research were exemplified by the work of Elstein *et al.* (1978). What has united all the investigations of clinical reasoning carried out since the work of Elstein and colleagues is the use of the contrastive method, in which performance of experts is compared to that of novices. This method is a legacy of De Groot's (1965) work on chess masters, which subsequently influenced the research of Chase and Simon (1973) and Larkin *et al.* (1980) on physics problem solving.

It is recognized that the study of medical cognition in its current form started with the publication by Elstein *et al.* (1978) of their pioneering work, covering more than a decade. This work was largely influenced by the study of problem solving that Newell and Simon had carried out during the late 1950s and that was changing the way research was done in psychology.

Some characteristics serve to differentiate the new, cognitive, from the old, behaviouristic, approaches. One characteristic that differentiates this work from earlier work is that it was aimed at developing a characterization of clinical reasoning, in line with work that was being conducted in other areas of research, such as chess and physics. As in these other areas, one of the aims of the new cognitive research in the health sciences was to specify the knowledge structures and processes used during clinical reasoning. This research posed questions about the cognitive strategies and the type of knowledge used in diagnosing patient problems. In contrast, the aim of earlier research was mainly to develop assessment instruments for health care professionals. Another characteristic of the new cognitive approach is that this research was developed under the guidance of theoretical models of the development of expertise and clinical reasoning. Whereas the previous work started by defining the aspects of clinical reasoning in purely behavioural terms, the new approach was based on a theory of the cognitive processes used in clinical reasoning.

The methodology that was used by Elstein *et al.* (1978) consisted of several methods, which varied in terms of their fidelity to real-life clinical situations. They developed these methods in order to maximize the information available, as no one method could provide all the information needed to investigate clinical reasoning and problem solving. Whereas some high-fidelity methods (e.g. use of simulated patients) capture some real-life aspects of the process, they may fail to capture some hidden cognitive processes. Low-fidelity methods (e.g. recall tasks) have the advantage of allowing specific aspects of the clinical reasoning process to be isolated and studied in more depth. This work exemplifies the methodological pluralism that is encountered today in the study of clinical reasoning.

Following the theoretical and experimental approach of Newell and Simon (1972), Feltovich *et al.* (1984) investigated the clinical reasoning process. In their research, they uncovered some of the characteristics that differentiate novices from experts. The main difference identified was in terms of the quality of knowledge structures of experts.

The study of some conceptual aspects of clinical reasoning was investigated by Bordage and Zacks (1984). Borrowing from the traditional methods of cognitive psychology used by Bruner *et al.* (1956), these researchers investigated the nature of diagnostic categories used by physicians and medical students. Their research was influenced by the work of Rosch (1978), who investigated the psychological nature of categories. Although this work is influenced by a different tradition, its basic concepts and methods are compatible with the information processing approach to cognition. This research is still an active area of inquiry (e.g. Brooks *et al.*, 1991).

A line of research which has also been influenced by the work of Chase and Simon has been conducted by Patel and Groen (Patel and Groen, 1986; Patel *et al.*, 1990) at McGill University in Montreal and by Schmidt and his collaborators at the University of Limburg in Maastricht, Holland (Schmidt *et al.*, 1988). These two research teams have investigated several aspects of expertise using

somewhat similar methodologies derived from propositional analysis (Kintsch, 1974). Their research has focused on the knowledge differences between novices and experts and on the kinds of inductive inferences they use. Of particular importance has been the investigation of the intermediate effect (i.e. the finding that intermediate subjects, those between novice and experts, often perform more poorly than either experts or novices) and the identification of different kinds of expertise (e.g. general and specific expertise).

In conclusion, the study of clinical reasoning has diversified to include very different methodological commitments and techniques. From purely behaviouristic and psychometric roots, it has developed into a multiplicity of methods and continues to do so. This has had a profound impact on the quantity and quality of the research. Various topics such as conceptual understanding (Feltovich *et al.*, 1992) and collaboration in naturalistic environments (Patel *et al.*, 1996), which until not long ago were non-existent, are now active and promising areas of study.

Methods of studying clinical reasoning in the health sciences

There have been basically two main traditions in the study of clinical reasoning in the health sciences. One tradition has emphasized the study of clinical decision making. This tradition uses quantitative methodologies and models to describe or prescribe clinical decision making. Descriptive decision making has been based on simple input/output models such as linear regression, on the assumption that such models can account for the decision making of clinicians. Prescriptive decision making has been based on decision theory, with the assumption that this theory is a normative guide for successful action (as a prescriptive guide to how decision making ought to be done).

The second major tradition has aimed at an understanding of the cognitive processes used during problem solving. It differs from the first approach in that it describes the knowledge structures used during problem solving. Instead of looking at clinical reasoning only at the points of decisions between alternatives, it examines the whole process from the formulation of hypotheses to the reaching of a solution to the problem. It also examines the nature of the knowledge used and the cognitive operations used to reach the solution. This second tradition has been highly influenced by the field of Artificial Intelligence (AI). AI aims at developing machines capable of reproducing some human cognitive functions, such as perception, reasoning and problem solving (Barr and Feigenbaum, 1981).

A third research tradition emphasizes the study of interactions as a form of reasoning and understanding. This is the interpretive tradition, which has been applied mostly in nursing research (Benner, 1984). The interpretive tradition has also influenced a newer research approach, given such diverse labels as situated cognition, situated action and interactionism (Greeno, 1998). This approach also borrows from the AI approach some of its concepts and its problematics, but interprets cognitive functions as part of an interaction between the human and its environment, rather than something happening inside someone's head. Probably the major movement in the field has been in the direction of relating reasoning (as a mental process) with action in dynamic environments.

Quantitative methods

Experimental methods

Quantitative experimental methodologies have been widely used in the field of medical cognition in various clinical tasks. One of the tasks most widely used by these researchers involves the study of perceptual aspects of expertise (Lesgold *et al.*, 1988; Norman *et al.*, 1989a,b). In such studies, subjects are presented a series of slides (e.g. X-rays, photographs of dermatological affections) and then, after some period, are asked to interpret or recall the information in the slides. The goal is to show how variations in the subjects' interpretations (e.g. verbal protocols, recalls) relate to the variations of the experimental conditions (e.g. types of slide, X-ray). These data are then quantified and subjected to statistical analysis. The basic model underlying this type of research is an input–output model, where the output is accounted for in terms of the input. The same methods have been employed by others (e.g. Patel and Frederiksen, 1984; Schmidt and Boshuizen, 1993) using verbal materials such as clinical case descriptions or 'think aloud' protocols.

Although the most commonly used research strategy is to investigate groups (i.e. samples of subjects), there is a fundamental reason for also investigating individual subjects, namely the search for invariants (i.e. what is similar across *all* individuals). If the overall goal of research is to understand the functioning of human beings, how they are organized such that they are capable of producing what we observe them producing, then that organization must be the same for everyone. The basic idea is that humans operate according to a set of principles that must be known in order to give an accurate account of human performance in detail. Once that is known, it is possible to investigate how individuals differ.

Approaches consistent with the single-subject approach have been associated mostly with research in AI (e.g. Clancey, 1997). Although unfortunately little use has been made of such methods, their addition to the methodological toolbox of the clinical reasoning researcher is welcome. These approaches are various (e.g. control theoretic and systems dynamics approaches), but all view the process of thinking and reasoning as part of people's attempts to engage in interaction with the external environment (or the perceived consequences of such engagement), which occurs as part of a person–environment feedback loop. This characteristic (its feedback loop nature) separates them from the traditional approaches, since feedback loops involve a dialectical relationship between input and outputs, where outputs are not a function of inputs, but they mutually change one another.

Decision-making methods

The study of decision making has been carried out in a variety of domains and is an active area of research. Typically, decision-making researchers start with a formal model of decision making and then collect data which are compared to the model. The models can be of various types, such as simple regression models, Bayesian estimation models and decision–theoretic models. The latter are the most mathematically sophisticated (Christensen *et al.*, 1991).

Decision theory has its roots in the work of von Neumann and Morgenstern (1944) on game theory. The theory deals with making decisions in situations of uncertainty. The basic principle of the theory is that a rational person should maximize his or her expected utility, which is defined as the product of probability by utility. Hammond (1967) gives the following example: a businessman faces the decision of either winning $500 000 or losing $100 000, both of which have the same probability, 0.5. The expected utility in this case would be of $200 000 [0.5 (500 000) – 0.5 (100 000)]. Decision theory has been used mostly as a model for rational decision making. Previously, the theory was thought to describe actual human decision making, but empirical research on the psychological bases of decision making has falsified its claims as a descriptive theory (Tversky and Kahneman, 1974). The theory also has been used as a normative theory under the assumption that the maximization of the expected utilities is rational. Under this assumption, to be rational, people's decisions must mirror those derived from the model. If people's decisions depart from those specified by the model, it is taken as evidence that they are not behaving rationally. This assumption, and therefore, the normative character of the theory, have also been severely questioned (Allais and Hagen, 1979; Bunge, 1985; Hammond, 1967). In short, critics argue that it is not always rational to maximize one's expected utility and therefore the theory cannot be taken as a prescription for action.

Whatever its merits either as a descriptive or a prescriptive theory, decision theory has stimulated a great deal of research in medicine (Weinstein *et al.*, 1980) and various other domains (Carroll and Johnson, 1990; Dawes, 1988). The research on decision theory uses a model that serves as comparison for the empirical studies. The model is assumed to be a model of rationality such that lack of agreement between the subjects' responses and the model is taken as evidence that the subjects do not make decisions rationally. The model assumes the maximization of expected utilities as the criterion for rationality.

Decision theory, as well as other statistical approaches to investigating decision making, makes use of explicit numerical models for the evaluation of human decisions. The most used models, beside the expected utility model, are the regression and the Bayesian models. These are called weighted additive models because of the assumption that the decision process has the form of an additive function, $Y_i = f(X_{ij})$, in which i represents the alternative, j represents the number of attributes and f is the function that relates the decision to the set of weighted attributes.

Typically, in a decision-making study, the subject is asked to generate a series of attributes that are of most importance for a given situation (e.g. a clinical case) and rank them in order of importance or preference. Once this is done, a set of weights is gathered for each of the attributes. The data are then combined into a decision formula (i.e. the decision model) and a decision is generated from the model. This is then used either to help the human decision maker arrive at a good decision or as a description of the decision maker's behaviour.

These models, also called input–output models, do not consider any mediating process between the attributes and the decision. Most of them also assume that the decision function is linear. The methods used within these approaches consist of collecting a series of responses to a limited set of choices. The models assume that all the alternatives and their consequences are known. The subject's task is to choose among these alternatives.

It is important to note that for such models to apply, all the information has to be available to the subject (and to the model). Also note that only the selection of alternatives (e.g. diagnoses) is illustrated by these models. This has provoked some researchers (Fox, 1988) to argue for an expansion in the study of decision making to include also the intermediate processes between the selection of attributes and the reaching of the decision. The argument supports the developing of knowledge-based decision methods based on the techniques of artificial intelligence, which calls for the inclusion of heuristics (e.g. means–ends analysis) and knowledge structures in the decision model.

Although decision models have been used to describe human behaviour, psychological research (Tversky and Kahneman, 1974) has shown that subjects do not behave according to the models. People show various kinds of biases that depart systematically from the models' predictions.

Summary of quantitative methods

Quantitative methods, as they are used in the study of clinical reasoning, cover a large variety of techniques. There are some similarities among them, however. Their use involves the collection of easily scorable responses, and they mostly investigate input–output connections with no direct examination of the processes mediating these connections. This does not mean that they do not allow claims about what goes on between stimulus and responses, but there is no direct consideration of mediating reasoning processes. The emerging methodologies based on control theory offer a quantitative approach that allows inquiry into people's inner processes, but that departs significantly from the standard quantitative approaches. Other methodologies, however, have dealt with mental processes in qualitative terms.

Qualitative methods

This section deals with what are considered to be, overall, qualitative methods. The methods described in this section vary widely in terms of their origins and applications and cover methods such as the generation of think-aloud protocols, discourse analysis methods and ethnographic methods. The first originates in the study of clinical reasoning and the computer simulation of thought processes, the second in the analysis of text comprehension and conversation, and the third in the analysis of complex, mostly social, situations. A common theme to all these methods is that they deal with real-life, or as close to real-life as possible, situations. Another common aspect is that they have only recently become accepted as methods of scientific study by scientists. A third common feature is that they are applied to unique situations. By this we mean that each case, consisting of a physician solving a case or a pair of nurses discussing a patient problem, is taken as a unit. In contrast to the quantitative methods discussed in the previous section, qualitative researchers attempt to describe single episodes in detail rather than obtaining gross average measures of many situations (Newell and Simon, 1972). A precursor of such a method is the clinical interview method exemplified in the research carried out by Piaget (1950). This method has been one of the more fruitful in psychology and has had a tremendous influence on current research in thinking.

Verbal reports

A common method of data gathering used by psychologists at the turn of the century was the introspective method. This consisted of asking a previously trained subject to report on his or her thoughts while engaged in carrying out a cognitive task. With the advent of behavioural psychology, however, the method lost its appeal. The problem was that the method required the subject to theorize about his or her own thought processes. This theorizing introduces new information and cognitive processes that the subject may have not used at the time of performance, resulting in a distortion of the thinking process underlying performance.

Although during the behaviourist era introspection was much attacked for its unscientific character and verbal report methods were not much used, some of the most influential behaviourists recognized the value of verbal data in the study of thinking (e.g. Watson, 1920) and some form of verbal data were used during that era, even by behaviourists. There are several kinds of verbal reports. One of the earliest in psychological research was the use of recall to investigate memory phenomena. A second kind is the retrospective protocol, such as stimulated recall (Elstein *et al.*, 1978). A third kind is the 'think-aloud' method used in clinical reasoning and expertise research (Kassirer *et al.*, 1982). Still another kind is a form of retrospective protocol, called explanation protocol, used to study knowledge structures (Patel and Groen, 1986).

In its accepted modern form, research that uses verbal reports as data deals with the study of pieces of discourse about a problem or a situation, without introspection. That is, the subject is asked to verbalize his or her thoughts without 'theorizing' about his or her cognitive processes. Any theorizing is the responsibility of the experimenter and not of the subject. Verbalizations are considered as any other behavioural data. A further difference with introspection is that the method is supported by a theory of the human information processing system (Ericsson and Simon, 1984; Newell and Simon, 1972).

In summary, we can distinguish between simultaneous or think-aloud protocols and retrospective protocols. In both cases subjects report only whatever comes to their minds. The difference is that in simultaneous protocols subjects are reporting their thoughts while solving a task, whereas in retrospective protocols subjects are asked to report a previous situation. Analysis methods can be found in Ericsson and Simon (1984).

In typical think-aloud research, subjects are presented with a clinical case, most frequently in written form, which may contain anything from a single sentence to a whole patient record including the clinical interview, the physical examination results and the laboratory results. The subject is asked to read the information and verbalize whatever thoughts come to mind. If the subject pauses for a few seconds, the experimenter intervenes with questions such as 'What are you thinking about?' or demands such as 'Please, continue', which encourage the subject to carry on talking.

Once the protocol has been collected, it is subjected to an analysis aimed at uncovering the cognitive processes and the information that were used. The analysis of the protocol is then compared to a reference or domain model of the task to be solved. This model is frequently taken either from an expert collaborator in the study or from printed information about the topic, such as textbooks or scholarly expositions. For instance, Kuipers and Kassirer (1984), in their study of causal reasoning, used a model of the Starling equilibrium mechanism which was compared to the protocols from subjects at different levels of expertise: medical students, residents and expert physicians. In the same vein, Patel and her colleagues (Joseph and Patel, 1990; Patel and Groen, 1986) used a reference model of the clinical cases, which served as a standard for comparison with subjects' protocols.

For verbal reports to be valid, it is necessary that some conditions be met. The conditions pertain to the type of task that should be used, the kinds of instruction given to the subject and the familiarity of the subject with the task. Ericsson and Simon (1984) have developed an extensive description of these conditions and there is also independent research that has shown the validity of the methods (White, 1988). The theory of protocol analysis is based on the idea that, in problem solving, the verbalizations are interpreted as a search through a problem space of hypotheses and data.

Retrospective protocols

Retrospective protocols are collected after the situation described has already happened. In most situations, they are collected and analysed in the same manner as think-aloud protocols but with different goals in mind. They differ in that in think-aloud protocols subjects are asked to report whatever comes to mind without making any evaluation of their thinking. In this sense the verbalizations at time t are hypothesized to be the contents of short-term memory at time t_1. In retrospective protocols, verbalizations do not refer to the contents in short-term memory alone but are probably a mixing of short-term and long-term memory information (Newell and Simon, 1972). Therefore, whereas think-aloud protocols can be reliably used to characterize clinical reasoning, retrospective protocols can be used to characterize processes that are not dependent on the concurrent presentation of the stimulus materials. They may be used as a complement to think-aloud protocols or to investigate other cognitive aspects associated with reasoning such as comprehension, meta-cognitive activities and the use of knowledge.

Explanation protocols

One of the more interesting types of verbal data collection and analysis is the explanation task. This has been used by Patel and Groen (1986), Schmidt

et al. (1988) and Norman *et al.* (1989a,b). The research by Patel and her colleagues began by collecting recall protocols with the aim of obtaining expert/novice differences akin to those obtained in previous research in other domains such as physics (Larkin *et al.*, 1980). Research into expert/novice differences in medicine had failed to detect differences between subjects at different levels of expertise. Patel, influenced by the research on text comprehension (Frederiksen, 1975; Kintsch, 1974), attempted to use the concept of the proposition (i.e. an idea unit) as a cognitive unit rather than the 'chunk'. It is important to note that the proposition had been used in comprehension research and was found to be the most useful unit for the analysis of linguistic discourse. By applying these methods, using the standard free-recall method of cognitive psychology, similar results were obtained to those of Chase and Simon in the study of chess expertise (e.g. use of chunking and forward reasoning).

Subsequently, Patel and colleagues developed the explanation protocol method. This method consists of asking the subject to explain the pathophysiology of a case. The explanation is then represented in the form of a propositional structure (see Table 9.1). Analysis consists of several steps: (a) segment the subject protocol (the explanation of the case) into clauses according to the clause analysis method of Winograd (1972); (b) determine the propositions in each clause, by taking each idea unit separately as a proposition; (c) relate the propositions in a semantic network in which the relations between propositions are labelled following the propositional grammar developed by Frederiksen (1975). A semantic network is a structure of concepts and relations among concepts. Concepts are represented as nodes and relations are represented as links between nodes, according to graph theoretic notions (Sowa, 1984). The relations in the semantic networks contain mostly conditional and causal links. Thus a semantic network is a connected graph in which the connections among concepts as well as the direction of reasoning are represented. A graph is connected if there exists a path, directed or undirected, between any two nodes. The types of nodes correspond either to data given in the problem or to hypothesized information. Reasoning is characterized in the following form. When the direction of the relations are from the given data in the problem to the hypothesized node, it is coded as forward, or data-driven reasoning. When the link is from the hypothesized node to explain

Table 9.1 Example of propositional analysis

Sentence: Painless recurrent haematuria suggests a possible tumour of the urinary tract

	Propositional analysis	
Proposition number	*Predicate*	*Arguments*
1.0	COND	[1.1], [1.2]
1.1	HAEMATURIA	ATT: Painless, ASPECT:ITER (recurrent)
1.2	SUGGEST	THM: 1.3
1.3	TUMOUR	LOC: Tract, MOD:QUAL (Possible)
1.4	TRACT	ATT:Urinary

Propositions are numbered within segments and consist of a predicate and a series of labelled arguments. A predicate may be an action (e.g. examine), an object (e.g. system) or a relation which connects propositions (e.g. COND, a conditional relation). Arguments may be case relations, such as PAT, the patient of a progressive action; AGT, the agent of the resultive action; THM, the theme of a cognitive process and RSLT, the result of an action. Arguments can also be relations such as LOC, the location of an object or action, and TNS, the tense, ASPECT, the aspect or MOD, the modality. ATT expresses an attribute of an object or an act; ITER expresses an iterative, repeatable event or act; QUAL, qualified relationship indicating a probabilistic truth value (between 0 and 1).

the data in the problem, it is coded as backward reasoning, or hypothesis-driven reasoning. A series of inferences between the two is coded as an elaboration. With this methodology it has been possible to investigate some aspects of expert and novice reasoning in diagnostic tasks. More specifically, the method has been used to uncover the kinds of reasoning pattern used by expert physicians, which has served to identify several kinds of expertise, such as general and specific expertise (Groen and Patel, 1988).

Discourse analysis

As is the case with protocol analysis, discourse analysis techniques have been used to analyse verbal data. The theoretical tradition of discourse analysis originates in linguistics and psycholinguistics, more specifically in the study of texts. Discourse analysis developed against the traditional emphasis on simple forms of linguistic performance, such as morphemes and lexical units. The idea was to begin to investigate larger bodies of language in order to tackle issues hardly dealt with by traditional theories, such as text semantics. What started as a research program in linguistics was extended to other forms of human performance, such as memory and reasoning in medicine (Patel and Frederiksen, 1984), and later to the investigation of reasoning and decision making in multi-agent interacting settings.

Another methodology influenced by the theories of discourse is the phenomenological or phenomenographic approach (Marton and Saljo, 1976). The emphasis in this method is on investigating general approaches and knowledge that individuals use to learn and understand a situation or problem. Thus, the emphasis is on finding individual differences in the way people approach the phenomena around them. Methodologically, the work has been influenced by Piaget's clinical method in which subjects (thus far mostly students) are asked a series of questions and are also asked to externalize their cognitive process by solving a problem task. This approach has been applied to medicine by Ramsden *et al.* (1989). The data are collected by asking subjects to study patient records, taking as much time as they need. They are then asked questions in a non-directed way with the aim of eliciting information about their understanding of the problem and their ways of solving it. The analysis consists of generating categories that can meaningfully characterize what subjects are doing from their perspective.

Interpretive methods

With the increasing acceptance of qualitative methodologies, scholars in the behavioural sciences have begun to be receptive to new forms of conducting research that stress the interpretive aspect of inquiry. Instead of taking quantitative measures and subjecting them to statistical analyses, ethnographic researchers attempt to describe whole real-life situations in order to grasp their meaning (Benner, 1984). These researchers argue that quantitative research produces a great deal of meaningless numbers while more important aspects are neglected or misunderstood. They also argue that the behavioural sciences need rich descriptive data that take into account the context of behaviour. Without this context, interpretation of human action cannot be done in a meaningful way. This context-dependence of action requires a methodology that takes a more descriptive approach to research.

Some philosophers (Taylor, 1971) and researchers in the social sciences (Suchman, 1987) have argued that the traditional scientific approach to research, based on the natural sciences such as physics, is inadequate for investigating human issues. These require a new conceptualization of science that takes into account the 'social construction of shared meaning'. An analogy is the reading of texts. That is, just as a word in a text obtains its meaning from the context provided by other words, situations involving human action are not comprehensible without the context in which they occur. In both cases, the reader/observer's task is to 'interpret' the meaning of the text/actions. Because of this contextual character, human action cannot be studied by using wholly objective methods.

Rather than investigating from the outside, in an objective manner, the researcher is a participant of the 'community' he or she is studying. Rather than attempting to minimize interaction with the subject, the interpretive researcher attempts to maximize it, since it is this very interaction which comprehensively informs the researcher about the phenomenon under investigation.

In a study by Benner (1984) on nursing expertise, paired interviews were conducted with novice and expert nurses about a situation that was common to both. Benner's research is based on the models of skill acquisition and expertise developed by Dreyfus and Dreyfus (1986), whose work is, in turn, inspired by the phenomenological philosophy of Martin Heidegger (1962). Benner's method consists of interpreting each situation by independent observer/interpreters and then comparing their interpretations and reaching a consensus about the meaning of the situations. The idea behind this method is to capture subjects' experiences in terms of their interpretations of the problem.

Interpretive research has had a somewhat long history in educational research (Glaser and Strauss, 1967). During the last 10 or so years, this kind of research endeavour has been growing in popularity among people dissatisfied with the traditional research approaches. It has been mostly applied to investigate processes that involve social interaction, such as classroom instruction. Its acceptance in medical education has been somewhat late, but it may also grow, as medical educators become familiar with it.

Situated cognition methods

In recent years, an approach to thinking and reasoning has developed that emphasizes the contextual aspect of cognition. Although indirectly related to the interpretive approach, it has been developed by independent researchers. Greeno (1989), in an exposition of the new approach, complains that contrary to the standard, domain-based view of thinking in specific tasks such as diagnostic and arithmetic tasks, the study of critical, productive thinking has not produced major advances. He cites several of the framing assumptions of the standard view of thinking as causes of this slow progress (Greeno, 1989, p. 134):

> First, the locus of thinking is assumed to be in an individual's mind, rather than in interaction between an agent and a physical and social situation. Second, processes of thinking and learning are assumed to be uniform across persons and situations. Different individuals are more or less capable of critical or creative thinking, and different situations are assumed to have approximately the same character wherever and in whomever they occur. Third, resources for thinking are assumed to be knowledge and skills that are built up from simple components, socially through instruction in school, rather than general conceptual capabilities that children may have as a result of their everyday experience or native endowment.

In the situated approach, the methods involve rich ethnographic description of persons acting in their environment, as reasoning is conceived of taking place in interaction with situations, rather than conceiving of it as a set of processes occurring inside someone's mind (e.g. as a set of knowledge structures and operations on them). The shift proposed by the situated cognition approach involves a new consideration of the environmental aspect in theories of cognition.

The methodologies used in situated cognition research have some similarities with those used in information processing psychology research, in the sense of consisting of 'thick' descriptions. However, since proponents consider any thinking to occur in a situation, they record not only verbal data, but also the actions and the tasks subjects perform. Methods have been developed to record and analyse videotapes that capture the situated character of reasoning and thinking.

Video-coding and analysis

Videotaping and videoanalysis software (e.g. Roschelle and Goodman, 1991; Roschelle and

Sibley, 1992) are essential methodological tools in the situated perspective (Greeno, 1989; Jordan and Henderson, 1995), but have also been extensively used within other cognitive approaches (e.g. Frederiksen *et al.*, 1992). The selection of such tools is in keeping with the emphasis on analysing the context of action as part of the subject/environment, where reasoning is treated as a relation between persons and the environment where they act. In fact, the method allows a better characterization of cognitive processing by providing extra nonverbal information, such as gestures, movements and gazes, which complements the information obtained from the subjects' verbal protocols. In this way, video data (e.g. behavioural data from the subject, the environmental situation, visible aspect of the task) can be used to support hypotheses made from verbal data or can suggest new hypotheses. Furthermore, video data are helpful in analysing tasks designed to externalize subjects' thought processes. In such tasks, both verbalizations and physical actions (e.g. pointing, gazing) can be analysed in a more complete fashion. Methods of analysis often involve the classification of streams of behaviour into a coding scheme that is developed beforehand, based typically on a theoretical understanding of the phenomenon under consideration (e.g. Frederiksen *et al.*, 1992).

Methods for the study of group reasoning in naturalistic environments

Reasoning in naturalistic settings, such as organizations and institutions, is an increasingly important topic of research (Patel *et al.*, 1996). The transition from studying individual subjects in controlled experimental situations to investigations of group interaction in naturalistic environments requires an expanded methodological framework that captures cognition and action in complex settings. These settings are characterized (Orasanu and Connoly, 1993) as dynamic and ill-structured, where ambiguous and incomplete information is the rule and where unpredictable changes may occur resulting in high stress and sometimes high risk situations. Finally, they most often involve multiple players, where decisions are distributed over a set of co-operating individuals who try to coordinate their activities. In such settings, verbal protocols must be complemented by other techniques of data collection, such as video recording or note-taking, other materials (e.g. patient charts and records) and interviews

(e.g. with the hospital staff), in order to capture the whole event that is occurring.

Summary of qualitative methods

The last 20 years of research in clinical reasoning have seen an explosion of approaches for the study of cognition. Methodologically, it has meant a multiplication of methods and techniques, with a somewhat beneficial effect on research. More topics in and related to clinical reasoning have been investigated in this period than ever before. A large arsenal of methodologies suitable for the study of clinical reasoning has accumulated, from constrained experimental studies of perceptual aspects of reasoning, to the study of cognitive operations, to the investigations of shared understandings in social situations. On the other hand, this multiplicity should also be a stimulus for reflecting on what has been accomplished and where the field is moving, as well as for gathering a taxonomy of findings and a summary evaluation of the various theories and hypotheses developed to account for those findings.

Still unsolved issues

In their 1990 article reviewing the progress of the field of medical cognition, Elstein *et al.* foresaw several orientations that could be taken by the study of clinical reasoning in the health sciences. Despite their earlier optimism regarding the unification of the decision-making and the information-processing approaches (see also Berner, 1984; Elstein *et al.*, 1978), the field has moved in different directions and has branched into several somewhat disconnected approaches. This has, in turn, generated a multiplicity of methodologies ranging from the more traditional psychometric-based methods still in much use to the newer developments such as the phenomenological approach (Ramsden *et al.*, 1989), the interpretive approach (Benner, 1984), the naturalistic approach, as well as research based on experimental psychology (Norman *et al.*, 1989a,b). This methodological pluralism is healthy as long as it is accompanied by the development of a theory of expertise, of which a theory of reasoning would be a major component. Pluralism brings also a needed awareness of what the methods are designed for, what questions they should answer and what their limitations are.

Among the issues that remain to be solved is clarification of the goal that a particular methodological approach is supposed to accomplish. It is common to criticize an investigation for failing to give answers that are relevant to that study. An objection frequently made about qualitative research concerns the generalizability of its research results. However, this criticism misses the point of qualitative research, which uses either a single or a few subjects. Such research has as its goal a detailed description of a series of phenomena. Most research using qualitative methods attempts this in one way or other. Whereas some attempt only a description of a phenomenon, others go further by trying to develop more or less formal representations of the structures and processes involved. The basic idea behind these research studies, however, is to provide evidence for the existence of the phenomenon in question, not to determine its generality. This should, in turn, help develop theories which include what Simon (1990) has called 'laws of qualitative structure'.

Questions about generalizability of results can be meaningfully asked of studies that are based on statistical comparisons, because they invariably are designed to answer such questions. The interest in carrying out such studies is not in determining whether or not a phenomenon exists but how general it is. They are unsuitable for answering questions regarding the mechanisms underlying performance.

A second issue concerns the external validity of the research. Some critics argue that the artificiality of research conditions places serious doubts on the quality of research studies. This artificiality would severely distort what actually happens in real-life situations, enough to make this kind of research meaningless. However, maybe because of the extreme empiricist biases of many behavioural scientists, these critics fail to see the point of artificiality. The claim is that it is the results of an experiment that should be judged as valid or invalid. But conducting research in artificial environments implies a different view of what is valid or not. It is not the results of the study *per se*, but the theoretical conclusions that are logically tied to such results. Let us present an example. In a study carried out by Coughlin (1985; see also Vicente and Wang, 1998) in which a clinical text describing a patient was presented with the sentences scrambled, it was found that expert physicians were able to reorganize the text in a way that novices were unable to do. Of course, this study could be criticized for failing to approximate the conditions

where expert physicians work; after all, they are unlikely to read patient reports in which the information has been scrambled. But criticizing the study for this reason would totally miss the point of the study. The conclusion of this study was not that expert physicians were better at unscrambling clinical cases, but rather that their memory for clinical information was organized differently from that of novices. Only this theoretical conclusion can be meaningfully made.

The major goal of science is to generate laws that account for the phenomena under consideration. Some researchers believe that laws of behaviour and cognition are impossible to achieve; others, that these laws are not universal as in the case of the mature sciences (Simon, 1990). Others hold the belief that it is by inductive generalizations that laws are obtained. Empirical generalizations, if strongly confirmed, then become laws of the discipline. Although there is some truth to the last position, most laws in the hard sciences are much more than empirical generalizations. They are theoretical propositions that possess referential universality and that have no counterpart in empirical terms. That is, they explain, but are not, empirical regularities themselves. Rather, they refer to the unobservable underlying processes that produce the empirical regularities. The solution is to acknowledge that science admits several kinds of laws. We mentioned the laws of qualitative structure (Simon, 1990), which can be uncovered by proposing models and then testing them by comparing them with human performance. The advantage of laws of this kind is that they not only describe a phenomenon, but also account for it.

Different methodologies serve different purposes. Early research on reasoning was too monolithic, giving primacy to the standard methods typically studied in research design courses. As research becomes more sophisticated, new methods and techniques become increasingly used and new approaches to research tried out. To be effective, methodological pluralism needs to be accompanied by a real effort in developing rigorous theories of reasoning. Theorizing about such a complex field of clinical reasoning is a challenging task, but one that cannot be postponed.

Conclusion: a look at the future

Despite promises of unification, the study of clinical reasoning has branched into diverse methodological and substantial areas. This diversity has been welcomed to the extent that it has encouraged investigators to study reasoning more freely. It has also obviously resulted in some lack of communication among researchers involved in different research programs. There is, however, the hope of providing some unification to the field, as witnessed by attempts outside the area of clinical reasoning (Clancey, 1997; Greeno, 1998; Patel *et al.*, 1995). This unification involves a plethora of methodologies, each serving the purpose of investigating all aspects of cognition, including mental heuristics, knowledge generation and utilization, the process of discovery and interpretation of evidence, and collaborative reasoning. It is time for clinical reasoning researchers to take steps in this direction. This requires that researchers of clinical reasoning with diverse backgrounds, from artificial intelligence to psychology to education, help promote the development of a unified theory of clinical reasoning and decision making.

Acknowledgements

The updating of this chapter was supported by grants from the Social Sciences and Humanities Research Council of Canada (nos 41095206 and 410951208).

References

Allais, M. and Hagen, O. (1979) *Expected Utility Hypothesis and the Allais Paradox*. Dordrecht: Reidel.

Barr, A. and Feigenbaum, E. A. (1981) *The Handbook of Artificial Intelligence*. Los Altos, CA: Kaufmann.

Barro, A. R. (1973) Survey and evaluation of approaches to physician performance measurement. *Journal of Medical Education*, **48**, 1048–1093.

Benner, P. (1984) *From Novice to Expert: Excellence and Power in Clinical Nursing Practice*. Menlo Park, CA: Addison-Wesley.

Berner, E. (1984) Paradigms and problem solving: A literature review. *Journal of Medical Education*, **59**, 625–633.

Bordage, G. and Zacks, R. (1984) The structure of medical knowledge in memories of medical students and practitioners: Categories and prototypes. *Medical Education*, **18**, 406–416.

Brooks, L. R., Norman, G. R. and Allen, S. W. (1991) The role of similarity in a medical diagnostic task. *Journal of Experimental Psychology: General*, **120**, 278–287.

Bruner, J. S., Goodnow, J. J. and Austin, G. A. (1956) *A Study of Thinking*. New York: Wiley

Bunge, M. (1985) *Philosophy of Social Sciences and Technology (Treatise on Basic Philosophy: Vol. 7)*. Dordrecht: Reidel.

Carroll, J. S. and Johnson, E. S. (1990) *Decision Research*. Newbury Park, CA: Sage.

Chase, W. G. and Simon, H. A. (1973) Perception in chess. *Cognitive Psychology*, **4**, 55–81.

Christensen, C., Elstein, A. S., Bernstein, L. M. and Balla, J. I. (1991) Formal decision support in medical practice and education. *Teaching and Learning in Medicine*, **3**, 62–70.

Clancey, W. J. (1997) *Situated Cognition: On Human Knowledge and Computer Representations*. Cambridge: Cambridge University Press.

Coughlin, L. D. J. (1985) *The Effects of Randomization on the Free Recall of Medical Information by Experts and Novices*. Department of Educational Psychology, McGill University, Montreal, Quebec.

Dawes, R. M. (1988) *Rational Choice in an Uncertain World*. New York: Harcourt Brace Jovanovich.

De Groot, A. D. (1965) *Thought and Choice in Chess*. The Hague: Mouton.

Dreyfus, H. L. and Dreyfus, S. E. (1986) *Mind over Machine: The Power of Human Intuition and Expertise in the Era of the Computer*. New York: Free Press.

Elstein, A. S., Shulman, L. S. and Sprafka, S. A. (1978) *Medical Problem Solving. An Analysis of Clinical Reasoning*. Cambridge, MA: Harvard University Press.

Elstein, A. S., Shulman, L. S. and Sprafka, S. A. (1990) Medical problem solving: A ten year retrospective. *Evaluation and the Health Professions*, **13**, 5–36.

Ericsson, A. and Simon, H. A. (1984) *Protocol Analysis: Verbal Reports as Data*. Cambridge, MA: MIT Press.

Feltovich, P. J., Coulson, R. L., Spiro, R. J. and Dawson-Saunders, B. K. (1992) Knowledge application and transfer for complex tasks in ill-structured domains: Implications for instruction and testing in biomedicine. In *Advanced Models of Cognition for Medical Training and Practice* (D. A. Evans and V. L. Patel, eds), pp. 213–244. NATO ASI. Series F: Computer and Systems Sciences, Vol. 97. Heidelberg: Springer.

Feltovich, P. J., Johnson, P. E., Moller, J. H. and Swanson, D. B. (1984) LCS: The role and development of medical knowledge in diagnostic expertise. In *Readings in Medical Artificial Intelligence: The First Decade* (W. J. Clancey and E. H. Shortliffe, eds), pp. 275–319. Reading, MA: Addison-Wesley.

Fox, J. (1988) Formal and knowledge-based methods in decision technology. In *Professional Judgment: A Reader in Clinical Decision Making* (J. Dowie and A. Elstein, eds), pp. 226–252. Cambridge: Cambridge University Press.

Frederiksen, C. H. (1975) Representing logical and semantic structure of knowledge acquired from discourse. *Cognitive Psychology*, **7**, 371–458.

Frederiksen, J. R., Sipusic, M., Gamoran, M. and Wolfe, E. (1992) *Video Portfolio Assessment: A Study for the National Board for Professional Teaching Standards*. Princeton, NJ: Educational Testing Service.

Glaser, B. and Strauss, A. (1967) *The Discovery of Grounded Theory*. Chicago: Aldine.

Greeno, J. (1989) A perspective on thinking. *American Psychologist*, **44**, 134–141.

Greeno, J. (1998) The situativity of knowing, learning, and research. *American Psychologist*, **53**, 5–26.

Groen, G. J. and Patel, V. L. (1988) The relationship between comprehension and reasoning in medical expertise. In *The Nature of Expertise* (M. Chi, R. Glaser and M. Farr, eds), pp. 287–310. Hillsdale, NJ: Lawrence Erlbaum.

Hammond, J. S. (1967) Better decision with preference theory. *Harvard Business Review*, **45**, 123–141.

Heidegger, M. (1962) *Being and Time* (translated by J. Macquarrie and E. Robinson). New York: Harper & Row.

Hovland, C. I. (1960) Computer simulation of thinking. *American Psychologist*, **15**, 687–693.

Jordan, B. and Henderson, A. (1995) Interaction Analysis: Foundations for practice. *Journal of the Learning Sciences*, **4**, 39–103.

Joseph, G. M. and Patel, V. L. (1990) Domain knowledge and hypothesis generation in diagnostic reasoning. *Medical Decision Making*, **10**, 31–46.

Kassirer, J. P., Kuipers, B. J. and Gorry, G. A. (1982) Toward a theory of clinical expertise. *American Journal of Medicine*, **73**, 251–259.

Kintsch, W. (1974) *The Representation of Meaning in Memory*. Hillsdale, NJ: Lawrence Erlbaum.

Kuipers, B. J. and Kassirer, J. P. (1984) Causal reasoning in medicine: Analysis of a protocol. *Cognitive Science*, **8**, 363–385.

Larkin, J. H., McDermott, J., Simon, H. A. and Simon, D. S. (1980) Expert and novice performance in solving physics problems. *Science*, 208, 1335–1342.

Lesgold, A., Rubinson, H., Feltovich, P., Glaser, R., Klopfer, D. and Wang, Y. (1988) Expertise in a complex skill: Diagnosing X-ray pictures. In *The Nature of Expertise* (M. T. H. Chi, R. Glaser and M. J. Farr, eds), pp. 311–342. Hillsdale, NJ: Lawrence Erlbaum.

Marton, F. and Saljo, R. (1976) Qualitative differences in learning: I. Outcome and process. *British Journal of Educational Psychology*, **46**, 4–11.

McGuire, C. H. (1985) Medical problem solving: A critique of the literature. *Journal of Medical Education*, **60**, 587–595.

Newell, A., Shaw, J. C. and Simon, H. A. (1958) Elements of a theory of human problem solving. *Psychological Review*, **65**, 151–166.

Newell, A. and Simon, H. A. (1972) *Human Problem Solving*. Englewood Cliffs, NJ: Prentice-Hall.

Norman, G., Brooks, L. R. and Allen, S. W. (1989a) Recall by expert medical practitioners and novices as a record of processing attention. *Journal of Experimental Psychology: Learning, Memory, and Cognition*, **15**, 1116–1174.

Norman, G., Brooks, L. R., Rosenthal, D., Allen, S. W. and Muzzin, L. J. (1989b) The development of expertise in dermatology. *Archives of Dermatology*, 125, 1063–1068.

Orasanu, J. and Connoly, T. (1993) The reinvention of decision making. In *Decision Making in Action: Models and Methods* (G. A. Klein, J. Orasanu, R. Calderwood and C. E. Zsambok, eds), pp. 3–20. Norwood, NJ: Ablex.

Patel, V. L. and Frederiksen, C. H. (1984) Cognitive processes in comprehension and knowledge acquisition by medical students and physicians. In *Tutorials in Problem-Based Learning* (H. G. Schmidt and M. L. De Volder, eds), pp. 143–157. Assen: van Gorcum.

Patel, V. L. and Groen, G. J. (1986) Knowledge-based solution strategies in medical reasoning. *Cognitive Science*, **10**, 91–116.

Patel, V. L., Groen, G. J. and Arocha, J. F. (1990) Medical expertise as a function of task difficulty. *Memory and Cognition*, **18**, 394–406.

Patel, V. L., Kaufman, D. R. and Arocha, J. F. (1995) Steering through the murky waters of a scientific conflict: Situated and symbolic models of clinical cognition. *Artificial Intelligence in Medicine*, **7**, 413–438.

Patel, V. L. Kaufman, D. R. and Magder, S. A. (1996) The acquisition of medical expertise in complex dynamic environments. In *The Road to Excellence: The Acquisition of Expert Performance in the Arts and Sciences, Sports and Games* (K. A. Ericsson ed.), pp. 127–165. Hillsdale, NJ: Lawrence Erlbaum.

Piaget, J. (1950) *The Psychology of Intelligence* (Translated by M. Piercy and E. Berlyne). London: Routledge & Kegan Paul.

Ramsden, P., Whelan, G. and Cooper, D. (1989) Some phenomena of medical students' diagnostic problem solving. *Medical Education*, **23**, 108–117.

Rimoldi, H. J. A. (1961) The test of diagnostic skills. *Journal of Medical Education*, **36**, 73–79.

Rosch, E. (1978) Principles of categorization. In *Cognition and Categorization* (E. Rosch and B. B. Lloyd, eds), pp. 27–48. Hillsdale, NJ: Lawrence Erlbaum.

Roschelle, J. and Goldman, S. (1991) Videonoter: A productivity tool for video data analysis. *Behavior, Research Methods, Instruments and Computers*, **23**, 219–224.

Roschelle, J. and Sibley, J. W. (1992) *Video User Guide* (Computer Program). San Francisco, CA: Envisionology.

Schmidt, H., Boshuizen, H. P. A. and Hobus, P. P. M. (1988) Transitory stages in the development of medical expertise: The 'intermediate effect' in clinical case representation studies. In *Proceedings of the 10th Annual Conference of the Cognitive Science Society* (V. L. Patel and G. J. Groen, eds), pp. 139–145. Hillsdale, NJ: Lawrence Erlbaum.

Schmidt, H. G. and Boshuizen, H. P. (1993) On the origin of intermediate effects in clinical case recall. *Memory and Cognition*, **21**, 338–351.

Simon, H. A. (1990) Invariants of human behavior. *Annual Review of Psychology*, **41**, 1–19.

Sowa, J. F. (1984) *Conceptual Structures: Information Processes in Mind and Machine*. Reading, MA: Addison-Wesley.

Suchman, L. (1987) *Plans and Situated Action: The Problem of Human/Machine Communication*. Cambridge, MA: Cambridge University Press.

Taylor, C. (1971) Interpretation and the sciences of man. *Review of Metaphysics*, **25**, 3–51.

Tversky, A. and Kahneman, D. (1974) Judgment under uncertainty: Heuristics and biases. *Science*, **185**, 1124–1131.

Vicente, K. J. and Wang, J. H. (1998) An ecological theory of expertise effects in memory recall. *Psychological Review*, **105**, 33–57.

von Neumann, J. and Morgenstern, O. (1944) *Theory of Games and Economic Behavior*. Princeton: Princeton University Press.

Vu, N. V. (1979) Medical problem solving assessment: A review of methods and instruments. *Evaluation and the Health Professions*, **2**, 281–307.

Watson, J. B. (1920) Is thinking merely the action of language mechanisms? *British Journal of Psychology*, **11**, 87–104.

Weinstein, M. C., Fineberg, H. V., Elstein, A. S., Frazier, H. S., Neuhauser, D., Neutra, R. R. and McNeil, B. J. (1980) *Clinical Decision Analysis*. Philadelphia, PA: Saunders.

White, P. (1988) Knowing more about what we can tell: 'Introspective access' and causal report accuracy 10 years later. *British Journal of Psychology*, **79**, 13–45.

Winograd, T. (1972) Understanding natural language. *Cognitive Psychology*, **3**, 1–191.

Section Two

Clinical reasoning in the health professions

10

Clinical reasoning in medicine

Arthur S. Elstein and Alan Schwartz

How do physicians solve diagnostic problems? What is known about the process of diagnostic clinical reasoning? This chapter sketches our current understanding of answers to these questions by reviewing the cognitive processes involved in diagnostic reasoning in clinical medicine. We describe and analyze the psychological processes and mental structures employed in identifying and solving diagnostic problems of varying degrees of complexity and review common errors and pitfalls in diagnostic reasoning. We will not consider the parallel sets of issues in selecting a treatment or developing a management plan. For theoretical background, we draw upon two approaches that have been particularly influential in research in this field: (a) problem solving, exemplified in the work of Newell and Simon (1972), Elstein *et al.* (1978), and Bordage and his colleagues (Bordage and Lemieux, 1991; Bordage and Zacks, 1984; Friedman *et al.*, 1998; Lemieux and Bordage, 1992), and (b) decision making, illustrated in the work of Kahneman *et al.* (1982), Baron (1988) and the research reviewed by Mellers *et al.* (1998).

Problem-solving research has usually focused on how an ill-structured problem situation is defined and structured (as by generating a set of diagnostic hypotheses). Psychological decision research has typically looked at factors affecting diagnosis or treatment choice in well-defined, tightly controlled problems. A common theme in both approaches is that human rationality is limited. Nevertheless, the problem-solving paradigm has concentrated on identifying the strategies of experts in a field, with the aim of facilitating the acquisition of these strategies by learners. It thus focuses on the wisdom of practice. Research in this tradition emphasizes how experts generally function effectively despite limits on their rational capacities which may cause some mistakes. Behavioural decision research, on the other hand, contrasts human performance with a normative statistical model of reasoning under uncertainty. It emphasizes errors in reasoning about uncertainty, typically demonstrating that even experts in a domain are not immune from these errors, and thus raising the case for some type of decision support.

Problem solving: diagnosis as hypothesis selection

To solve a clinical diagnostic problem means first to recognize a malfunction and then to set about tracing or identifying its causes. The diagnosis is thus an explanation of disordered function, where possible a causal explanation.

In most cases, not all of the information needed to identify and explain the situation is available in the early stages of the clinical encounter. Physicians must decide what information to collect, what aspects of the situation need attention, and what can be safely set aside. Thus, data collection is both sequential and selective. Experienced physicians often go about this task almost automatically, sometimes very rapidly; novices struggle to develop a plan. But both approach a problem by collecting detailed information and drawing inferences about the underlying causes from these observations.

The hypothetico-deductive method

Early hypothesis generation and selective data collection

Elstein *et al.* (1978) found that diagnostic problems are solved by a process of generating a limited number of hypotheses or problem formulations early in the workup and using them to guide subsequent data collection. Each hypothesis can be used to predict what additional findings ought to be present if it were true and then the workup is a guided search for these findings; hence, the method is hypothetico-deductive. The process of problem structuring via hypothesis generation begins with a very limited data set and occurs rapidly and automatically, even if clinicians are explicitly instructed not to generate hypotheses. Given the complexity of the clinical situation, the enormous amount of data that could potentially be obtained and the limited capacity of working memory, hypothesis generation is a psychological necessity. It transforms an unstructured problem into a structured problem by generating a small set of possible solutions; this is a very efficient way to solve diagnostic problems. Novices and experienced physicians alike attempt to generate hypotheses to explain clusters of findings, although the content of the experienced group's productions is of higher quality.

Other clinical researchers have concurred with this view (Kassirer and Gorry, 1978; Kuipers and Kassirer, 1984; Pople, 1982). It has also been favored by medical educators (e.g. Barrows and Pickell, 1991; Kassirer and Kopelman, 1991), while researchers in cognitive psychology have been more sceptical. We will examine these conflicting interpretations later.

Data collection and interpretation

Next, the data obtained must be interpreted in the light of the hypotheses being considered. How much should previous diagnostic opinions or hunches be revised? To what extent do the data strengthen or weaken belief in the correctness of a particular diagnostic hypothesis?

Accuracy of data interpretation and thoroughness of data collection are separate issues. A clinician could collect data quite thoroughly but could nevertheless ignore, misunderstand or misinterpret a significant fraction. In contrast, a clinician might be overly economical in data collection but could interpret whatever is available quite accurately. Elstein *et al.* (1978) found no statistically significant association between thoroughness of data collection and accuracy of data interpretation. This was an important finding for two reasons:

(a) *Increased emphasis upon interpretation of data.* It is possible to study clinical reasoning either by allowing physicians to collect their own database or by controlling the content of the case and examining differences in interpretation. Most early research allowed subjects to select items from a large array or menu of items. This approach, exemplified in Patient Management Problems (Feightner, 1985), facilitated investigation of the amount and sequence of data collection but offered less insight into data interpretation and problem formulation. The use of standardized patients (SPs) (Swanson *et al.*, 1995; van der Vleuten and Swanson, 1990) offers researchers considerable latitude in how much to focus the investigation (or student assessment) on data collection or on hypothesis generation and testing. To deepen understanding of reasoning processes, investigators in the problem-solving tradition have asked subjects to think aloud while problem solving and have then analysed their verbalizations as well as their data collection (Barrows *et al.*, 1982; Elstein *et al.*, 1978; Friedman *et al*, 1998; Joseph and Patel, 1990; Neufeld *et al.*, 1981; Patel and Groen, 1986). Considerable variability in acquiring and interpreting data has been found, increasing the complexity of the research task. One way to minimize this variability is to control the data base. Consequently, some researchers switched to controlling what data were presented to subjects in order to concentrate on data interpretation and problem formulation (e.g. Feltovich *et al.*, 1984; Kuipers *et al.*, 1988). This shift led naturally to the second major change in research tactics.

(b) *Study of clinical judgement separated from data collection.* Controlling the database facilitates analysis at the price of fidelity to clinical realities. This strategy is the most widely used in current research on clinical reasoning, the shift reflecting the influence of the paradigm of decision making research. Sometimes clinical information is presented sequentially to a subject, so that the case unfolds in a simulation of real time, but the subject is given few or no options in data collection (Chapman *et al.*, 1996). The analysis can focus on memory organization, knowledge utilization, data interpretation, or problem representation (e.g. Bordage and Lemieux, 1991; Joseph and Patel, 1990; Moskowitz *et al.*, 1988). In other studies, clinicians are given all the data at once and asked to make a diagnostic or treatment decision (Patel and Groen, 1986; Elstein *et al.*, 1992).

Emphasizing problem representation and diagnosis reflects the assumption that once a diagnosis is correctly made, treatment planning follows almost automatically. Matters are actually more complex. The management of common conditions varies for many reasons, including perhaps disagreements about the balance of risks and benefits of plausible strategies. Practice guidelines have been developed in response to the widely replicated finding of practice variation. The recent literature accepts practice variation as a given and concentrates on identifying and remedying barriers to physicians' adopting and using practice guidelines (Inouye *et al.*, 1998; James *et al.*, 1997).

Case specificity

Problem solving expertise varies greatly across cases and is highly dependent on the clinician's mastery of the particular domain. Differences between clinicians are to be found more in their understanding of the problem and their problem representations than in the reasoning strategies employed (Elstein *et al.*, 1978). Thus it makes more sense to talk about reasons for success and failure in a particular case than about generic traits or strategies of expert diagnosticians.

For the community of evaluators in medical and other fields of health professional education, this information raises the practical problem of how many case simulations would be needed in a case-based examination for a reliable and valid assessment of a student's problem solving skill. Test developers are now much more concerned about the number and content of clinical simulations in an examination than they were prior to this discovery (e.g. Page *et al.*, 1990). (For discussion of psychometric properties of clinical simulations, see van der Vleuten and Swanson, 1990.)

Diagnosis as categorization or pattern recognition

The finding of case specificity also challenged the hypothetico-deductive model as an adequate account of the process of clinical reasoning. Both successful and unsuccessful diagnosticians employed a hypothesis-testing strategy. Diagnostic accuracy depended more on mastery of the content in a domain than on the strategy employed. So, by the mid-1980s, the view of diagnostic reasoning as complex and systematic generation and testing of hypotheses was being criticized. Patel, Norman and their associates (e.g. Brooks *et al.*, 1991; Eva *et al.*, 1998; Groen and Patel, 1985; Schmidt *et al.*, 1990) pointed out that the clinical reasoning of experts in familiar situations frequently does not display explicit hypothesis testing. It is rapid, automatic, and often non-verbal. The speed, efficiency and accuracy of experienced physicians suggested that they might not even use the same reasoning processes as novices, and that experience itself might make hypothesis-testing unnecessary. Not all cases seen by an experienced physician appear to require hypothetico-deductive reasoning (Davidoff, 1998). Once a physician has seen a case of chicken pox, it is a relatively simple matter to diagnose the next case by recalling the characteristic appearance of the rash.

For experienced physicians, much of daily practice consists of seeing new cases that strongly resemble patients previously seen. For this reason, expert reasoning in non-problematic situations looks more like pattern recognition or direct automatic retrieval from a well-structured network of stored knowledge (Groen and Patel, 1985). Even the use of the hypothetico-deductive method could be plausibly affected by previous experience: since experienced clinicians have a better sense of clinical realities and therefore of the likely diagnostic possibilities, they can more efficiently generate an early set of plausible hypotheses so as to avoid fruitless and expensive pursuit of unlikely diagnoses. These arguments, and the evidence supporting them, suggested that experts use pattern recognition or direct retrieval of needed strategies from a well-organized network of stored information and knowledge as much as or more than hypothesis testing. The research emphasis shifted from the problem-solving process to the organization of knowledge in the long-term memory of experienced clinicians (Norman, 1988).

Categorization of a new case can be based either on retrieval of and matching to specific instances (instance-based or exemplar-based recognition) or on a more abstract prototype. In instance-based recognition, a new instance is classified by resemblance to memory of a past case (Brooks *et al.*, 1991; Medin and Schaffer, 1978; Norman *et al*,

1992; Schmidt *et al.*, 1990). This model is supported by the fact that clinical diagnosis is strongly affected by the context of events (e.g. the location of a skin rash on the body), even when this context is normatively irrelevant. These context effects suggest that clinicians are matching a new case to a previous case, not to an abstraction from several cases, since an abstraction should not include irrelevant features. Expert–novice differences are mainly explicable in terms of the size of the knowledge store of prior instances available for pattern recognition. This theory of clinical reasoning has been developed with particular reference to pathology, dermatology and radiology, all medical specialties where the clinical data are predominantly visual and where verbal or quantitative representation of knowledge is less than in, say, internal medicine, nephrology or endocrinology.

The prototype model (and its variants) holds that clinical experience facilitates the construction of abstractions or prototypes (Bordage and Zacks, 1984; Rosch and Mervis, 1975). Differences between stronger and weaker diagnosticians are explicable mainly in terms of variation in the content and complexity of their prototypes. Better diagnosticians have constructed more diversified and abstract sets of semantic relations, ways of representing the links between clinical features or aspects of the problem (Bordage and Lemieux, 1991; Lemieux and Bordage, 1992). Support for this view of knowledge organization is found in the fact that experts in a domain are more able to relate findings to each other and to potential diagnoses, and to identify what additional findings are needed to complete a picture (Elstein *et al.*, 1993). These capabilities suggest that experts are working with more abstract representations and are not simply trying to match a new case to a previous instance, although that matching process may occur with simple cases.

Norman *et al.* (1994) found that experienced physicians use a hypothetico-deductive strategy with difficult cases only, a view supported by Davidoff (1998). When a case is perceived to be simple or not very challenging, quicker and easier methods are used, such as pattern recognition or feature matching. Thus, controversy about the methods used in diagnostic reasoning can be resolved by realizing that the method selected depends upon the perceived characteristics of the problem. There is an interaction between the clinician's level of skill and the perceived difficulty of the task (Elstein, 1994). Easy cases are solved by pattern recognition and going directly

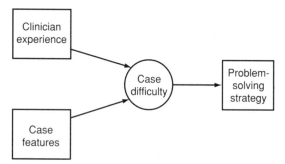

Figure 10.1 Factors affecting problem-solving strategy. Clinician exprience and case features interact to determine case difficulty. Difficulty determines choice of hypothesis testing or pattern recognition strategies

from data to diagnostic classification [what Groen and Patel (1985) call forward reasoning]. Difficult cases need systematic hypothesis generation and testing. Whether a problem is easy or difficult depends in part on the knowledge and experience of the clinician who is trying to solve it (see Figure 10.1).

Errors in hypothesis generation and restructuring

Clinical reasoning can proceed either by pattern recognition or by hypothesis testing. Neither is an error-proof strategy, nor are they always consistent with statistical rules of inference with imperfect information. Errors that can occur in difficult cases in internal medicine are illustrated and discussed by Kassirer and Kopelman (1991). The frequency of errors in actual practice is unknown, but considering a number of studies as a whole, an error rate of 15% might be a good first approximation.

Looking at an instance of diagnostic reasoning retrospectively, it is easy to see that a clinician could err either by oversimplifying a complex problem or by taking a problem that could appropriately have been dealt with routinely and using the much more effortful strategy of multiple competing hypotheses. It has been far more difficult for researchers and teachers of diagnostic reasoning to prescribe the appropriate strategy in advance. Because so much depends on the interaction between case and clinician, prescriptive guidelines for the proper amount of hypothesis generation and testing are still unavailable for the student clinician. Perhaps the most useful advice is to emulate the hypothesis-testing strategy used by experienced clinicians when they are having difficulty, since novices will experience as problematic many situations that the former solve by routine pattern-recognition methods. Gathering more data without having hypotheses in mind is less likely to pay off. Occasionally these searches are successful, but more often than not they waste money and time with little return. In an era that emphasizes cost-effective clinical practice, gathering data unrelated to diagnostic hypotheses will be discouraged.

Many diagnostic problems are so complex that the correct solution is not contained within the initial set of hypotheses. Restructuring and reformulating must occur through time as data are obtained and the clinical picture evolves. However, as any problem solver works with a particular set of hypotheses, psychological commitment takes place and it becomes more difficult to restructure the problem (Janis and Mann, 1977). Ideally, one might want to work purely inductively, reasoning only from the facts, but this strategy is never employed because it is inefficient and produces high levels of cognitive strain (Elstein *et al.*, 1978). A purely inductive approach to clinical reasoning would be inefficient in two ways. (a) Early findings could lead to a long list of preliminary hypotheses. The problem space would become steadily larger as new clusters of data are obtained, rather than becoming better structured. (b) Exhaustive data collection would be required until enough evidence had been obtained to point conclusively to one candidate. It is much easier to solve a problem where some boundaries and hypotheses provide the needed framework. On the other hand, early problem formulation may also bias the clinician's thinking (Barrows *et al.*, 1982; Voytovich *et al.*, 1985). Errors in interpreting the diagnostic value of clinical information have been found by several research teams (Elstein *et al.*, 1978, Friedman *et al.*, 1998; Gruppen *et al.*, 1991; Wolf *et al.*, 1985).

Decision making: diagnosis as opinion revision

Bayes' theorem

In the literature on medical decision making, reaching a diagnosis is conceptualized as a process of reasoning about uncertainty, updating an opinion with imperfect information (the clinical evidence). As new information is obtained, the probability of each diagnostic possibility is continuously revised. Each post-test probability becomes the pre-test probability for the next stage of the inference process. Bayes' theorem, the formal mathematical rule for this operation (Sox *et al.*, 1988; Weinstein *et al.*, 1980), states that in taking new diagnostic information into account, the post-test probability is a function of two variables, pre-test probability and the strength of the evidence. The pre-test probability can be either the known prevalence of the disease or the clinician's belief about the probability of disease before new information is acquired. The strength of the evidence is measured by a 'likelihood ratio', the ratio of the probabilities of observing a particular finding in patients with and without the disease of interest. This framework directs attention to two major classes of errors in clinical reasoning: in a clinician's beliefs about pre-test probability or in assessing the strength of the evidence. Bayes' theorem is a normative rule for diagnostic reasoning; it tells us how we should reason, but it does not claim that we actually revise our opinions in this way. Indeed, from the Bayesian viewpoint, the psychological study of diagnostic reasoning centres on errors in both components.

Errors in probability estimation

Availability

People are prone to overestimate the frequency of vivid or easily recalled events and to underestimate the frequency of events that are either very ordinary or difficult to recall (Tversky and Kahneman, 1981). Diseases or injuries which receive considerable media attention (e.g. injuries due to shark attacks) are often considered more probable than their true prevalence. This psychological principle is exemplified clinically in overemphasizing rare conditions. Unusual cases are more memorable than routine problems (Nisbett *et al.*, 1982).

Representativeness

People overestimate the frequency of events that fit their ideas of a prototypical or representative case (Tversky and Kahneman, 1974). When this heuristic comes into play, the probability of a disease given a finding can be confused with the probability of a finding given the disease (Eddy, 1982).

Probability distortions

Small probabilities tend to be overestimated and large probabilities tend to be underestimated (Tversky and Kahneman, 1981). This results in strange discontinuities when probabilities are very close to 0 or 1. Cumulative prospect theory (Tversky and Kahneman, 1992) and similar rank- and sign-dependent utility theories provide formal descriptions of how people distort probabilities in risky decision making. The distortions are exacerbated when the probabilities are vague and not precisely known (Einhorn and Hogarth, 1986).

Support theory

Many of the biases in probability estimation are captured by support theory (Redelmeier *et al.*, 1995; Rottenstreich and Tversky, 1997; Tversky and Koehler, 1994), which posits that subjective estimates of the frequency or probability of an event are influenced by how detailed the description is. More explicit descriptions yield higher probability estimates than do compact, condensed descriptions, even when the two would refer to exactly the same events (such as 'probability of death due to a car accident, train accident, plane accident, or other moving vehicle accident' versus 'probability of death due to a moving vehicle accident'). This theory can explain availability (when memories of an available event include more detailed descriptions than those of less available events) and representativeness (when a typical case description includes a cluster of details that 'fit' while a less typical case lacks some of these features).

Errors in probability revision

Conservatism

In clinical case discussions, data are commonly presented sequentially. In this circumstance, people often fail to revise their diagnostic probabilities as much as is implied by Bayes' theorem. This 'stickiness' has been called 'conservatism' and was one of the earliest cognitive biases identified (Edwards, 1968).

Anchoring and adjustment

One explanation of conservatism is that people revise their diagnostic opinion up or down from an initial anchor, which is either given in the problem or subjectively formed. Anchoring and adjustment mean that final opinions are sensitive to the starting point (the 'anchor') and that the revision up or down from this anchor is typically insufficient (the 'adjustment'), so the final judgement is closer to the initial anchor than would be implied by Bayes' theorem (Tversky and Kahneman, 1974).

Confounding probability and value of an outcome

It is difficult for everyday judgement to keep separate accounts of the probability of a particular disease and the benefits that accrue from detecting it. Probability revision errors that are systematically linked to the perceived cost of mistakes demonstrate the difficulties experienced in separating assessments of probability from values (Poses *et al.*, 1985; Wallsten, 1981).

Acquiring redundant evidence

In collecting data, there is a tendency to seek information that confirms a hypothesis rather than data that facilitate efficient testing of competing hypotheses. This tendency has been called 'pseudodiagnosticity' (Kern and Doherty, 1982) or 'confirmation bias' (Wolf *et al.*, 1985).

Incorrect interpretation

The most common error in interpreting findings is over-interpretation: data which should not support a particular hypothesis, and which might even suggest that a new alternative be considered, are interpreted as consistent with hypotheses already under consideration (Elstein *et al.*, 1978; Friedman *et al.*, 1998). The data best remembered tend to be those that support the hypotheses generated. Where findings are distorted in recall, it is generally in the direction of making the facts more consistent with typical clinical pictures. Positive findings are overemphasized and negative findings tend to be discounted (Elstein *et al.*, 1978; Wason and Johnson-Laird, 1972). From a Bayesian standpoint, these are all errors in assessing the diagnostic value of information, i.e. errors in subjective assessments of the likelihood ratio. The principle of bounded rationality helps us understand the adaptive function of these errors: (a) a problem must be structured, so hypotheses are required, and (b) the representation must be simpler than the problem; generating more hypotheses would make matters more complex and require more information processing. In general, efforts are continually made to keep matters simple and within the capacity of working memory. Even when clinicians agree on the presence of certain clinical findings, wide variations have been found in the weights assigned to these findings in the course of interpreting their meaning (Bryant and Norman, 1980; Wigton *et al.*, 1986).

Base-rate neglect

The basic principle of Bayesian inference is that a posterior probability is a function of two variables, the prior probability and the strength of the evidence. Research has shown that unless trained to use Bayes' theorem and to recognize when it is appropriate, physicians are just as prone to misusing or neglecting base rates in diagnostic inference as anyone else (Elstein, 1988).

Order effects

Bayes' theorem implies that clinicians given identical information should reach the same diagnostic opinion, regardless of the order in which information is presented. Order effects mean that final opinions are also affected by the order of presentation of information. The information presented late in a case is given more weight than information presented earlier (Bergus *et al.*, 1995; Chapman *et al.*, 1996).

Educational implications

What can be done to help learners acquire expertise in clinical reasoning? Each of these approaches offers some direction.

Problem solving: Educational implications

Consider first the hypothetico-deductive model. Even if experts in non-problematic situations do not routinely generate and test hypotheses and instead retrieve a solution (diagnosis) directly from their structured knowledge, they clearly do generate and evaluate alternatives when confronted with problematic situations. For novices, most situations will initially be problems, not solvable by routine methods, and generating a small set of hypotheses is a useful procedural guideline. Second, since much expert hypothesis-generation and testing is implicit, a model that explicitly calls it to

the novice's attention will aid learning. Thirdly, the hypothetico-deductive model directs the learner's attention toward forming a conception of the problem and using this plan to guide the workup. This plan will include a set of competing diagnoses and the semantic relationships that make it possible to order the diagnostic candidates as similar and different. This plan will make it possible to reduce unnecessary and expensive laboratory testing, a welcome emphasis in an era that stresses cost containment.

The instance-based model implies that clinical experience is needed in contexts closely related to future practice, because transfer from one context to another is limited. The implicit message is that expertise is complex, and is acquired with time and practice in the relevant context. In one way, this model reinforces a very traditional doctrine in medical education: practical arts are learned by supervised practice and rehearsal combined with progressively increasing professional responsibility, supplemented by instruction in case conferences, clinical rounds, reading and the like. In another way, it conflicts with traditional training, since the model argues that trainees will not generalize as much from one context (say, hospitalized patients) to another (say, ambulatory patients) as has traditionally been thought.

The prototype position offers a more optimistic view of the instructional potential of cognitive science approaches, since it implies that clinical experience is necessary but needs to be reviewed and analysed so that the correct general models and principles are abstracted from the experience. Although the desired level of elaboration and structure generally develops, one ought not to count upon its spontaneous occurrence. Well-designed educational experiences can facilitate the development of the desired cognitive structures. Given the emerging consensus about characteristics distinguishing experts from novices, an effective route to the goal would be extensive focused practice and feedback with a variety of problems. (Bordage, 1987; Lemieux and Bordage, 1992). Similarly, Rabinowitz and Glaser (1985) proposed that an adequate understanding of the expert's knowledge structure would lead to more effective instruction to assist novices in acquiring that structure.

The emphasis in internal medicine training on formally constructing and analysing a set of diagnostic alternatives, called the differential diagnosis, is a useful heuristic strategy, rather than one that guarantees success, because instructions to develop a differential diagnosis generally omit clearly defined rules stating the best alternatives for a given situation or even how many alternatives should be in the differential list. Everyday clinical reasoning would insist that such rules are too rigid and that some artistry is needed. Room should be left for common sense, intuition and flexibility. Thus, the strategy of working through a differential diagnosis can prevent premature closure on a single salient alternative, but it cannot guarantee that the correct diagnostic alternative is included on the list. The longer and more exhaustive the list, the more likely it is to include the correct diagnosis, but the workup will become correspondingly more inefficient, expensive and time-consuming.

Decision making: Educational implications

If expert clinicians are not consistent in their approach across cases, what formal generalizable logic or operations can or should be taught to learners? In this section, we review some recent efforts to teach the logic of clinical decision making that have been strongly influenced by decision theoretic principles and research results.

Evidence-based medicine

Until recently, medical educators paid little attention to formal quantitative methods for dealing with these problems. It was implicitly assumed that the problems would become insignificant as clinical experience was acquired. Criticisms of clinical practice and efforts at controlling costs have both led to the rise of evidence-based medicine (EBM), an approach to clinical education and practice which reflects growing interest in applying formal quantitative methods to diagnosis and treatment choice (Evidence-based Medicine Working Group, 1992; Sackett *et al.*, 1997). EBM emphasizes using the clinical literature to find answers to questions arising in clinical practice. The approach involves formulating a well-structured clinical question focused on such matters as the diagnostic value of a particular test or the expected outcomes of alternative treatments for well-defined conditions. Answers to these questions are sought in the medical literature. Individual studies are rigorously evaluated to determine how well the study responds to the clinical question that prompted the inquiry. This assessment considers soundness of research design, whether the findings apply to the patient of concern, trustworthiness of the conclusions, and limitations of the evidence. For integrating the

results of diverse studies into a treatment recommendation or overall judgement of effectiveness of various treatments, EBM strongly prefers meta-analysis (L'Abbe *et al.*, 1987; Oxman *et al.*, 1994; Rosenthal, 1991), a more structured, quantitative form of literature review, to the traditional narrative review that embodies the subjective judgement of the experts who wrote the review. Meta-analyses have been particularly useful in integrating the results of clinical trials of new therapies because they use statistical measures, such as effect size, that can be combined across several studies to produce an overall estimate of effect. Whether meta-analyses will ultimately replace traditional reviews remains to be seen.

EBM is particularly relevant for the diagnostic inference process discussed in this chapter because it is, in our opinion, currently the most popular vehicle explicitly advocating a Bayesian approach to clinical evidence. Textbooks of EBM (Sackett *et al.*, 1991; Sackett *et al.*, 1997) show how to use prevalence rates and likelihood ratios to calculate posterior probabilities of diagnostic alternatives (predictive value of a positive or negative test). Formal statistical reasoning and decision analysis are likewise explained and advocated in an ever-growing number of works aimed at physicians (Albert *et al.*, 1988; Glass, 1996; Goldman, 1998; Kassirer and Kopelman, 1991; Panzer *et al.*, 1991; Pauker, 1996; Sox *et al.*, 1988; Weinstein *et al.*, 1980). Decision theory, decision analysis, and evidence-based medicine seem to be on their way to becoming standard components of clinical education and training.

Decision support systems

Computer programs that run on microcomputers and can provide decision support have been developed (Applied Informatics, 1990; de Bliek *et al.*, 1988). The role of these programs in medical education and in future clinical practice is still to be determined. Broader use of these programs, at least as instructional tools if not in routine clinical practice, may be anticipated as the cost of microcomputers declines while the machines and programs become steadily more powerful.

Debiasing

A number of researchers have proposed methods for debiasing judgements without resorting to formal methods of probability estimation and revision (Arkes, 1991; Keren, 1990; Mumma and

Wilson, 1995). Debiasing methods include educating judges about common biases, encouraging judges to consider the opposite hypothesis carefully and making judges more accountable for errors. The evidence on the effectiveness of these methods is mixed.

Nomograms

A program that calculates posterior probabilities can be implemented on any microcomputer using a simple spreadsheet. Convenient graphical nomograms have also been developed to simplify the application of Bayes' Theorem. In a Bayesian nomogram, a line drawn from the prior probability through the test's likelihood ratio intersects the posterior probability, thus collapsing the calculation of prior odds, multiplication of likelihood ratio and calculation of posterior probability into a single operation. Fagan (1975) published the best known nomogram, which is widely available on a pocket-sized card. Schwartz (1998) provides an on-line version at http://araw.mede.uic.edu/cgi-bin/testcalc.pl.

Conclusion

Research on the clinical reasoning of physicians has a broad range, including but not limited to differences between expert and novice clinicians, psychological processes in judgement and decision making, non-normative biases in judgement and decision making and factors associated with their production and maintenance, improving instruction and training to enhance acquisition of good reasoning, and the development, evaluation and implementation of decision support systems and guidelines. Many recent studies of physicians' decision making have used statistical decision theory as a standard by which to assess unaided, intuitive clinical decisions. The aims of these studies have included understanding the process of clinical reasoning, improving instructional programs designed for medical students and clinical training, assessing competence at the level of medical licensure and certification, analysing the cognitive processes employed in specific clinical situations, and developing practice guidelines and standards.

Clinicians have been understandably reluctant to share their decision-making authority with impersonal guidelines. Yet the expansion of biomedical knowledge and the growth of technological capability have vastly increased both the range of possible actions for diagnosis and treatment and their associated costs. These forces have led to pressure to control the costs of medical care, and to involve patients and families more meaningfully in decision making. Thus, these forces imply some limitation of professional authority, while simultaneously increasing the scope of professional capability. Research on reasoning in medicine thus stands at the intersection of the interests of psychologists, medical sociologists, health policy planners, economists, patients and clinicians. Given this conjunction, both normative and descriptive studies of clinical reasoning in medicine, as well as studies to find practical methods of improving the level of reasoning, are still needed.

Acknoledgements

Preparation of this review was supported in part by grant RO1 LM5630 from the National Library of Medicine.

References

Albert, D. A., Munson R. and Resnik, M. D. (1988) *Reasoning in Medicine*. Baltimore, MD: Johns Hopkins University Press.

Applied Informatics (1990) *ILIAD User Manual*. Salt Lake City, UT: Applied Informatics.

Arkes, H. (1991) Costs and benefits of judgment errors: Implications for debiasing. *Psychological Bulletin*, **110**, 486–498.

Baron J. (1988) *Thinking and Deciding*. New York: Cambridge University Press.

Barrows, H. S., Norman, G. R., Neufeld, V. R. and Feightner, J. W. (1982) The clinical reasoning process of randomly selected physicians in general practice. *Clinical and Investigative Medicine*, **5**, 49–56.

Barrows, H. S. and Pickell, G. C. (1991) *Developing Clinical Problem-Solving Skills: A Guide to More Effective Diagnosis and Treatment*. New York: Norton.

Bergus, G. R, Chapman, G. B., Gjerde, C., Elstein, A. S. (1995) Clinical reasoning about new symptoms in the face of pre-existing disease: Sources of error and order effects. *Family Medicine*, **27**, 314–320.

Bordage G. (1987) The curriculum: Overloaded and too general? *Medical Education*, **21**, 183–188.

Bordage, G. and Lemieux, M. (1991) Semantic structures and diagnostic thinking of experts and novices. *Academic Medicine*, **66**(9), S70–S72.

Bordage, G. and Zacks, R. (1984) The structure of medical knowledge in the memories of medical students and general practitioners: Categories and prototypes. *Medical Education*, **18**, 406–416.

Brooks, L. R., Norman, G. R. and Allen, S. W. (1991) Role of specific similarity in a medical diagnostic task. *Journal of Experimental Psychology, General*, **120**, 278–287.

Bryant, G. D. and Norman, G. R. (1980) Expressions of probability: Words and numbers. *New England Journal of Medicine*, **302**, 411.

Chapman, G. B., Bergus, G. R. and Elstein, A. S. (1996) Order of information affects clinical judgment. *Journal of Behavioral Decision Making*, **9**, 201–211.

Davidoff, F. (1998) Is basic science necessary? In *Who Has Seen a Blood Sugar? Reflections on Medical Education*, pp. 18–23. Philadelphia, PA: American College of Physicians.

de Bliek, R., Miller, R. A. and Masarie, F. E. (1988) *QMR User Manual*. Pittsburgh, PA: University of Pittsburgh.

Eddy, D. M. (1982) Probabilistic reasoning in clinical medicine: Problems and opportunities. In *Judgment Under Uncertainty: Heuristics and Biases* (D. Kahneman, P. Slovic and A. Tversky, eds), pp. 249–267. New York: Cambridge University Press.

Edwards, W. (1968) Conservatism in human information processing. In *Formal Representation of Human Judgment* (B. Kleinmuntz, ed.), pp. 17–52. New York: Wiley.

Einhorn, H. J. and Hogarth, R. M. (1986) Decision making under ambiguity. *Journal of Business*, **59**, S225–S250.

Elstein, A. S. (1988) Cognitive processes in clinical inference and decision making. In *Reasoning, Inference and Judgment in Clinical Psychology* (D. C. Turk and P. Salovey, eds), pp. 17–50. New York: Free Press/Macmillan.

Elstein A. S. (1994) What goes around comes around: The return of the hypothetico-deductive strategy. *Teaching and Learning in Medicine*, **6**, 121–123.

Elstein, A. S., Holzman, G. B., Belzer, L. J. and Ellis, R. D. (1992) Hormonal replacement therapy: Analysis of clinical strategies used by residents. *Medical Decision Making*, **12**, 265–273.

Elstein, A. S., Kleinmuntz, B., Rabinowitz, M., McAuley, R., Murakami, J., Heckerling, P. S. and Dod, J. M. (1993) Diagnostic reasoning of high- and low-domain knowledge clinicians: A re-analysis. *Medical Decision Making*, **13**, 21–29.

Elstein, A. S., Shulman, L. S. and Sprafka, S. A. (1978) *Medical Problem Solving: An Analysis of Clinical Reasoning*. Cambridge, MA: Harvard University Press.

Eva, K. W., Neville, A. J. and Norman, G. R. (1998) Exploring the etiology of content specificity: Factors influencing analogic transfer and problem solving. *Academic Medicine*, **73**, S1–S5 (October 1998 supplement)

Evidence-based Medicine Working Group (1992) Evidence-based medicine: A new approach to teaching the practice of medicine. *Journal of the American Medical Association*, **268**, 2420–2425.

Fagan, T. J. (1975) Nomogram for Bayes' theorem. *New England Journal of Medicine*, **293**, 257.

Feightner, J. W. (1985) Patient management problems. In *Assessing Clinical Competence* (V. R. Neufeld and G. R. Norman, eds), pp. 183–200. New York: Springer.

Feltovich, P. J., Johnson, P. E., Moller, J. H. and Swanson, D. B. (1984) LCS: The role and development of medical knowledge in diagnostic expertise. In *Readings in Medical Artificial Intelligence: The First Decade* (W. J. Clancey and E. H. Shortliffe, eds), pp. 275–319. Reading, MA: Addison-Wesley.

Friedman, M. H., Connell, K. J., Olthoff, A. J., Sinacore, J. and Bordage, G. (1998) Medical student errors in making a diagnosis. *Academic Medicine*, **73**, S19–S21 (October 1998 Supplement)

Glass, R. D. (1996) *Diagnosis: A Brief Introduction*. New York: Oxford University Press.

Goldman, L. (1998) Quantitative aspects of clinical reasoning. In *Harrison's Principles of Internal Medicine*, 14th edn (A. S. Fauci, E. Braunwald, K. J. Isselbacher, J. D. Wilson, J. B. Martin, D. L. Kasper, S. L. Hauser and D. L. Longo, eds), pp. 9–14. New York: McGraw-Hill.

Groen, G. J. and Patel, V. L. (1985) Medical problem-solving: Some questionable assumptions. *Medical Education*, **19**, 95–100.

Gruppen, L. D., Wolf, F. M. and Billi, J. E. (1991) Information gathering and integration as sources of error in diagnostic decision making. *Medical Decision Making*, **11**, 233–239.

Inouye, J., Kristopatis, R., Stone, E., Pelter, M., Sandhu, M. and Weingarten, S. (1998) Physicians' changing attitudes toward guidelines. *Journal of General Internal Medicine*, **13**, 324–326.

James, P. A., Cowan, T. M., Graham, R. P. and Majeroni, B. A. (1997) Family physicians' attitudes about and use of clinical practice guidelines. *Journal of Family Practice*, **45**, 341–347.

Janis, I. L. and Mann, L. (1977) *Decision-Making*. New York: Free Press.

Joseph, G. M. and Patel, V. L. (1990) Domain knowledge and hypothesis generation in diagnostic reasoning. *Medical Decision Making*, **10**, 31–46.

Kahneman, D., Slovic, P. and Tversky, A. (eds) (1982) *Judgment Under Uncertainty: Heuristics and Biases*. New York: Cambridge University Press.

Kassirer, J. P. and Gorry, G. A. (1978) Clinical problem solving: A behavioral analysis. *Annals of Internal Medicine*, **89**, 245–255.

Kassirer, J. P. and Kopelman, R. I. (1991) *Learning Clinical Reasoning*. Baltimore, MD: Williams & Wilkins.

Keren, G. (1990) Cognitive aids and debiasing methods: Can cognitive pills cure cognitive ills? In *Advances in Psychology: Vol. 68. Cognitive Biases* (J. Caverni and J. Fabre, eds), pp. 523–552. Amsterdam: North-Holland.

Kern, L. and Doherty, M. E. (1982) 'Pseudodiagnosticity' in an idealized medical problem-solving environment. *Journal of Medical Education*, **57**, 100–104.

Kuipers, B. J. and Kassirer, J. P. (1984) Causal reasoning in medicine: Analysis of a protocol. *Cognitive Science*, **8**, 363–385.

Kuipers, B., Moskowitz, A. J. and Kassirer, J. P. (1988) Critical decisions under uncertainty: Representation and structure. *Cognitive Science*, **12**, 177–210.

L'Abbe, K. A, Detsky, A. S. and O'Rourke, K. (1987) Meta-analysis in clinical research. *Annals of Internal Medicine*, **107**, 224–233.

Lemieux, M. and Bordage, G. (1992) Propositional versus structural semantic analyses of medical diagnostic thinking. *Cognitive Science*, **16**,185–204.

Medin, D. L. and Schaffer, M. M. (1978) A context theory of classification learning. *Psychological Review*, **85**, 207–238.

Mellers, B. A, Schwartz, A. and Cooke, A. D. J. (1998) Judgment and decision making. *Annals of Review in Psychology*, **49**, 447–477.

Moskowitz, A. J., Kuipers, B. J. and Kassirer, J. P. (1988) Dealing with uncertainty, risks, and tradeoffs in clinical decisions: A cognitive science approach. *Annals of Internal Medicine*, **108**, 435–449.

Mumma, G. H. and Wilson, S. B. (1995) Procedural debiasing of primacy/anchoring effects in clinical-like judgments. *Journal of Clinical Psychology*, **51**, 841–853.

Neufeld, V. R., Norman, G. R., Feightner, J. W. and Barrows, H. S. (1981) Clinical problem-solving by medical students: A cross-sectional and longitudinal analysis. *Medical Education*, **15**, 315–322.

Newell, A. and Simon, H. A. (1972) *Human Problem Solving*. Englewood Cliffs, NJ: Prentice-Hall.

Nisbett, R. E., Borgida, E., Crandall, R. and Reed, H. (1982) Popular induction: Information is not always informative. In *Judgment Under Uncertainty: Heuristics and Biases*. (D. Kahneman, P. Slovic and A. Tversky, eds), pp. 101–116. New York: Cambridge University Press.

Norman, G. R. (1988) Problem-solving skills, solving problems and problem-based learning. *Medical Education*, **22**, 279–286.

Norman, G. R., Coblentz, C. L., Brooks, L. R. and Babcock, C. J. (1992) Expertise in visual diagnosis: A review of the literature. *Academic Medicine*, **66**, S78–S83.

Norman, G. R., Trott, A. L., Brooks, L.R. and Smith, E. K. M. (1994) Cognitive differences in clinical reasoning related to postgraduate training. *Teaching and Learning in Medicine*, **6**, 114–120.

Oxman, A. D., Cook, D. J. and Guyatt, G. H. (1994) Users' guides to the medical literature: VI. How to use an overview. *Journal of the American Medical Association*, **272**, 1367–1371.

Page, G., Bordage, G., Harasym, P., Bowmer, I. and Swanson, D. (1990) A revision of the Medical Council of Canada's Qualifying Examination: Pilot test results. In *Teaching and Assessing Clinical Competence* (W. Bender, R. Hiemstra, A. Scherpbier, R. Zwierstra, eds), pp. 403–407. Groningen: BoekWerk Publications.

Panzer, R. J., Black, E. R. and Griner, P. F. (1991) *Diagnostic Strategies for Common Medical Problems*. Philadelphia, PA: American College of Physicians.

Patel, V. L. and Groen, G. (1986) Knowledge-based solution strategies in medical reasoning. *Cognitive Science*, **10**, 91–116.

Pauker, S. G. (1996) Clinical decision making: Handling and analyzing clinical data. In *Cecil Textbook of Medicine*, 20th edn (J. C. Bennett and F. Plum, eds), pp. 78–83. Philadelphia: Saunders.

Pople, H. E. (1982) Heuristic methods for imposing structure on ill-structured problems: The structuring of medical diagnostics. In *Artificial Intelligence in Medicine* (P. Szolovits, ed.), pp. 119–190. Boulder, CO: Westview Press.

Poses, R. M., Cebul, R. D., Collins, M. and Fager, S. S. (1985) The accuracy of experienced physicians' probability estimates for patients with sore throats. *Journal of the American Medical Association*, **254**, 925–929.

Rabinowitz, M. and Glaser, R. (1985) Cognitive structure and process in highly competent performance. In *The Gifted and Talented: Developmental Perspectives* (F. D. Horowitz and M. O'Brien, eds), pp. 75–98. Washington, DC: American Psychological Association.

Redelmeier, D. A., Koehler, D. J., Liberman, V. and Tversky, A. (1995) Probability judgment in medicine: Discounting unspecified probabilities. *Medical Decision Making*, **15**, 227–230.

Rosch, E. and Mervis, C. B. (1975) Family resemblances: Studies in the internal structure of categories. *Cognitive Psychology*, **7**, 573–605.

Rosenthal R. (1991) *Meta-analytic Procedures for Social Research*, 2nd edn. Newbury Park, CA: Sage.

Rottenstreich, Y. and Tversky, A. (1997) Unpacking, repacking, and anchoring: Advances in support theory. Psychological Review, **104**, 406–415.

Sackett, D. L., Haynes, R. B., Guyatt, G. H. and Tugwell, P. (1991) *Clinical Epidemiology: A Basic Science for Clinical Medicine*, 2nd edn. Boston, MA: Little, Brown.

Sackett, D. L., Richardson, W. S., Rosenberg, W. and Haynes, R. B. (1997) *Evidence-based Medicine: How to Practice and Teach EBM*. New York: Churchill Livingstone.

Schmidt, H. G., Norman, G. R. and Boshuizen, H. P. A. (1990) A cognitive perspective on medical expertise: Theory and implications. *Academic Medicine*, **65**, 611–621.

Schwartz, A. (1998) *Nomogram for Bayes' theorem.* http://araw.mede.uic.edu/cgi-bin/testcalc.pl

Sox, H. C., Jr, Blatt, M. A., Higgins, M. C. and Marton, K. I. (1988) *Medical Decision Making*. Stoneham, MA: Butterworths.

Swanson, D. B, Norman, G. R. and Linn, R. L. (1995) Performance-based assessment: Lessons from the health professions. *Educational Researcher*, **24**, 5–11.

Tversky, A. and Kahneman, D. (1974) Judgment under uncertainty: Heuristics and biases. *Science*, **185**, 1124–1131.

Tversky, A. and Kahneman, D. (1981) The framing of decisions and the psychology of choice. *Science*, **211**, 453–458.

Tversky, A. and Kahneman, D. (1992), Advances in prospect theory: Cumulative representation of uncertainty. *Journal of Risk and Uncertainty*, **5**, 297–323.

Tversky, A. and Koehler, D. J. (1994) Support theory: A nonextensional representation of subjective probability. *Psychol. Review*, **101**, 547–567.

van der Vleuten, C. P. M. and Swanson, D. B. (1990) Assessment of clinical skills with standardized patients: State of the art. *Teaching and Learning in Medicine*, **2**, 58–76.

Voytovich, A. E., Rippey, R. M. and Suffredini, M. D. (1985) Premature conclusions in diagnostic reasoning. *Journal of Medical Education*, **60**, 302–307.

Wallsten, T. S. (1981) Physician and medical student bias in evaluating information. *Medical Decision Making*, **1**, 145–164.

Wason, P. C. and Johnson-Laird, P. N. (1972) *Psychology of Reasoning: Structure and Content*. Cambridge, MA: Harvard University Press.

Weinstein, M. C., Fineberg, H. V., Elstein, A. S., Frazier, H. S., Neuhauser, D., Neutra, R. R. and McNeil, B. J. (1980) *Clinical Decision Analysis*. Philadelphia, PA: Saunders.

Wigton, R. S, Hoellerich, V. L and Patil, K. D. (1986) How physicians use clinical information in diagnosing pulmonary embolism: An application of conjoint analysis. *Medical Decision Making*, **6**, 2–11. Reprinted in *Professional Judgment: A Reader in Clinical Decision Making* (J. Dowie and A. Elstein, eds), pp. 130–149 New York: Cambridge University Press (1988).

Wolf, F. M, Gruppen, L. D. and Billi, J. E. (1985) Differential diagnosis and the competing hypotheses heuristic: A practical approach to judgment under uncertainty and Bayesian probability. *Journal of American Medical Association*, **253**, 2858–2862. Reprinted in *Professional Judgment: A Reader in Clinical Decision Making* (J. Dowie and A. Elstein, eds), pp. 349–359. New York: Cambridge University Press (1988).

11

Clinical reasoning in nursing

Marsha E. Fonteyn and Barbara J. Ritter

Why seek to understand nurses' clinical reasoning? The answer to this question may seem obvious to many, but is nonetheless worthy of consideration at the beginning of a chapter devoted to this topic. Clinical reasoning represents the essence of nursing practice. It is intrinsic to all aspects of care provision, and its importance pervades nursing education, research and practice. An understanding of nurses' clinical reasoning is important to nursing research because of the need for a scientific basis to evaluate nursing practice and education, and a need to develop and test theories of nurses' cognitive processes and reasoning skills. Research is also needed to describe and explain the relationship between nurses' reasoning and patient outcomes, in order to demonstrate to society the essential role that nursing plays in the health care delivery system.

Knowledge about clinical reasoning is important to nursing education because education is expensive, and teaching that is based on inappropriate or irrelevant models of reasoning can lead to waste and can also result in graduates who are ill-prepared to reason well in practice. Clinical reasoning is also important to nursing practice because patient care provision is becoming increasingly more complex and difficult, requiring sound reasoning skills to maintain patient stability, provide high quality care with positive outcomes, and avoid the costly, even deadly, mistakes that can occur from faulty reasoning and errors in decision making.

Definition of clinical reasoning

The literature provides several definitions of nurses' clinical reasoning. Fonteyn (1991) defines nurses' clinical reasoning as the cognitive processes that nurses use when reviewing and analyzing patient data to plan care and make decisions for positive patient outcomes. Gordon *et al.* (1994) see nurses' reasoning as a form of clinical judgement that occurs in a series of stages: encountering the patient, gathering clinical information, formulating possible diagnostic hypotheses, searching for more information to confirm or reject these hypotheses, reaching a diagnostic decision and determining actions. Ritter (1998) views clinical reasoning as a process involving inclusion of evidence to facilitate optimum patient outcomes. Therefore, nurses' clinical reasoning can be defined as the cognitive processes and strategies that nurses use to understand the significance of patient data, to identify and diagnose actual or potential patient problems, to make clinical decisions to assist in problem resolution, and to achieve positive patient outcomes.

Distinguishing between nurses' reasoning process and the nursing process

Johnson (1959) used the term nursing process to describe the series of steps that comprise the process of nursing. All the steps require reasoning skills. This concept of a five-step process, consisting of assessment, diagnosis, planning, implementation and evaluation, has become entrenched in both nursing practice and education. In what has become a classic treatise, Henderson (1982) cautioned that the nursing process should not be confused with the process of clinical reasoning.

Although fundamental to providing care, nurses' reasoning and decision making has yet to be fully described in nursing research literature, but the descriptive work that has been done reveals a distinction between how nurses reason in practice and how they first learn to reason as an academic endeavour. In their classic study of nurses' clinical judgement, Benner and Tanner (1987) found that with experience, nurses develop a method of reasoning that provides them with an 'intuitive grasp' of the whole clinical situation, without having to rely on the step-by-step analytic approach of the nursing process. They advocated for nursing curricula to include activities that would foster students' skills in intuitive judgement.

Grobe *et al.* (1991) found that experienced nurses link patient problems and interventions to resolve problems more efficiently. Because the nursing process method teaches students to focus on individual patient problems and associated interventions separately, it may promote a less efficient way of reasoning and does not always reflect the realities encountered in actual practice, where one patient problem is often associated with another. In summary, when discussing the cognitive processes and strategies that nurses use to reason about patient care, it is important to clearly distinguish them from the nursing process, which represents one of the many approaches that nurses use in problem solving.

Theoretical perspectives

Several different theoretical perspectives have helped provide an understanding of nurses' clinical reasoning: information processing, decision analysis and hermeneutics.

Information processing theory (IPT)

IPT was first described by Newell and Simon (1972) in their seminal work examining how individuals with a great deal of experience in a specific area (domain expertise) reasoned during a problem solving task. A fundamental premise of

IPT is that human reasoning consists of a relationship between an information processing system (the human problem solver) and a task environment (the context in which problem solving occurs). A postulate of this theory is that there are limits to the amount of information that one can process at any given time and that effective problem solving is the result of being able to adapt to these limitations. Miller's (1956) earlier classic work had demonstrated that an individual's working, short-term memory (STM) can hold only 7 ± 2 symbols at a time. Newell and Simon's (1972) research showed that the capacity of STM could be greatly increased, however, by 'chunking' simple units into familiar patterns. Individuals with a great deal of knowledge and experience in a particular domain can more easily chunk information pertaining to that domain, and thus can make more efficient use of their STM during reasoning.

Another memory bank identified by Newell and Simon (1972) is long-term memory (LTM), which has infinite storage space for information. The theory proposes that information gained from knowledge and experience is stored throughout life in LTM and that it takes longer to access LTM information than the small amount of information temporarily stored in STM. This theory also proposes that the information stored in LTM may need to be accessed by associating it with related information, which helps explain why experts reason so well within their domain. Indeed, cognitive research has demonstrated that experts possess an organized body of domain-specific conceptual and procedural knowledge that can be easily accessed using reasoning strategies (heuristics), and specific reasoning processes that are gradually learned through academic learning and through clinical experience (Fonteyn, 1998; Glaser and Chi, 1988; Joseph and Patel, 1990; Norman, 1988).

Decision analysis theory (DAT)

DAT was introduced in medicine about 20 years ago as a method of solving difficult clinical problems. DAT methods include use of Bayes' theorem, use of decision trees, sensitivity analysis and utility analysis. Bayes' theorem application involves the use of mathematical formulas, tabular techniques, nomograms and computer programs to determine the likelihood of meaning of clinical data.

Several nursing studies have demonstrated the applicability of decision theory to nurses' decision making. In her classic study examining the relationship between the expected value (anticipated outcome) nurses assign to each of their outcomes and their ranking of nursing actions, Grier (1976) demonstrated that nurses select actions that are consistent with their expected values, which seems to support the use of decision trees in some instances of nurses' reasoning and decision making. In a more recent study, Lipman and Deatrick (1997) found that nurse practitioner students who used a decision tree made better decisions about diagnosis and treatment choices for both acute and chronic conditions.

Lauri and Salantera (1995) studied decision-making models and the variables related to them. Findings were that the nature of nursing tasks and the context yielded the greatest difference in decision-making approach. Lewis (1997) found that conflict and ambiguity significantly increased task complexity. Therefore, recommendations are to consider task complexity during model design when developing decision models for use in nursing.

Hermeneutics

Hermeneutics is based on the phenomenological tradition that maintains that meaning is subjective and contextually constructed. The intent of studies of nurses' reasoning guided by this method is to understand the clinical world of nurses, including their reasoning as they make decisions about patient care. Benner *et al.* (1992) used a hermeneutic approach to study the development of expertise in critical care nursing practice. Their findings indicated that nurses at different levels of expertise 'live in different clinical worlds, noticing and responding to different directives for action' (Benner *et al.*, 1992, p. 13). Findings from a later study by the same authors (Benner *et al.*, 1996) indicate that this clinical world is shaped by experience that teaches nurses to make qualitative distinctions in practice. They also found that beginner nurses were more task-oriented, while those with more experience focused on understanding their patients and their illness states.

Research findings of studies related to clinical reasoning

Studies of nurses' clinical judgement, problem solving, decision making and intuition have contributed to the understanding of nurses' clinical reasoning.

Clinical judgement studies

Nurses' clinical judgement represents a composite of traits that assists them in reasoning (Tanner, 1987). The previously cited hermeneutic study of Benner *et al.* (1992) described characteristics of clinical judgement exhibited by critical care nurses with varying levels of practice experience when they reasoned about patient care. Characteristics of clinical judgement identified in the most experienced subjects included (a) the ability to recognize patterns in clinical situations that fit with patterns they had seen in other similar clinical cases; (b) a sense of urgency related to predicting what lies ahead; (c) the ability to concentrate simultaneously on multiple, complex patient cues and patient management therapies; and (d) an aptitude for realistically assessing patient priorities and nursing responsibilities.

The characteristics of clinical judgement identified by Benner and Tanner (1987) and Benner *et al.* (1992) assist in our understanding of nurses' clinical reasoning by identifying and describing some of the cognitive traits or skills that nurses use during reasoning. Benner and Tanner's subsequent work with Chesla (1996) helps further the theoretical understanding of nurses' judgement that is needed to improve educators' ability to teach their students to reason better, and to provide nurses in practice with knowledge that will help them to problem-solve and to make better decisions about patient care.

Problem-solving and decision-making studies

One of the primary objectives of clinical reasoning is to make decisions to resolve problems. Thus, research into nurses' problem solving and decision making provides understanding about the processes involved in their clinical reasoning. Fonteyn and Fisher (1995) examined nurses' decision making when monitoring unstable clients immediately after major surgery. The nurses used three types of reasoning in this situation: predictive reasoning (anticipating patient responses and outcomes based on the current status of a client and on previous experience with similar client cases), backward reasoning (searching the available data for support or substantiation of a clinical hunch when the working plan of care fails to provide an explanation for new data) and forward reasoning (incorporating new data into the working plan of care, while persisting with that plan that nurses commonly use to make clinical decisions). de la Cruz (1994) studied the problem-solving skills of home health nurses, and identified three types of thinking styles: skimming, surveying, and sleuthing. de la Cruz defines skimming as a decision-making style that is used by experienced nurses who draw upon their previous knowledge and experience to quickly assess a clinical situation to expedite a pre-determined and well-defined task. Surveying is a decision-making style that focuses on addressing distinct and specific patient problems which can be resolved using standardized nursing interventions. Sleuthing, a third decision-making style described by de la Cruz, is used by experienced nurses when managing ambiguous, uncertain, complex problems, and involves the use of heuristics and inferencing (de la Cruz, 1994, pp. 223–224).

Studies that identify the specific processes that nurses commonly use during problem solving further overall theoretical understanding of nurses' clinical reasoning.

Intuition studies

Several investigators have proposed that intuition is an important part of nurses' reasoning processes. A classic study that continues to guide nursing research on intuition was conducted by Pyles and Stern (1983) to explore the reasoning of a group of critical care nurses with varying levels of expert-ise. The investigators identified a 'gut feelings' experienced by the more seasoned nurse subjects, which they believed was as important to nurses' reasoning as their formal knowledge about patient cases. Subjects said they used these gut feelings to temper information from specific clinical cues; they also emphasized the importance of previous clinical experience in developing intuitive skills. Rew (1990) demonstrated the important role that intuition played in nurses' reasoning and decision making. Subjects described their intuitive experi-ences as strong feelings or perceptions about their patients, about themselves and responding to their patients, or about anticipated outcomes, that they sensed without going through an analytical reason-ing process. The applicability of findings from studies about nurses' use of intuition to theoretical understanding of nurses' clinical reasoning is limited because of an incomplete description of nurses' intuition.

Clinical reasoning studies

Fonteyn and Grobe (1993) showed that, unlike physicians' reasoning, most of nurses' reasoning tasks are not aimed at diagnosis and hypotheses generation. Rather, nurses reason to distinguish between relevant and irrelevant patient data, to determine the significance of patient data, and to make decisions that assist in accomplishing the overall treatment plan for each patient. Their study also provided a description of nurses' reasoning-thinking strategies (heuristics).

Heuristics are mental rules of thumb that assist in reasoning and are acquired over time through multiple experiences with similar patient cases (Fonteyn and Fisher, 1995; Fonteyn and Grobe, 1993). In a later study, Fonteyn (1998) provided more complete description of the heuristics nurses use when reasoning about clinical dilemmas. They include recognizing a pattern, setting priorities, searching for information, generating hypotheses, making predictions, forming relationships, stating a proposition, asserting a practice rule, making choices, judging the value, drawing conclusions and providing explanations. Additional, less-com-mon thinking strategies were pondering, posing a question, making assumptions, and qualifying and making generalizations. This evidence strengthens and expands previous clinical reasoning studies of nurses' use of heuristics.

The seminal studies of heuristic use were conducted by the cognitive psychologists Tversky and Kahneman (1974, 1977, 1981). They revealed that although the use of heuristics may facilitate efficiency in reasoning and usually results in more effective decision making, heuristic use can also lead to biases and result in reasoning errors. Cioffi and Markham (1997) found that advanced practice nurses relied on heuristics in clinical decision making when uncertainty was not resolved by information collected during an assessment or to simplify task complexity which could lead to inaccurate diagnoses and treatment. Further research remains to be done on biases associated with nurses heuristics use.

Future directions of research examining nurses' clinical reasoning

Despite the research that has already been done, the nature of nurses' clinical reasoning remains unclear. One explanation for the lack of clarity may be the continued propensity for investigators to study nurses' clinical reasoning outside the clinical arena, using simulation, questionnaires or interviews. The fullest and most accurate descrip-tion of nurses' clinical reasoning will be obtained when reasoning is studied in the clinical arena at the time it is occurring during care provision. Until recently, however, investigators have avoided this approach because it was thought to be either logistically impossible or a risk to patient care.

Fonteyn and Fisher (1995) demonstrated that it is both logistically possible and safe to study nurses' clinical reasoning in the clinical setting during the time that care is being given. Using a triangulated method, consisting of guided interviews, participant observation and think-aloud technique, the investigators collected data from a group of expert critical care nurses while they were providing postoperative care to critically ill patients. Findings from this pilot study suggest that a tremendous amount of rich, relevant data about nurses' reasoning can be obtained using this method. Moreover, studying nurses' reasoning in the clinical setting does not appear to compromise patient care nor disrupt either subject or unit functioning. Narayan and Corcoran-Perry (1997) demonstrated the feasibility of this methodological approach in a recent study examining how nurses with varying levels of expertise use knowledge to make a particular clinical decision.

Future studies of nurses' clinical reasoning that use methods that examine reasoning in the clinical setting while care is being given to real (not simulated) patients will assist in completing the description of this phenomenon. Subsequently studies should be initiated that examine the relationship between nurses' clinical reasoning and other variables, such as level of expertise, domain knowledge, the climate in which the reasoning and decision making take place, patient stability, and patient outcomes. Some of the important questions are: How is nurses' reasoning related to their sense of autonomy and job satisfaction? How is clinical reasoning related to expertise and level of knowledge within a domain? What factors are associated with optimal reasoning? What is the relationship between nurses' clinical reasoning and patient outcomes? Later, as the state of the science evolves from research that provides answers to these questions, experimental studies can be undertaken to provide answers to additional questions, such as: Is nurses' reasoning improved with increased autonomy or job satisfaction? Can nurses be taught strategies that will improve their reasoning? Can methods be devised to improve nurses' reasoning outside their domain knowledge? Does improvement in nurses' reasoning result in improved patient outcomes?

Educational focus on clinical reasoning

Critical thinking (CT)

Nurses increasingly need well-developed reasoning skills to assist them in understanding and resolving the complex patient problems encountered in practice. In their text entitled *Developing Clinical Problem-Solving Skills*, Barrows and Pickell (1991, p. 3) remind us that 'ambiguities and conflicting or inadequate information are the rule in medicine'. This is equally true in nursing, where dealing with complex patient problems with uncertain and unpredictable outcomes requires continuous astute reasoning and accurate and efficient decision making. Thus, the ability to think critically is essential.

The roots of CT can be traced to the time of Aristotle and Socrates. Since that time, various authors have constructed definitions of CT. The American Philosophical Association (APA) consensus panel (1990) recognized that divergent conceptualizations of CT have hindered research and education efforts. The expert panel worked toward development of a clear conceptualization of CT, as well as other critical factors such as expertise that have an influence on CT. A key result of the project was the conceptualization of CT in two dimensions, cognitive skills and affective dispositions. Firstly, the experts were virtually unanimous on including analysis, evaluation and inference as central to CT cognitive skills. Secondly, one must have the affective dispositions to think critically about issues. Affective dispositions that characterize good critical thinkers include inquisitiveness, self-confidence in one's ability to reason, open mindedness regarding divergent world views, flexibility, honesty, diligence and reasonableness.

Facione and Facione (1996) contend that the description of the ideal critical thinker resembles the descriptions of a nurse with expert clinical judgement. In the clinical context, the expert nurse adept in clinical reasoning draws judiciously on developed nursing knowledge in forming, evaluating or re-evaluating a purposeful clinical judgement. An expert nurse uses an organized and exhaustive approach to reflectively analyse, interpret, evaluate, infer, and explain evidence and hypotheses.

The Faciones point out that the APA consensus definition is consistent with descriptions of the nursing knowledge base which include carefully examining and delineating key concepts, constructing meaning, categorizing phenomena, identifying assumptions, testing relationships, hypotheses and theories, while formulating alternatives for justifying procedures and stating findings. All are manifestations of CT skills needed for clinical decision making in situations that are often vital and time limited. In addition, the Faciones indicate that the APA consensus definition of CT integrates consideration of contexts, criteria and evidence that are relevant to a given problem, as well as organization of new information and reorganization of previously learned material into forms leading to new responses which can be applied to new situations. Thus, reasoned responses and actions are formulated for anticipated and unanticipated situations. This consensus definition aligns the conceptual definition of CT to nursing, as the definition incorporates descriptions of nursing practice wherein nurses need to make effective practice decisions, utilizing good judgement, in the context of uncertainty.

Gordon *et al.* (1994) realized the complexities of operationalizing a broad concept such as CT and proposed a nursing model in which nursing judgement is the outcome of CT. Like the APA definition, the model focuses on CT as a process of purposeful judgement with emphasis on decision making, which can be placed in the context of the nursing process as an identified problem, goal, and desired outcome. This conceptualization of CT as a cognitive skill and a disposition has implications for nursing curriculum and instruction.

The cognitive skills that today's nursing students need to learn in order to reason accurately and make decisions effectively in practice are causing nurse educators to adjust their teaching methods. They are beginning to shift from reliance on the more traditional didactic methods of teaching to more creative teaching methods designed to improve students' reasoning skills and to furnish them with a repertoire of creative approaches to care (Curry and Makoul, 1996; Graham, 1996; Norman and Schmidt, 1993; Sivam *et al.*, 1995).

Much of nursing education literature has begun to focus on ways to teach CT. Fonteyn and Flaig (1994) proposed using case studies to improve nursing students' reasoning skills by teaching them to identify potential patient problems, suggest nursing actions, and describe outcome variables that would allow them to evaluate the effectiveness of their actions. Case studies provide the advantage of allowing nurse educators to give continuous feedback in the safe environment of simulation and many others have supported their use (Haffer and Raingruber, 1998; Manning *et al.*, 1995; Neill *et*

al., 1997; Ryan-Wenger and Lee, 1997). Lipman and Deatrick (1997) found that beginning nurse practitioner students tended to formulate diagnoses too early in the data gathering phase, thus precluding consideration of all diagnostic options. When they used a case study approach incorporating algorithms to guide the decision-making process, students developed a broader focus and diagnostic accuracy improved. To increase realism, case studies can be designed to provide information in chronological segments that more closely reflect real-life cases, in which clinical events and outcomes evolve over time (Fonteyn, 1991).

Other methods that have been suggested by nurse educators to improve students' CT skills include clinical experience, conferences, computer simulations, clinical logs, collaboration, decision analysis, discussion, E-mail dialogue, portfolios, reflection, role modelling, role playing, and writing position papers (Baker, 1996; Fonteyn and Cahill, 1998; Girot, 1995; Sorrell *et al.*, 1997; Todd, 1998; Weis and Guyton-Simmons, 1998).

Videbeck (1997b) indicates that as well as being effectively taught, CT must be assessed in an appropriate manner. She points out that standardized paper-and-pencil tests are often selected as an evaluation measure since normative data are available and reliability has been established. However, none of the available instruments is specific to nursing, and there is not a consistent relationship between scores on this type of test and clinical judgement. The use of faculty-developed instruments to assess student outcomes is strongly recommended. Videbeck states that course-specific measures, such as clinical performance criteria or written assignments, have the advantage of being specific to nursing practice. One effective evaluation method which incorporates the time needed for accurate assessment is the capstone project, which requires students to use knowledge and abilities from many courses and occurs toward the completion of the major. Hence, the term capstone, which is the finishing stone of a structure, is used to indicate a summary course which refines and 'finishes' the formal academic preparation of a student prior to their entry into practice. Videbeck (1997a) suggests that a model which integrates CT in all aspects of the program (definition, course objectives and evaluation) be used. Similarly, Dexter *et al.* (1997) describe a model for teaching and evaluating CT that could provide a framework to guide nursing faculty at all levels (associate, baccalaureate, master's and doctoral). The model focuses on the CT competencies of interpretation, analysis, evaluation, inference, explanation and self-regulation described by Facione (1992), and measured by the California Critical Thinking Skills Test (CCTST) (Facione, 1993).

Kataoka-Yahiro and Saylor (1994) point out that evaluation of CT should be based on safe, competent, and professional standards which are required for practice. Page *et al.* (1995) support the use of key feature problem (case scenario) examinations to assess clinical decision-making skills. The format consists of providing clinical scenarios which include essential features in a problem followed by questions that focus on the critical steps. A scoring rubric, which includes content considered by experts to be essential, is used for assessment. Jacobs *et al.* (1997) and others recommend further studies to establish reliability for using a case study approach for evaluation of CT.

Future directions of educational efforts related to nurses' clinical reasoning

In the future, educators must strive to devise additional methods to develop and improve nurses' clinical reasoning. Further changes will be required in the structure and function of nursing curriculum. Students need to learn to improve the ways in which they identify significant clinical data and determine the meaning of data in regard to patient problems. They also need to learn how to reason about patient problems in ways that facilitate decisions about problem resolution.

Educators are realizing that the body of clinical knowledge and information is increasing too rapidly to expect that students can possibly remember all the information they will need for practice. Moreover, possessing an encyclopaedic memory of facts and concepts will not ensure effective clinical reasoning.

O'Sullivan *et al.* (1997) indicate that teaching strategies which promote clinical reasoning are ones in which the educator designs classroom activities to engage the students. Meleis and Price (1988) suggest that teaching modalities which would incorporate active involvement and allow information to be transformed into knowledge are those which allow the student to construct and solve problems specific to the domain of nursing. In this regard Paul and Heaslip (1995) advocate that students need to reason their way critically through nursing principles, concepts and theories frequently, so that accurate application and transfer of knowledge occurs in an integrated and intuitive way. Glen (1995) advocates implementing a model

such as problem-based learning (PBL). She believes this a teaching methodology would promote conceptual understanding and development of the reasoning skills for effective clinical judgement and would encourage students to be active creators rather than passive receptors of knowledge.

PBL develops students' ability to reflect continuously on their reasoning and decision making during patient care, and leads to self-improvement through practice. Evidence exists that PBL significantly increases CT, clinical reasoning, problem solving and transfer of knowledge gained (Khoiny, 1995; Schmidt, 1993; Sobral, 1995). Once students have developed their reasoning skills in this manner, they can then apply them while caring for real patients in the clinical setting. Fonteyn and Flaig (1994) advocate that educators temper the practice of requiring nursing students to write lengthy care plans focusing on the nursing process. Rather, they suggest teaching students to reason and plan care in the same manner as practising nurses. In practice, nurses first identify (from data initially obtained in report form and confirmed by patient assessment) the most important patient problems on which to focus during their nursing shift. Information from the patient, the family and other members of the health care team should be included in a plan of care that will assist in resolving the problems identified. As the shift progresses, nurses continuously evaluate and refine their plan of care based on additional data obtained from further patient assessment, additional clinical data and information from all individuals involved in carrying out the plan of care.

Computer-assisted instruction (CAI) can also improve students' reasoning skills (Perciful and Nester, 1996). CAI programs can save educators time and effort, while at the same time providing high-quality instruction that is intellectually challenging (Junge and Assal, 1993). CAI offers another means of providing problem-based learning for students, using the computer to combine self-paced individual and small-group learning. Technological advances such as the Internet, with access to online video conferencing, journals, web-sites, interactive programs and distance learning, hold rich promise for promoting creative and effective teaching environments (Fetterman, 1996).

Practice

The ultimate goal of both research and educational endeavours related to clinical reasoning in nursing is to improve nurses' reasoning in practice and, ultimately, to achieve more positive patient outcomes. Nursing literature suggests that nurses' reasoning and interventions have a significant effect on patient outcome (Chase, 1995; Fowler, 1994; Nielsen, 1992). The relationship between nurses' reasoning and patient outcome will remain unclear, however, until the specific patient outcome indicators associated with nurses' reasoning have been identified, until the measurements of these indicators have been explicated, and until their impact on patient mortality and morbidity has been demonstrated through research. If nursing is to continue to play a proactive role in health care provision, it is essential to identify the role of nurses' reasoning and decision-making in overall patient outcome.

A major difficulty in demonstrating the influence of nurses' reasoning on patient outcomes is the complex nature of the outcomes, which span a broad range of effects or presumed effects that are influenced not only by nursing and other health care providers, but by many other variables, including time, environmental conditions, support systems and patient history.

Decision support systems and expert systems are currently being developed to assist nurses in practice to reason more efficiently and to make better clinical decisions. Expert system development began in research laboratories in the mid-1970s and was first implemented in commercial and practical endeavours in the early 1980s (Frenzel, 1987). The HELP Patient Care Information System, an interactive computerized health information system, facilitates diagnostic and therapeutic decisions via critiquing and suggesting modification for diagnosis and care delivery (Haug *et al.*, 1994). CompuHx is an Interactive Health Appraisal System, used in the examination room to record patient information, assist in diagnosis, as well as provide a legible summary of findings (Aydin *et al.*, 1994).

Fonteyn and Grobe (1994) suggest that an expert system could be designed to represent the knowledge and reasoning processes of experienced nurses, and could then be used to assist less experienced nurses to improve their reasoning skills and strategies. 'Illiad' is one such expert system case-based teaching program, which has been shown by Lange *et al.* (1997) to be effective in improving nurse practitioner students' diagnostic abilities.

Until recently, expert systems required special programming languages and were designed to cover broad, rather than specific, domains in nursing. Both these factors made development complicated, expensive, and time consuming. Expert system shells, coupled with a trend to focus on the more concise nursing problems encountered within a specific area of nursing practice and a common taxonomy, will provide a means to expedite and facilitate the growth and development of expert systems for use in nursing practice (Bowles, 1997).

Future directions in practice related to nurses' clinical reasoning

The relationship between nurses' reasoning and patient outcomes should receive greater attention in future research, to demonstrate the important role that nurses play in health care delivery. There will be increasing need to develop meaningful data sets related to patient outcomes. These data sets should contain the nursing actions that nurses commonly choose after reasoning about specific patient problems and their associated patient outcomes. Prior to the development of these data sets, the indicators of patient outcome that are related to nurses' reasoning and decision making need to be identified and described in a manner that facilitates their measurement.

Computerized support systems will play an increased role in assisting nurses to reason, make decisions about appropriate nursing actions, and evaluate their impact on patient outcome. Although only a select portion of the nursing profession will be directly involved in system development, all nurses need to be knowledgeable enough about these systems to be able to be actively involved in their design and implementation in practice. Additionally, all nurses should understand enough about these systems to use them effectively in their practice.

Conclusion

The information presented in this chapter, although not intended to be all-inclusive, nonetheless provides a perspective on what is currently known about nurses' clinical reasoning. The ultimate goal for understanding nurses' clinical reasoning is to improve problem solving and decision making in practice, with the assumption that improvement will result in optimal patient outcomes.

References

American Philosophical Association (APA) (1990) *Critical thinking: A statement of expert consensus for purposes of educational assessment and instruction.* Recommendations prepared for the Committee on Pre-College Philosophy. ERIC ED 315–423.

Aydin, C. E., Rosen, P. N. and Felitti, V. J. (1994) Transforming information use in preventive medicine: Learning to balance technology with the art of caring. In *Proceedings of Annual Symposium of Computer Application in Medical Care*, pp. 563–567.

Baker, C. (1996) Reflective learning: A teaching strategy for critical thinking. *Journal of Nursing Education*, **35**, 19–22.

Barrows, H. and Pickell, G. (1991) *Developing Clinical Problem-Solving Skills.* New York: Norton.

Benner, P. and Tanner, C. (1987) Clinical judgement: How expert nurses use intuition. *American Journal of Nursing*, **87**, 23–31.

Benner, P., Tanner, C. and Chesla, C. (1992) From beginner to expert: Gaining a differentiated clinical world in critical care nursing. *Advances in Nursing Science*, **14**, 13–28.

Benner, P., Tanner, C. and Chesla, C. (1996) *Expertise in Nursing Practice: Caring, Clinical Judgement and Ethics.* New York: Springer.

Bowles, K. H. (1997) The barriers and benefits of nursing information systems. *Computers in Nursing*, **15**, 197–198.

Chase, S. (1995) The social context of critical care clinical judgment. *Heart and Lung*, **24**, 154–162.

Cioffi, J. and Markham, R. (1997) Clinical decision-making by midwives: Managing case complexity. *Journal of Advanced Nursing*, **25**, 265–272.

Curry, R. and Makoul, G. (1996) Active learning approach to basic clinical skills. *Academic Medicine*, **71**, 41–44.

de la Cruz, F. (1994) Clinical decision making styles of home healthcare nurses. *Image: The Journal of Nursing Scholarship*, **26**, 222–226.

Dexter, P., Applegate, M., Backer, J., Claytor, K., Keffer, J., Norton, B. and Ross, B. (1997) A proposed framework for teaching and evaluating critical thinking in nursing. *Journal of Professional Nursing*, **13**, 160–167.

Facione, N. and Facione, P. (1996) Externalizing the critical thinking in knowledge development and clinical judgment. *Nursing Outlook*, **44**, 129–136.

Facione, P. (1992) *Critical Thinking: What It is and Why It Counts.* Milbrae, CA: California Academic Press.

Facione, P. (1993) *Critical Thinking: A Statement of Expert Consensus for Purposes of Educational Assessment and Instruction.* Milbrae, CA: California Academic Press.

Fetterman, D. (1996) Videoconferencing on-line: Enhancing communication over the internet. *Educational Researcher*, **24**(4), 23–27.

Fonteyn, M. (1991) A descriptive analysis of expert critical care nurses' clinical reasoning. *Doctoral dissertation.* University of Texas, Austin, TX.

Fonteyn, M. (1998) *Thinking Strategies for Nursing Practice.* Philadelphia, PA: Lippincott.

Fonteyn, M. and Cahill, M. (1998) The use of clinical logs to improve students metacognition. *Journal Advanced Nursing*, **28**, 149–154.

Fonteyn, M. and Fisher, A. (1995) An innovative methodological approach for examining nurses' heuristic use in clinical practice. *Journal of Scholarly Inquiry*, **9**, 263–276.

Fonteyn, M. and Flaig, L. (1994) The written nursing process: Is it still useful to nursing education? *Journal of Advanced Nursing*, **19**, 315–319.

Fonteyn, M. and Grobe, S. (1993) Expert critical care nurses' clinical reasoning under uncertainty: Representation, structure and process. In *Sixteenth Annual Symposium on Computer Applications in Medical Care* (M. Frisse, ed.), pp. 405–409, New York: McGraw-Hill.

Fonteyn, M. and Grobe, S. (1994) Expert system development in nursing: Implications for critical care nursing practice. *Heart and Lung*, **23**, 80–87.

Fowler, L. (1994) *Clinical reasoning of home health nurses: A verbal protocal analysis. Doctoral dissertation.* University of Southern Carolina, Los Angeles, CA.

Frenzel, L. (1987) *Understanding Expert Systems.* Indianapolis, IN: H. W. Sama .

Girot, E. (1995) Preparing the practitioner for advanced academic study: The development of critical thinking. *Journal of Advanced Nursing*, **21**, 387–394.

Glaser, R. and Chi, M. (1988) Overview. In *The Nature of Expertise* (M. Chi, R.Glaser and M. Farr, eds), pp. xv–xxxvi. Englewood Cliffs, NJ: Lawrence Erlbaum.

Glen, S. (1995) Towards a new model of nursing education. *Nurse Education Today*, **15**, 90–95,

Gordon, M., Murphy, C., Candes, D. and Hiltunen, E. (1994) Clinical judgment: An integrated model. *Advances in Nursing Science*, **16**(4), 55–70.

Graham, C. (1996) Conceptual learning processes in physical therapy students. *Physical Therapy*, **76**, 856–865.

Grier, M. (1976) Decision making about patient care. *Nursing Research*, **25**, 105–110.

Grobe, S., Drew, J. and Fonteyn, M. (1991) A descriptive analysis of experienced nurses' reasoning during a planning task. *Research in Nursing and Health*, **14**, 305–314.

Haffer, A. and Raingruber, B. (1998) Discovering confidence in clinical reasoning and critical thinking development in baccalaureate nursing students. *Journal of Nursing Education*, **37**, 61–70.

Haug, P. J., Gardner, R. M., Tate, K. E., Evans, R. S., East, T. D., Kuperman, G., Pryor, T. A., Huff, S. M. and Warner, H. R. (1994) Decision support in medicine: Examples from the HELP system. *Computer Biomedical Research*, **27**, 396–418.

Henderson, V. (1982) The nursing process – Is the title right? *Journal of Advanced Nursing*, **7**, 103–109.

Jacobs, P., Ott, B., Sullivan, B., Ulrich, Y. and Short, L. (1997) An approach to defining and operationalizing critical thinking. *Journal of Nursing Education*, **36**, 19–22.

Johnson, D. (1959) A philosophy for nursing diagnosis. *Nursing Outlook*, **7**, 198–200.

Joseph, G. and Patel, V. (1990) Domain knowledge and hypothesis generation in diagnostic reasoning. *Medical Decision Making*, **10**, 31–46.

Junge, C. and Assal, J. (1993) Designing computer assisted instruction programs for diabetic patients: How can we make them really useful? In *Proceedings of the 16th Annual*

Symposium on Computer Applications in Medical Care (ed. M. Frisse), pp. 215–219. New York: McGraw-Hill.

Kataoka-Yahiro, M. and Saylor, C. (1994) A critical thinking model for nursing judgment. *Journal of Nursing Education*, **33**, 351– 356.

Khoiny, F. (1995) The effectiveness of problem-based learning in nurse practitioner education. *Doctoral dissertation*. University of Southern California, Los Angeles, CA.

Lange, L., Haak, S., Lincoln, M., Thomspon, C., Turner, C., Weir, C., Foerster, V., Nilasena, D. and Reeves, R. (1997) Use of Illiad to improve diagnostic performance of nurse practitioner students. *Journal of Nursing Education*, **36**, 35–45.

Lauri, S. and Salantera, S. (1995) Decision-making models of Finnish nurses and public health nurses. *Journal of Advanced Nursing*, **21**, 520–527.

Lewis, M. (1997) Decision-making task complexity: Model development and initial testing. *Journal of Nursing Education*, **36**, 114–120.

Lipman, L. and Deatrick, J. (1997) Preparing advanced practice nurses for clinical decision making in specialty practice. *Nurse Educator*, **22**(2), 47–50.

Manning, J., Broughton, V. and McConnel, E. (1995) Reality based scenarios facilitate knowledge network development. *Contemporary Nurse*, **4**, 16–21.

Meleis, A. and Price, M. (1988) Strategies and conditions for teaching theoretical nursing: An international perspective. *Journal of Advanced Nursing Science*, **13**, 112–117.

Miller, G. (1956) The magical number seven, plus or minus two: Some limits on our capacity to process information. *The Psychological Review*, **63**, 81–97.

Narayan, S. and Corcoran-Perry, S. (1997) Line of reasoning as a representation of nurses' clinical decision making. *Research in Nursing and Health Care*, **20**(4), 353–364.

Neill, K., Lachat, M. and Taylor-Panek, S. (1997) Enhancing critical thinking with case studies and nursing process. *Nurse Educator*, **22**(2), 30–32.

Newell, A. and Simon, H. (1972) *Human Problem Solving*. Englewood Cliffs, NJ: Prentice-Hall.

Nielsen, P. (1992) Quality of care: Discovering a modified practice theory. *Journal of Nursing Care Quality*, **6**, 63–76.

Norman, G. (1988) Problem-solving, solving problems, and problem-based learning. *Medical Education*, **22**, 279–286.

Norman, G. and Schmidt, H. (1993) The psychological basis of problem based learning: A review of the evidence. *Academic Medicine*, **67**, 557–565.

O'Sullivan, P., Bevins-Stephens, W., Smith, F. and Vaughn-Worbel, B. (1997) Addressing the National League for Nursing critical thinking outcome. *Nurse Educator*, **22**(1), 23–29.

Page, G., Bordage, G. and Allen, T. (1995) Developing key-feature problems and examinations to assess clinical decision-making skills. *Academic Medicine*, **70**, 194–201.

Paul, R. and Heaslip, P. (1995) Critical thinking and intuitive nursing practice. *Journal of Advanced Nursing Practice*, **22**, 40–47.

Perciful, E. and Nester, P. (1996) The effect of an innovative clinical teaching method on nursing students' knowledge and critical thinking skills. *Journal of Nursing Education*, **35**, 23–28.

Pyles, S. and Stern, P. (1983) Discovery of nursing gestalt in critical care nursing: The importance of the grey gorilla syndrome. *Image: The Journal of Nursing Scholarship*, **15**(2), 51–57.

Rew, L. (1990) Intuition in critical care nursing practice. *Dimensions of Critical Care Nursing*, **9**, 30–37.

Ritter, B. (1998) Why evidence-based practice? *CCNP Connection*, **11**(5), 1–8.

Ryan-Wenger, N. and Lee, J. (1997) The clinical reasoning case study: A powerful teaching tool. *The Nurse Practitioner*, **22**(5), 66–70.

Schmidt, H. (1993) Foundations of problem based learning: Some explanatory notes. *Medical Education*, **27**, 422–432.

Sivam, S., Iatridis, P. and Vaughn, S. (1995) Integration of pharmacology into a problem based learning curriculum for medical students. *Medical Education*, **29**, 289–296.

Sobral, D. (1995) Diagnostic ability of medical students in relation to their learning characteristics and preclinical background. *Medical Education*, **29**, 278–282.

Sorrell, J., Brown, H., Silva, M. and Kohlenberg, E. (1997) *Nursing Forum*, **32**(4), 12–24.

Tanner, C. (1987) Teaching clinical judgement. In *Annual Review of Nursing Research* (J. Fitzpatrick and R. Tauton, eds), pp. 153–174. New York: Springer.

Todd, N. (1998) Using e-mail in an undergraduate nursing course to increase critical thinking skills. *Computers in Nursing*, **16**, 115–118.

Tversky, A. and Kahneman, D. (1974) Judgement under uncertainty: Heuristics and biases. *Science*, **285**, 1124–1131.

Tversky, A. and Kahneman, D. (1977) Features of similarity. *Psychological Review*, **84**, 327–351.

Tversky, A. and Kahneman, D. (1981) The framing of decisions and the psychology of choice. *Science*, **211**, 453–458.

Videbeck, S. (1997a) Critical thinking: Prevailing practice in baccalaureate schools of nursing. *Journal of Nursing Education*, **36**, 5–10.

Videbeck, S. (1997b) Critical thinking: A model. *Journal of Nursing Education*, **36**, 23–28.

Weis, P. and Guyton-Simmons, J. (1998) A computer simulation for teaching critical thinking skills. *Nurse Educator*, **23**(2), 30–33.

12

Clinical reasoning in physiotherapy

Mark Jones, Gail Jensen and Ian Edwards

This chapter presents physiotherapy research and theory in clinical reasoning, as well as findings and views outside of physiotherapy, to consider the nature of clinical reasoning in physiotherapy. Significant revision has been made to this chapter from its first edition, with greater attention paid to the collaborative nature of the reasoning process and a new description of clinical reasoning strategies as used in physiotherapy practice.

The current focus on clinical reasoning in physiotherapy is consistent with physiotherapy's continued growth as a profession. Autonomy, one of the key traits of a profession, implies a defined body of knowledge and expertise in a domain. Professional expertise is not merely application of theoretical or research-based knowledge in practice. Expertise evolves from professionals' use of critical analysis during and after their interaction with their patients, often in unclear or indeterminate situations (Kennedy, 1987). For physiotherapists, expertise develops in part through clinical reasoning.

Clinical reasoning refers to the thought processes associated with a clinician's examination and management of a patient or client. Clinical reasoning is influenced by attributes of the therapist (e.g. needs and goals, values and beliefs, knowledge, cognitive, interpersonal and technical skills), the patient (e.g. values and beliefs, individual physical, psychological, social and cultural presentation) and the environment (e.g. resources, time, funding, and any externally imposed requirements). Physiotherapists work with a multitude of problem situations, many of which can be characterized by complexity, uniqueness and ambiguity. The goal of physiotherapists' reasoning is wise action. Wise action means making the best judgement in a specific context (Cervero, 1988).

The clinical reasoning process in physiotherapy – hypothesis oriented and collaborative

Understanding the clinical reasoning underlying a physiotherapist's assessment and management of a patient requires consideration of the thinking process of the therapist, the patient and the shared decision making between the two. Figure 12.1 presents a model of the collaborative clinical reasoning process between physiotherapists and patients as proposed by Jones (1995). This model is intended to provide a simple pictorial representation of clinical reasoning in physiotherapy. In all physiotherapy settings, the physiotherapist's reasoning begins with the initial data/cues obtained. For example, in a rehabilitation setting it may be a referral, case notes, observation of the patient in the waiting room, as well as opening introductions and inquiries with the patient. This preliminary information will evoke a range of impressions or working interpretations. While typically not thought of as such, they can be considered hypotheses. The cognition involved in hypothesis generation includes a combination of specific data interpretations or inductions and the synthesis of multiple clues or deductions. In most settings the initial hypotheses will be quite broad, e.g. in an outpatient setting ('looks like a back or hip problem') or in a domiciliary care setting ('appears the carer may not be coping'). Initial hypotheses may be physical, psychological or socially related, with or without a 'diagnostic' implication.

All physiotherapists have an element of routine to their examination. Individual therapists will have identified through experience the categories of information which they have found to be particularly useful for problem identification and management decisions (e.g. site, behaviour and history of symptoms, family and social information, function and structure, specific tests of cognition, perception and the neuro-musculoskeletal system, ergonomic and environmental analysis). While a degree of routine commonly exists, specific inquiries and tests are tailored to each patient's unique presentation. Initial hypotheses will lead to certain inquiries and tests specific to that patient. This cognitive activity of hypothesis testing ideally includes the search for both supporting and negating evidence. The resulting data are then interpreted for their fit with previously obtained data and the hypotheses considered. Even routine inquiries, tests and spontaneous information offered by the patient will be interpreted in the context of initial hypotheses. In this way the physiotherapist acquires an evolving understanding of the patient and the patient's problem. Initial hypotheses will be modified and new hypotheses considered. This hypothesis generation and testing process continues until sufficient information is obtained to make a diagnostic decision (identification of the source and underlying cause of the patient's disabilities) and a management decision.

The clinical reasoning process continues throughout ongoing patient management. In particular, physiotherapy intervention serves as another test of hypotheses. Re-assessment either provides support for the hypotheses and chosen course of action or signals the need for hypothesis modification/generation or further data collection and problem clarification (e.g. additional physiotherapy examination or referral for other specialist consultation). At the micro level therapists are constantly reading patient responses (listening, observing, feeling) and using these to build on their understanding and guide clinical decisions to modify and improve their interventions. At a macro level whole treatment sessions or even multiple treatments will be used to test management hypotheses.

Equally important to the therapist's thinking are the patient's thoughts about his/her problem, as reflected in the boxes on the right side of Figure 12.1. That is, patients begin their encounter with a physiotherapist with their own ideas of the nature of their problem, as shaped by personal experience and advice from medical practitioners, family and friends. Patients' understanding of their clinical problem has been shown to impact on their levels of pain tolerance, disability and eventual outcome (Borkan *et al.*, 1991; Feuerstein and Beatie, 1995; Malt and Olafson, 1995). Dysfunctional beliefs and feelings which are counterproductive to the patient's management and recovery can contribute to patients' inadequate involvement in the management process, poor self-efficacy and ultimately a poor outcome. Patients' self-efficacy and the responsibility they take for their management can be maximized through a collaborative reasoning process with their therapists. Through a process of evaluating patients' understanding of and feelings about their problems, through explanation, reassurance and shared decision making, the patient and the therapist jointly develop an evolving understanding of the problem and its management. Responsibility is shared between patient and therapist, with the patient taking a more active role in the management.

Patient learning (i.e. altered understanding and improved health behaviour) is a primary outcome sought in the collaborative reasoning approach. When the patient is recognized as a source of knowledge for the therapist, reflective therapists will also learn from the collaborative experience. That is, when patients are given the opportunity to tell their story rather than simply answer questions, reflective therapists, who attend to individual patient presentations noting features that appear to be linked (such as increased stress affecting one patient's symptoms but not another's), will learn the variety of ways in which patients' health, cognition, behaviour, movement and pain can interact. And just as patients can be taught to problem-solve to recognize various physical and psychological stressors, therapists must continually reflect on their working hypotheses and the effects of their interventions to 'validate' their clinical patterns and procedural knowledge.

The box to the left in Figure 12.1 highlights the strong relationship of the clinician's knowledge, cognition (e.g. data analysis and synthesis processes) and metacognition (i.e. awareness, self-monitoring, reflective processes) within the process of clinical reasoning. Double-headed arrows are used to convey that these factors influence all aspects of the clinical reasoning process and in turn

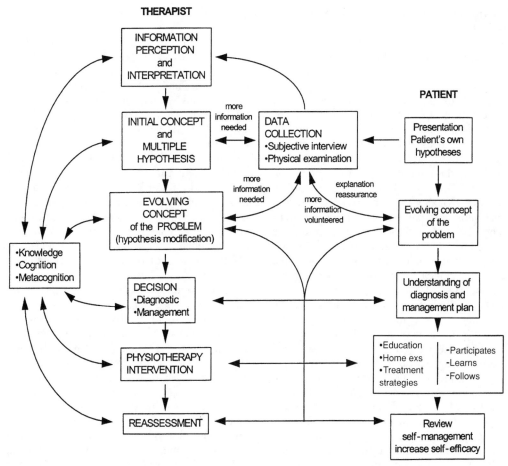

Figure 12.1 Collaborative clinical-reasoning process

are strengthened by clinical reasoning experience, particularly when clinicians think or reflect about what they do during and after a clinical encounter. Many clinicians, however, will be unaware of their use of these processes. They may reason through a problem without recognizing the various aspects of their reasoning. They may also have reached a stage where a systematic process of reasoning is no longer used for many problems, because past experience has enabled them to identify problems and treatments quickly. While awareness and understanding of one's clinical reasoning is not essential to clinical practice, it is our view that by promoting awareness, reflection and critical appraisal, clinical reasoning can be enhanced.

Clinical reasoning models such as the one described here need further investigation to establish their validity in relation to actual practice, and to identify how clinical reasoning differs between expert (highly effective and efficient managers of patient problems) and non-expert clinicians. Chapter 1 in this book presents a spiral analogy to further portray the integrated aspects of clinical reasoning which occur dynamically at varying process levels. The value of any conceptual model of clinical reasoning is to promote consideration, awareness and further exploration of the inherent elements of the process and the significance such a process has for patient care. At a time when some educators in physiotherapy are teaching and applying practice routines and protocols without adequate critical analysis and reflection, conceptual models of clinical reasoning that emphasize knowledge and professional judgement, make the less considered cognitive processes associated with those judgements more accessible, while challenging researchers, educators and clinicians to investigate, facilitate and strive to improve their clinical reasoning.

Hypothetico-deductive reasoning or pattern recognition

Physiotherapy research in clinical reasoning provides some evidence that similarity exists, at least at a broad level, with clinical reasoning in medicine (Payton, 1985; Thomas-Edding, 1987). While the process of clinical reasoning in medicine is still being studied and clarified, it appears to involve a process of hypothesis generation followed by either hypothesis evaluation (e.g. hypothesis testing) and/or pattern recognition (Barrows and Feltovich, 1987; Patel and Groen, 1986, 1991). Whether hypothesis testing (backward reasoning) or pattern recognition (forward reasoning) is used will depend in part on the clinician's level of practical experience, knowledge and method of education, as well as on the nature of the clinical task itself (Arocha *et al.*, 1993; Patel *et al.*, 1991).

Clinical reasoning in physiotherapy should similarly involve a combination of hypothesis testing and pattern recognition. Pattern recognition is required to generate hypotheses and hypothesis testing provides the means by which patterns are refined and proved reliable. However, this description may seem to over-simplify what occurs when clinicians are faced with complex, uncertain problem situations where physiotherapy management requires personal involvement (e.g. physical, emotional, social) in the patient's treatment. Problems often do not fit textbook presentations, and clinical rules of thumb do not always apply. Nor do all clinicians subscribe to the same rules. To better understand the way in which clinical patterns are acquired and the nature of clinical patterns relevant to physiotherapy, key factors including knowledge, cognitive skills and context are considered in the following section.

Key factors in clinical reasoning: considerations for physiotherapy

Clinical reasoning is influenced by factors relating to the specific task, the setting, the patient or client and the decision maker. For purposes of this discussion we will highlight certain critical aspects of those factors pertaining to the decision maker, including the knowledge base for decisions, the therapist's cognitive skills and assessment of context.

Knowledge

Elstein *et al.* (1978) found that clinical problem solving expertise varied greatly across cases and was dependent on clinicians' knowledge in particular areas. This finding highlighted the importance of clinicians' organization of knowledge rather than the process of reasoning which has been emphasized throughout the literature (e.g. Arocha *et al*, 1993; Bordage and Lemieux, 1991; Patel and Groen, 1986; Schmidt and Boshuizen, 1993). This view is exemplified by Custers *et al.* (1993, p. 3) who stated, 'for it is not the way problems are tackled, nor the thoroughness of the investigation, nor the use of problem solving strategies, but the ability to activate the pertinent knowledge as a consequence of situational demands, which distinguishes experienced from inexperienced physicians'.

In physiotherapy, Hislop (1985, p. 29) concurred that 'clinical decisions are based on knowledge readily understood, readily recalled and commonly encountered'. She cautioned that as therapists we must not allow the formidable growth of knowledge to subvert our interest in patients themselves. We must be critical of knowledge, and keep in perspective what we need to know versus what is nice, marginal or irrelevant to know (Hislop, 1985). One way to tackle this task is to consider what knowledge physiotherapists use for their evaluation and management of patients. Physiotherapists utilize various forms of knowledge in their clinical reasoning. These include basic science and biomedical knowledge, clinical knowledge (often in the form of recognized clinical patterns, 'if/then' rules of action and clinical procedures), everyday knowledge about life and social interactions, and tacit knowledge of the profession.

Procedural knowledge is not just recall of information but a transformation of information, requiring critical analysis and deliberate action (Cervero, 1988). The clinician must be able to critically analyse or recognize the situation in order to arrive at and apply the appropriate 'if/then' guides to action. Cervero (1988) emphasized that both *declarative* (e.g. theoretical, biomedical) knowledge ('knowing that') and *procedural* knowledge ('knowing how') are required for skilled performance and sound clinical reasoning. It is through reflective practice that declarative and procedural knowledge are transformed into clinical knowledge. Important to our ability to characterize the clinical reasoning of physiotherapists is the contention that in any field, a major difference between experts and non-experts is that experts have far more clinical knowledge (Cervero, 1988). Declarative knowledge initially provides the data to guide action. However, with experience and repetition clinicians are able to perform without having to access declarative knowledge in familiar cases. It is of educational importance that clinical knowledge is acquired predominantly through direct practical experience. That is, knowledge is made particularly meaningful and accessible when it is created or acquired in the context for which it must be used (Jensen *et al.*, 1999; Schön, 1987; Shepard and Jensen, 1990).

Similarly, Schön (1987) contended that the use of research-based knowledge does not differentiate the expert from the non-expert. Instead, Schön described three types of procedural knowledge that are inherent in professional expertise, 'knowing-in-action', 'reflection-in-action' and 'reflection-about-action'. Most spontaneous actions that professionals take are not elicited by a rule or plan that was consciously in the mind before acting (Cervero, 1988). Schön refers to this phenomenon as 'knowing-in-action'. That is, the actions, recognitions and judgements of professionals are often a function of their tacit knowledge, sometimes called intuition (Benner, 1984). Reflection-in-action refers to thinking about what you are doing while you do it. It is exemplified when the clinician encounters a problem and engages in a process of critical analysis that allows for self-correction or adaptation of practice. It is typically used in situations of uncertainty or when unexpected results are obtained. Reflection-about-action is a similar process that occurs retrospectively as the clinician thinks back about what happened in practice. Clinical reasoning that is reflective will eventually lead to recognition of patterns hidden within the ambiguity of the presentation or to the acquisition of new patterns not previously appreciated.

Cognitive skills

Along with the different forms of knowledge associated with decision making, cognitive skills (e.g. data analysis and synthesis and inquiry strategies) are essential for professionals. Practitioners must be able to identify and solve problems in ambiguous or uncertain situations (Barrows and Feltovich, 1987; Elstein *et al.*, 1990; Kennedy, 1987). In physiotherapy there is a growing interest in students' awareness, learning and development of cognitive skills (e.g. Higgs, 1992; Hislop, 1985; Jones, 1992; Shepard and Jensen, 1990). While

clinical expertise has been linked more to the clinician's organization of knowledge than the process of clinical reasoning used (see above), cognitive skills and knowledge are interdependent. For example, the inquiry strategy of hypothesis testing (including confirming and disconfirming strategies) plays a significant role in the acquisition of knowledge (Lawson *et al.*, 1991). While the expert may not need to engage in hypothesis testing with all problems, it provides the means by which textbook clinical patterns can be tested, refined and new patterns can be learned (Barrows and Feltovich, 1987). Novices, who lack sufficient knowledge to recognize clinical patterns, will rely on the slower hypothesis testing approach to work through a problem, where experienced clinicians are able to function more on pattern recognition. When confronted with a complex, unfamiliar problem, however, the expert, like the novice, will rely more on the hypothetico-deductive method of clinical reasoning (Barrows and Feltovich, 1987; Patel and Groen, 1991).

Errors in clinical reasoning are frequently related to errors in cognition. Examples of these include overemphasis on findings which support an existing hypothesis, misinterpretation of non-contributory information as confirming an existing hypothesis, rejection of findings which do not support a favoured hypothesis, and incorrect interpretation related to inappropriately applied inductive and deductive logic (Elstein *et al.*, 1978; Jones, 1992; Ramsden, 1985). An example of a cognitive error in data analysis and synthesis was demonstrated by Norman *et al.* (1992). These researchers demonstrated that both expert and resident radiologists could be biased to alter their disease probability ratings and reports of symptomatic features identified in both normal and abnormal films when the history was manipulated to bias toward a positive result. Bordage and colleagues suggest that most diagnostic errors are not the result of inadequate medical knowledge as much as an inability to retrieve relevant knowledge already stored in memory (Bordage and Allen, 1982; Bordage and Lemieux, 1991). Cognitive errors may contribute to the development of poorly organized knowledge. Thus any consideration of clinical reasoning in physiotherapy must incorporate attention to cognitive skills.

Context and the construction of meaning

An important distinction has been made by medical anthropology in differentiating between the biomedical entity of disease and the meaning-centred (or phenomenological) entity of illness experience (Kleinman, 1988). The presence of these entities in a patient presentation form a continuum of experience from the biomedical to the phenomenological poles: the world of the patient, as it were.

Physiotherapists, in dealing with their patients (or clients), need to be able to traverse and explore the terrain between these two poles, to be able to comprehend this world of the patient. According to Schön (1987, p. 3), there is a dilemma confronting professional practice between the 'high, hard ground of technical rationality' and 'the swampy lowland, messy, (where) confusing problems defy technical solution'. Technical rationality holds to a view of professional knowledge where 'practitioners are instrumental problem solvers' (Schön, 1987, p. 3), who through well selected technical and scientific means solve discrete, well-defined problems. Schön argues that the problems of actual professional practice present as complex and indeterminate situations, often with a quality of uniqueness about them.

Consider the scenario of maintenance or recurrence of pain in a long-standing shoulder problem. This pain may be judged to be a result of acquired incompetency of shoulder and/or scapular stabilizing muscles. In turn, it could be hypothesized that this poor muscle function, rather than being a result of inhibition in response to tissue damage (as at the time of injury), may be attributable to longer term disuse or central nervous system-driven maladaptive movement patterns, as a consequence of attitudinal factors such as loss of confidence or fear of further aggravation. These factors may have their genesis in other contributing factors such as depression about not being able to perform normal work, home duties or recreational pursuits, leading in turn to possible alterations in self-image and/or an increased pain experience for the patient. The normal equilibrium of relationships at home, socially or at work may be disturbed by a change in function or role on the part of the patient, resulting in altered attitudes and behaviour, further feeding back into and influencing the illness or pain experience. If one adds into this situation hypotheses of other possible influences such as age, educational and socio-economic levels (affecting employability) or ethnicity with particular personal values and belief systems, then the chronic shoulder problem is clearly multifactorial with the meaning for the patient constructed in

complexity. The extent to which these hypotheses are generated, from the inactivity of muscle through to personal and cultural beliefs, is a function of the therapist's ability to attribute meaning to the information being received. If the construction of meaning is not part of the therapist's inquiry and interaction with the patient, then critical hypotheses related to management and outcome may remain either unelicited or 'on the table', as it were, but not understood.

As important as this process of understanding patients in their world is in diagnostic terms, it is also vital to the wider interests of clinical practice. In physiotherapy, therapists are asking their patients to be active participants; to both learn and practice exercises, to understand and follow certain recommendations regarding movement techniques and postures in work, sport and other activities of daily life, and through these activities to work towards a goal or set of goals negotiated between patient and therapist. This orientation represents a genuine engagement of the patient in the therapeutic process, and achieving this collaboration requires a broader understanding and application of clinical reasoning than that associated with diagnosis alone.

The scope and organization of clinical reasoning in physiotherapy

Earlier physiotherapy research reflects the dominant influence of the medically developed model of reasoning, either through observation of its practitioners' reasoning as similar to that of physicians or by describing clinical reasoning in terms of being primarily a diagnostic process (Payton, 1985; Thomas-Edding, 1987). While it is important for physiotherapists to engage in diagnostic reasoning (Dekker *et al.*, 1993; Rose, 1989), subsequent physiotherapy literature (e.g. Jones, 1992) and further research (Beeston and Simons, 1996; Edwards *et al.*, in preparation; Embrey *et al.*, 1996; Jensen *et al.*, 1992) have both recognized and shown that clinical reasoning occurs in areas of physiotherapy practice outside of diagnosis. For example, in their qualitative study on the differentiating features of master and novice clinicians in orthopaedic settings, Jensen *et al.* (1992) reported that expert clinicians not only collected data related to pathology that helped validate or invalidate a diagnosis, but also gathered illness data which reflected how the patients' perceptions of their problem affected their lives. Similarly, an expert neurological physiotherapist in Beeston and Simons' (1996) interpretive study of the perspectives of expert therapists on their clinical practice, expressed a major approach to her work thus (Beeston and Simons, 1996, p. 236):

> I used to look at it much more from what their problem was in terms of spasticity or tight muscles or difficulty sitting or things, whereas now I'm much more aware of how it's affecting the patient's family; then themselves, and the implications . . . what sort of person are they? . . . what are they going back to?

It could be argued from observations such as these that clinical reasoning in physiotherapy is still essentially diagnostic in nature; that the information above represents merely a definition or understanding of diagnosis which is wider than that which deals exclusively with tissue derangement and pathology as the source of symptoms and/or dysfunction. In recent qualitative research in physiotherapy, Edwards *et al.* (in preparation) identified different patterns of clinical reasoning in expert physiotherapists in three different fields of physiotherapy (manipulative/orthopaedic, neurological and domiciliary care). They found that domiciliary care physiotherapists generated and tested hypotheses in aspects such as stressors affecting carers of patients. Pattern recognition in terms of recognizable carer behaviour was also demonstrated by the therapists. These can be considered forms of diagnosis. However, the same study also found that individual expert therapists in all three fields employed a range of clinical-reasoning strategies. These clinical reasoning strategies can be considered to be particular organizations of clinical reasoning (lines of inquiry, styles of dialogue or specific foci of thinking) related to various but specific activities of clinical practice:

- Positive and purposeful interaction with the patient.
- Accurate diagnostic assessment and treatment procedures.
- Collaborative decision making with the patient.
- Teaching of the patient on a number of different levels.
- Reliable prediction of outcomes including the provision of management or self-management options for the future.
- Recollection and purposeful use of patient stories, both recent and past, to further understand and manage a clinical situation.

- Engagement with and resolution of factors or circumstances (either moral, ethical or practical including economic) which impinge upon a particular therapist–patient treatment encounter or clinical practice in general.

The clinical reasoning strategies observed in the clinical practice of the expert therapists in the three fields of physiotherapy correspond with various clinical reasoning strategies which have been identified either by research, by theoretical proposition or by an exposition of the relevant skills in the literature of nursing, occupational therapy and physiotherapy. These are diagnostic or procedural reasoning (Fleming, 1991; Jones, 1988; Payton, 1985), interactive reasoning (Fleming, 1991), conditional or predictive reasoning (Fleming, 1991; Hagedorn, 1996), narrative reasoning (Benner *et al.*, 1992; Mattingly, 1991), pragmatic reasoning (Schell and Cervero, 1993) and ethical reasoning (Barnitt and Partridge, 1997; Gordon *et al.*, 1994; Neuhaus, 1988), teaching as reasoning (Sluijs, 1991a), and collaborative decision making (Beeston and Simons, 1996; Jensen *et al.*, in press; Mattingly and Hayes Fleming, 1994; Payton and Nelson, 1996). While these applications of reasoning are not mutually exclusive, they offer a conceptual framework to assist therapists' appraisal of their reasoning.

Diagnostic reasoning is that most familiar reasoning which aims at revealing the patient's disability and associated impairments, the underlying pain mechanisms, structures at fault, pathophysiology, and certain factors contributing to the development and maintenance of the dysfunction. Further possible contributing factors may be elicited in concert with other clinical reasoning strategies. Allied and closely related to diagnostic reasoning is *procedural reasoning,* which refers more to decision making in treatment, such as choosing one treatment technique over another, and to the intensity or frequency with which that particular treatment is carried out and then progressed. This reasoning is important since physiotherapists are not technicians carrying out set, unvarying treatments for specific conditions (although decision making may still take place at times within set treatment protocols).

Interactive reasoning occurs as positive and purposeful interaction between therapist and patient. Often appearing as social exchange, this interaction is used to build rapport and increase the therapist's understanding of the patient. It is more than the therapist being pleasant to the patient.

Whether it is the use of humour, general conversation or self-disclosure on the part of the therapist, this socializing provides an effective means of better understanding the context in which the patient's problem exists. Expert therapists vary their form of interaction according to the cues given by the patient (Jensen *et al.*, 1992).

Collaborative reasoning refers to the shared decision making between therapist and patient. Here the patient's opinions as well as information about the problem are valued and utilized. As patients' involvement in the therapeutic process is welcomed and encouraged, their capacity to contribute to this process increases through an enhanced understanding of their own problem and its proposed solutions (Jones, 1995). This form of reasoning is consistent with notions of patient responsibility and self-management.

Teaching as reasoning occurs in clinical practice on many levels, from the provision of simple advice from therapist to patient, to skill building or acquisition in any number of movement techniques or situations requiring muscle control, to situations such as counselling patients in modifying lifestyle (Sluijs, 1991a). In each of these situations the therapist makes judgements concerning the level and amount of teaching which is appropriate for an individual patient and the mode of delivery which is most suitable and likely to be accepted by the patient. Finally, the understanding of what has been taught must be assessed (Sluijs, 1991b). All this requires a reasoned response on the part of the therapist to the cues provided by the patient.

Predictive reasoning is employed by the therapist firstly to envisage and then to inform the patient of the estimated response to management and the implications for the patient of that likely outcome. Depending on the prognosis, the therapist may outline various options or courses of action available to the patient. These future scenarios are based not only on issues such as tissue healing and response to treatment, but on a weighting and synthesizing by the therapist of other factors in the psychological, social, work and/or recreational profile of the patient (Edwards *et al.*, in preparation).

Ethical/pragmatic reasoning involves the therapist wrestling with and coming to a resolution (what one might term 'urgent reflection' at times!) of those factors or circumstances which can impinge upon a particular therapist–patient treatment encounter or clinical practice in general. These factors which are external to the treatment encounter but affect the clinical reasoning therein become part of the clinical reasoning process itself (Schell and Cervero, 1993).

Narrative reasoning entails the recollection and purposeful use of patient stories, both recent and past, to further understand and manage a clinical situation. These stories, which emanate from memories of particular patients or treatments, may be told for different reasons. At certain times they reflect powerful lessons learned through negative or positive experiences in therapists' clinical practice. Such stories appear to encapsulate knowledge gained through clinical practice which significantly influences subsequent practice (Benner *et al.*, 1992). At other times, specifically chosen patient or treatment stories may be employed (in a confidential manner) in the context of interaction with the patient or for the purpose of teaching, predicting or illustrating an aspect of diagnosis or management (Edwards *et al.*, in preparation). There remains some debate about the nature of narrative reasoning (Mattingly and Fleming, 1994; Roberts, 1996) and whether it is a clinical reasoning process which is essentially different to hypothetico-deductive reasoning. Regardless of any conclusions which may arise from such a debate, the real contribution of narrative reasoning lies in its appeal to therapists to understand and be engaged in the unique 'story' or presentation of each patient, even when such a presentation has features which can be recognized or recalled from previous cases.

It is contended here that in each of these reasoning strategies the therapist is able to recognize the relevant cues (behavioural, psychological, social, cultural and environmental) and their significance and relationship. Then either confirmation of familiar, recognized clinical patterns or the generation and testing of hypotheses occurs in each area.

Like all good clinical reasoning, the clinical reasoning strategies described above are instrumental in the generation of further clinical knowledge; knowledge which informs and influences future clinical practice. For example, the process of ethical/pragmatic reasoning may be set in train because of a particular treatment situation: an instance such as the inability of an uninsured patient to afford the intensity of physiotherapy treatment which the therapist considers appropriate. Solutions to this dilemma, such as reconsideration of fee structure, or a different and greater emphasis on teaching the patient and carer treatment or self-management techniques, or providing open telephone access for the patient to contact and discuss questions or difficulties, or some combination of measures, add to the overall clinical repertoire of the therapist. Ethical/pragmatic reasoning achieves this not only by stimulating reflection on the therapist's underlying philosophy of practice, but by broadening understanding of the relevant issues and the repertoire of possible solutions for future situations.

Clinical reasoning strategies represent a means of applying and organizing clinical reasoning principles to the wide range of activities, both diagnostic and non-diagnostic, which make up clinical practice. It appears that these strategies are applicable to the many settings in which physiotherapists work (Edwards *et al.*, in preparation). And yet, as one considers the many different settings in which physiotherapists work, in the hospital ward or the community health centre; in the private clinic or the patient's home' or the sporting field or the factory floor, it is evident that the clinical skills and knowledge required are both vast and diverse. Technical skills apart, particular cultural, social and personal knowledge and understanding are required, together with diagnostic, teaching, collaborative, listening and counselling skills for each setting.

If clinical reasoning strategies can help in the organization of clinical reasoning for the various tasks in clinical practice, it is also important to consider how the clinical knowledge generated in and belonging to each of these settings is organized and thus made more explicit and accessible. There are implications for the teaching of students and inexperienced practitioners alike in each setting. Identification and organization of such knowledge would provide a framework from which experts in each field can share their clinical knowledge and insights, and through which existing clinical patterns can be questioned and new patterns learned.

This question of the way in which specialty knowledge is organized has been addressed is in the area of manual physiotherapy. Jones (1992) proposed that inquiries and clinical decisions made in manual therapy could be broadly categorized into discrete but related areas of information termed hypothesis categories. While diagnostic hypotheses are most easily recognized, other categories of hypothesis have also been proposed (Gifford, 1997; Gifford and Butler, 1997; Jones *et al.*, 1994) including:

- Dysfunction/disability (physical or psychological and the associated social consequences).
- Pathobiological mechanisms.

- Source of symptoms or dysfunction (often equated with diagnosis or impairment).
- Contributing factors.
- Precautions and contraindications.
- Prognosis.
- Management.

Identifying the most effective course of management in manual therapy requires reasoning about each of these hypothesis categories (Jones, 1992). Therapists recognize patient cues which in turn elicit hypotheses in one or more categories. Clinical patterns exist within all the hypothesis categories. As patient cues emerge and specific hypotheses are considered, the hypotheses should be tested for the remaining features of the pattern through further patient inquiry, physical tests and ultimately with the physiotherapy intervention. Although the concepts are still evolving, subsequent research (Rivett and Higgs, 1997) has validated the use of these hypotheses in the clinical practice of manipulative physiotherapists.

Thus the notion of clinical reasoning strategies, as a way of organizing the tasks of clinical practice, is complemented by the notion of hypothesis categories as a means of organizing the clinical knowledge required for those tasks. Other emerging knowledge, both theoretical and research based, can be included in this organization.

Regardless of any propositional or working conceptual models which may be elaborated to explain or teach clinical reasoning, clinical reasoning without self-monitoring and reflection on the part of the therapist is sterile. That is, assessment and treatment 'rules' and procedures may be followed correctly but remain unfruitful. This impasse is especially likely to occur in complex or ambiguous patient presentations, 'the swampy lowland . . . (where) confusing problems defy technical solution' of which Schön (1987, p. 3) speaks. These are precisely the indeterminate situations in which the experience and insights of experienced, senior and/ or expert clinicians are often called upon.

To grow in expertise, professionals need self-monitoring skills in order to plan, control and evaluate problem-solving knowledge and methods (Hassebrock *et al.*, 1993), while reflection is critical if practitioners are to learn from experience. While some clinicians learn little or nothing from their own experience, instead relying on literature and continuing education to acquire new information, others continually revise and expand their clinical knowledge through their reflective approach to patient care.

Conclusion

While a growing interest in physiotherapy clinical reasoning exists amongst physiotherapy clinicians and educators, physiotherapy research in clinical reasoning is still limited. This chapter has presented a conceptual model of clinical reasoning, describing research from both within and outside physiotherapy. An evolving model of clinical reasoning in physiotherapy has been described, that is broadly depicted as hypothetico-deductive, with consideration being given to the patient's entire illness or pain experience. This is particularly important in a profession like physiotherapy where clinicians are personally (physically, professionally, emotionally and socially) involved in the treatment. Clinicians must attend to and search for cues, both diagnostic (suggesting source and cause of the patient's impairment) and non-diagnostic (suggesting psychological, social and cultural aspects of the patient's problem), in order to arrive at management decisions that attend holistically to all relevant aspects of the individual's health. This process requires a highly advanced organization of both theoretical and clinical knowledge, and sound cognitive skills. Clinical reasoning strategies then serve as a means of organizing the tasks of clinical practice. In order to produce thinking therapists who have this phenomenological approach to patients, self-monitoring reflective skills are needed to complement a hypothetico-deductive method of clinical reasoning.

Acknowledgement

The authors would like to acknowledge the contribution of Jules Rothestein to the first edition of this chapter.

References

Arocha, J. F., Patel, V. L. and Patel, Y. C. (1993) Hypothesis generation and the coordination of theory and evidence in novice diagnostic reasoning. *Medical Decision Making*, **13**, 198–211.

Barnitt, R. and Partridge, C. (1997) Ethical reasoning in physical therapy and occupational therapy. *Physiotherapy Research International*, **2**, 178–192.

Barrows, H. S. and Feltovich, P. J. (1987) The clinical reasoning process. *Medical Education*, **21**, 86–91.

Beeston, S. and Simons, H. (1996) Physiotherapy practice: Practitioners' perspectives. *Physiotherapy Theory and Practice*, **12**, 231–242.

Benner, P. (1984) *From Novice to Expert: Excellence and Power in Clinical Nursing Practice*. Menlo Park, CA: Addison-Wesley.

Benner, P., Tanner, C. and Chesla, C. (1992) From beginner to expert: Gaining a differentiated clinical world in critical care nursing. *Advanced Nursing Science*, **14**, 13–28.

Bordage G. and Allen, T. (1982) The etiology of diagnostic errors: Process or content? An exploratory study. In *Proceedings of the 21st Annual Conference of Research in Medical Education*, pp. 171–176. Washington, DC: American Association of Medical Colleges.

Bordage, G. and Lemieux, R. (1991) Semantic structures and diagnostic thinking of experts and novices. *Academic Medicine*, **66**, S70–S72.

Borkan, J. M., Quirk, M. and Sullivan, M. (1991) Finding meaning after the fall: Injury narratives from elderly hip fracture patients. *Social Science and Medicine*, **33**, 947–957.

Cervero, R. M. (1988) *Effective Continuing Education for Professionals*. San Francisco: Jossey-Bass.

Custers, E. J. F. M., Boshuizen, H. P. A. and Schmidt, H. G. (1993) The influence of typicality of case descriptions on subjective disease probability estimations. Paper presented at the *Annual Meeting of the American Educational Research Association*, Atlanta, GA.

Dekker, J., van Baar, M. E., Chr Curfs, E. and Kerssens, J. J. (1993) Diagnosis and treatment in physical therapy: An investigation of their relationship. *Physical Therapy*, **73**, 10–22.

Edwards, I. C., Jones, M. A., Carr, J. and Jensen, G. (**in preparation**) Clinical reasoning in three different fields of physiotherapy: A qualitative study.

Elstein, A. S., Shulman, L. S. and Sprafka, S. S. (1978) *Medical Problem Solving: An Analysis of Clinical Reasoning*. Cambridge, MA: Harvard University Press.

Elstein, A. S., Shulman, L. S. and Sprafka, S. A. (1990) Medical problem solving: A ten year retrospective. *Evaluation and the Health Professions*, **13**, 5–36.

Embrey, D. G., Guthrie, M. R., White, O. R. and Dietz, J. (1996) Clinical decision making by experienced and inexperienced pediatric physical therapists for children with diplegic cerebral palsy. *Physical Therapy*, **76**, 20–33.

Feuerstein, M. and Beattie, P. (1995) Biobehavioral factors affecting pain and disability in low back pain: Mechanisms and assessment. *Physical Therapy*, **75**, 267–280.

Fleming, M. H. (1991) The therapist with the three track mind. *The American Journal of Occupational Therapy*, **45**, 1007–1014.

Gifford, L. S. (1997) Pain. In *Rehabilitation of Movement: Theoretical Bases of Clinical Practice* (J. Pitt-Brooke with H. Reid, J. Lockwood and K. Kerr, eds), pp. 196–232. London: Saunders.

Gifford, L. S. and Butler, D. (1997) The integration of pain sciences into clinical practice. *Journal of Hand Therapy*, **10**, 86–95.

Gordon, M., Murphy, C. P., Candee, D. and Hiltunen, E. (1994) Clinical judgement: An integrated model. *Advances in Nursing Science*, **16**, 55–70.

Hagedorn, R. (1996) Clinical decision making in familiar cases: A model of the process and implications for practice. *British Journal of Occupational Therapy*, **59**, 217–222.

Hassebrock, F., Jonas, A. P. and Bauer, L. (1993) Metacognitive aspects of medical problem solving. Paper presented to the *Annual Meeting of the American Educational Research Association*, Atlanta, GA.

Higgs, J. (1992) Developing knowledge: A process of construction mapping and review. *New Zealand Journal of Physiotherapy*, **20**, 23–30.

Hislop, H. J. (1985) Clinical decision making: Educational, data, and risk factors. In *Clinical Decision Making in Physical Therapy* (S. L. Wolf, ed.), pp. 25–60. Philadelphia, PA: F. A. Davis.

Jensen, G. M., Shepard, K. F. and Hack, L. M. (1992) Attribute dimensions that distinguish master and novice physical therapy clinicians in orthopedic settings. *Physical Therapy*, **72**, 711–722.

Jensen, G. M., Gwyer, J., Shepard, K. F. and Hack, L. M. (1999) *Expertise in Physical Therapy Practice*. Boston, MA: Butterworth-Heinemann.

Jones, J. A. (1988) Clinical reasoning in nursing. *Journal of Advanced Nursing*, **13**, 185–192.

Jones, M. A. (1992) Clinical reasoning in manual therapy. *Physical Therapy*, **72**, 875–884.

Jones, M. A. (1995) Clinical reasoning and pain. *Manual Therapy*, **1**, 17–24.

Jones, M. A., Christensen, N. and Carr, J. (1994) Clinical reasoning in upper quadrant dysfunction. In *Physical Therapy for the Cervical and Thoracic Spine*, 2nd edn (R. Grant, ed.), pp. 89–108. New York: Churchill Livingstone.

Kennedy, M. (1987) Inexact sciences: Professional education and the development of expertise. *Review of Research in Education*, **14**, 133–168.

Kleinman, A. (1988) *The Illness Narratives: Suffering, Healing and the Human Condition*. New York: Basic Books.

Lawson, A. E., McElrath, C. B., Burton, M. S., James, B. D., Doyle, R. P., Woodward, S. L., Kellerman, L. and Snyder, J. D. (1991) Hypothetico-deductive reasoning skill and concept acquisition: Testing a constructivist hypothesis. *Journal of Research in Science Teaching*, **28**, 953–970.

Malt, U. F. and Olafson, O. M. (1995) Psychological appraisal and emotional response to physical injury: A clinical, phenomenological study of 109 adults. *Psychiatric Medicine*, **10**, 117–134.

Mattingly, C. (1991) The narrative nature of clinical reasoning. *The American Journal of Occupational Therapy*, **45**, 998–1005.

Mattingly, C. and Hayes Fleming, M. (1994) *Clinical Reasoning: Forms of inquiry in a therapeutic practice*. Philadelphia, PA: F. A. Davis.

Neuhaus, B. E. (1988) Ethical considerations in clinical reasoning: The impact of technology and cost containment. *The American Journal of Occupational Therapy*, **42**, 288–294.

Norman, G. R., Brooks, L. R., Coblentz, C. L. and Babcock, C. J. (1992) The correlation of feature identification and category judgments in diagnostic radiology. *Memory and Cognition*, **20**, 344–355.

Patel, V. L. and Groen, G. J. (1986) Knowledge-based solution strategies in medical reasoning. *Journal of Cognitive Science*, **10**, 91–108.

Patel, V. L. and Groen, G. J. (1991) The general and specific nature of medical expertise: A critical look. In *Toward a General Theory of Expertise: Prospects and Limits* (A. Ericsson and J. Smith, eds), pp. 93–125. New York: Cambridge University Press.

Patel, V. L., Groen, G. J. and Norman, G. R. (1991) Effects of conventional and problem-based medical curricula on problem solving. *Academic Medicine*, **66**, 380–389.

Payton, O. D. (1985) Clinical reasoning process in physical therapy. *Physical Therapy*, **65**, 924–928.

Payton, O. D. and Nelson, C. E. (1996) A preliminary study of patients' perceptions of certain aspects of their physical therapy experience. *Physiotherapy Theory and Practice*, **12**, 27–38.

Ramsden, E. L. (1985) Basis for clinical decision making: Perception of the patient, the clinician's role, and responsibility. In *Clinical Decision Making in Physical Therapy* (S. L. Wolf, ed.), pp. 25–60. Philadelphia, PA: F. A. Davis.

Rivett, D. and Higgs, J. (1997) Hypothesis generation in the clinical reasoning behavior of manual therapists. *Journal of Physical Therapy Education*, **11**, 40–45.

Roberts, A. E. (1996) Approaches to reasoning in occupational therapy: A critical exploration. *British Journal of Occupational Therapy*, **59**, 233–236.

Rose, S. J. (1989) Physical therapy diagnosis: Role and function. *Physical Therapy*, **69**, 535–537.

Schell, B. A. and Cervero, R. M. (1993) Clinical reasoning in occupational therapy: An integrative review. *The American Journal of Occupational Therapy*, **47**, 605–610.

Schmidt, H. G. and Boshuizen, H. P. A. (1993) On acquiring expertise in medicine. *Educational Psychology Review*, **5**, 205–221.

Schön, D. (1987) *Educating the Reflective Practitioner*. San Francisco: Jossey-Bass.

Shepard, K. F. and Jensen, G. M. (1990) Physical therapist curricula for the 1990s: Educating the reflective practitioner. *Physical Therapy*, **70**, 566–577.

Shepard, K. F., Jensen, G. M., Schmoll, B. J., Hack, L. M. and Gwyer, J. (1993) Alternative approaches to research in physical therapy: Positivism and phenomenology. *Physical Therapy*, **73**, 88–101.

Sluijs, E. M. (1991a) Patient education in physiotherapy: towards a planned approach. *Physiotherapy*, **77**:503–508.

Sluijs, E. M. (1991b) A checklist to assess patient education in physical therapy practice: development and reliability. *Physiotherapy*, **71**, 561–569.

Thomas-Edding, D. (1987) Clinical problem solving in physical therapy and its implications for curriculum development. In *Proceedings of the Tenth International Congress of the World Confederation for Physical Therapy*, May 17–22, Sydney, pp. 100–104. World Confederation for Physical Therapy.

13

Clinical reasoning in occupational therapy

Chris Chapparo and Judy Ranka

Occupational therapy practice is undergoing evolution, particularly in recent years. Occupational therapy service provision has extended from medically based institutions to a variety of community, educational and social service agencies, and private practice. Demands of consumer groups, expectation of documentation, the need for accountability of services and government intervention in service delivery have made an impact on every therapist. Within this context occupational therapists have a mandate to develop and implement therapy programs aimed at promoting maximum levels of independence in life skills and optimal quality of life. The process of occupational therapy in this context consists of problem solving under conditions of uncertainty and change (Mattingly and Fleming, 1994; Rogers and Masagatani, 1982). The therapist collects, classifies and analyses information about client ability and life situation, and then uses the data to define client problems, goals and treatment focus. The fundamental process involved is clinical reasoning.

The importance of clinical reasoning in occupational therapy is clearly established (Mattingly and Fleming, 1994; Parham, 1987; Rogers, 1983). However, many elements of the content and process of reasoning still require further investigation. Several questions remain unanswered. What personal and contextual elements are involved with making clinical judgements? How do therapists combine science, practical knowledge and their personal commitments to make clinical decisions? What is the range of elements involved in making clinical judgements? Why are clinical decisions made the way they are?

The purpose of this chapter is to describe clinical reasoning in occupational therapy as it is portrayed in existing literature and by occupational therapy scholars researching the area. We examine clinical reasoning from three perspectives. First, an historical perspective of clinical reasoning in occupational therapy is outlined, and parallels with the development of the profession are drawn. Second, elements of therapist knowledge that have been found to influence the process of reasoning and ultimately determine occupational therapy action are examined. Third, alternative notions about the process of thinking that results in clinical decision making in occupational therapy are explored.

Clinical reasoning: an historical perspective

Throughout the development of the occupational therapy profession, elements of what is termed clinical reasoning have been referred to as treatment planning (Day, 1973; Pelland, 1987), the evaluative process (Hemphill, 1982), clinical thinking (Line, 1969), a subset of the occupational therapy process (Christiansen and Baum, 1997) and problem solving (Hopkins and Tiffany, 1988). The clinical-reasoning process has recently been described as a largely tacit, highly imagistic and deeply phenomenological mode of thinking, 'aimed at determining 'the good' for each particular client'(Mattingly and Fleming, 1994, p.13), 'thinking about thinking' (Schell, 1998, p. 90), and an example of behavioural intention that is based on salient beliefs, attitudes and expectancies held by the therapist (Chapparo, 1997). Current descriptions and definitions of clinical reasoning have been influenced by the diverse nature and goals of occupational therapy practice, the philosophy of the profession itself and the various epistemologies held by individual researchers. A brief review of the development of the profession illustrates how its history has influenced various reasoning strategies in current practice as well as the methods that have been employed for studying them.

Beliefs, values and humanism

Occupational therapy was founded on humanistic values (Meyer, 1922; Slagle, 1922; Yerxa, 1991). The view of occupation that was accepted by the profession early in its development centred around the relationship between health and the ability to organize the temporal, physical and social elements of daily living (Breines, 1990; Keilhofner, 1992). This view of occupation and occupational therapy treatment was influenced by theories and beliefs of the Moral Treatment movement of the 18th and 19th centuries (Harvey-Krefting, 1985) which acknowledged people's basic right to humane treatment (Pinel, 1948). A client-centred philosophy evolved which placed emphasis on the rights of all people to develop the skills and habits required for a balanced, wholesome life (Shannon, 1977).

The profession subscribed to a belief in the unity of mind and body in action, and developed a philosophical approach to health through active occupation (Breines, 1990). Influential in the creation of treatment principles was a thinking mode described by pragmatic theorist, John Dewey (1910), who claimed that actions of professionals depended on a unique mental analysis that sought to obtain an understanding of the significance and meaning in a person's everyday life. The criteria for judging this significance, meaning and worth were practical, largely arbitrary, qualitative rather than quantitative, non-specialized and purposive (Stanage, 1987). Clinical reasoning of the time took the form of commonsense inquiry and was structured around the goal of normalizing the activities and environments of people who had problems in daily living. This early pragmatic view of the subjective and individual reality of *knowing* is mirrored, not only in contemporary occupational therapy practice (Yerxa, 1991), but in contemporary methods employed to study clinical reasoning which have focused on the examination of personal

meaning of illness, disability and therapy action (Chapparo, 1997; Crepeau, 1991; Mattingly and Fleming, 1994).

Science and reductionism

During its early years, occupational therapy quickly expanded its services to a variety of medical facilities. Although everyday occupations remained the focus of therapy (Anderson and Bell, 1988), there was an increased alliance to medical trends that focused on isolated cause and effect principles of illness. Growing pressure from medicine for a more scientific rationale for practice (Licht, 1947) resulted in specialized interventions where scientific explanations and medical parallels existed (Keilhofner, 1992). Occupational therapists turned to kinesiologic, neurophysiological and psychodynamic explanations of human function and dysfunction (Barris, 1984; Keilhofner and Burke, 1977). During this period, the medical diagnosis permeated all aspects of occupational therapy clinical decision making. The client's problem was viewed in terms of physical or psychiatric diagnosis rather than occupational need (Spackman, 1968). Intervention focused on internal mechanisms (Jacob, 1964). Clinical decision making became reductionistic, as evidenced by examples of stated goals for intervention which were aimed at improving isolated units of function, such as particular physical or psychological attributes. The central concept of caring for self through a balanced sequence of activity found no place in the medical model and was discarded for many years. This type of reductionistic focus persists in a number of current clinical reasoning practices (Bissel and Mailloux, 1981; Neistadt and Crepeau, 1998; Rogers and Masagatani, 1982).

Elements of contemporary views of procedural reasoning emerged and reflected the scientific influence of the time. Reilly (1960), for example, proposed an early model of clinical reasoning for occupational therapy that was a type of procedural thinking process. She described its components using the formula: treatment plan equals the sum of the related raw data drawn from the data collecting instruments of observation, testing, interview and case history (Day, 1973; Reilly, 1960). During the 1970s this formula became formalized into the assessment and treatment planning part of the occupational therapy process.

From Reilly's work, and in keeping with the adoption of more scientific modes of thinking, systems approaches were applied to clinical reasoning (Line, 1969; Llorens, 1972). Day (1973), for example, created a model of decision making with the components of problem identification, cause, identification, treatment principle or assumption selection, activity selection and goal identification. The circular model created depended on generating and testing a series of hypotheses about client problems and reactions to intervention, and contributed to our understanding of procedural reasoning today (Bridge and Twible, 1997; Dutton, 1996; Rogers and Holm, 1991).

Theory development and conflict

Occupational therapy practice since the 1970s has been characterized by theoretical conflict, as the profession universally re-examined its direction and focus. A number of theories, models and frames of reference have emerged to explain the purpose of occupational therapy, with some emanating from other professions (Hagedorn, 1992; Reed, 1984). The result of this theoretical explosion is contemporary practice wherein various frames of reference are valued by different and substantial segments of the profession.

If theories, models and frames of reference are indeed the 'tools of thinking', as suggested by Parham (1987), the impact of this theoretical diversity on clinical reasoning is clear. By adhering to a specific frame of reference, therapists follow a particular line of thinking that translates knowledge into action. This specialized style of reasoning and action has been supported and fostered by current trends in health care, which has itself become divided into specialties over time. Occupational therapists in many instances refer to themselves as psychosocial therapists, physical disabilities therapists, hand therapists or sensory integration therapists, to designate the area of specialty (Schkade and Schultz, 1992). The existing pluralism appears to have defied attempts at synthesis (Katz, 1985) and creates problems for those who seek an encompassing view of occupational therapy practice (Christiansen, 1990; Van Deusen, 1991). The present position is perhaps best explained by Henderson (1988, p. 569) who urges the profession to 'be unified in . . . (its) fundamental assumptions, but diverse in . . . (its) technical knowledge'.

In summary, the nature of occupational therapy and the clinical-reasoning processes that continue to form a basis for its identity are founded in the history and humanistic philosophy that shaped the profession's beginning. Continuation of the profession's original belief in health through occupation is reflected in preoccupation with the form, function and meaning of *doing* in contemporary clinical reasoning (Zemke and Clark, 1996). The original belief in the client's right of choice and autonomy is reflected in current phenomenological approaches to studying clinical reasoning (Chapparo, 1997; Mattingly and Fleming, 1994; Neistadt and Crepeau, 1998).

The continuing impact of the reductionist and analytic orientation of medicine on current clinical reasoning in occupational therapy is illustrated by the prominent place that diagnosis and disease are still given in the clinical reasoning process (Bridge and Twible, 1997; Rogers and Masagatani, 1982). The influence of modes of scientific inquiry is reflected in a clinical reasoning style that involves systematic conceptualization and examination of clinical situations. Early scientific dogma has been tempered by the profession's emerging rejection of scientific dependency (Yerxa, 1991; Zemke and Clark, 1996), resulting in modification of current concepts of clinical reasoning as being more than applied science (Mattingly and Fleming, 1994).

Clinical reasoning is recognized as the core of occupational therapy practice. As a phenomenon for study, its contribution lies in describing the diversity, commonalities and complexities of therapists' thinking. Its importance in defining the professional identity of occupational therapy is summed up by Pedretti (1982, p. 12) who states, 'perhaps our real identity and uniqueness lies not as much in what we do, but in how we think'.

What do therapists think about?: The content of clinical reasoning

The therapy context, the client situation, theory, the personal individuality of the therapist, attitudes about therapy, and expectancies of therapy outcomes impose powerful internal and external influences on the decisions therapists make about their actions. One way to describe these influences is to consider them as sources of knowledge and motivation for decision making (Chapparo, 1997).

The therapy context

The organizational context contains powerful factors that establish conditions (e.g. organizational values) and constraints (e.g. human and financial resources, policies) of therapy. In many situations, these elements determine therapy action (Schell and Cervero, 1993). Within therapy contexts, therapists view themselves as autonomous individuals and reason according to their internalized values and theoretical perspectives, which may be consistent, or at odds, with the organizational influences. If practice beliefs and values held by therapists fail to account for prevailing institutional contexts, therapy goals can come into direct conflict with organizational goals. The resulting dilemma for clinical reasoning is one of conflict between what therapists perceive should be done, what the client wants done and what the system will allow.

Therapy experiences, including the organizational elements of therapy, contribute to the practical knowledge schemata that therapists develop. Therapy experiences are remembered by therapists as total contextual patterns of what is possible, involving people, actions, contexts and objects, rather than as decontextualized elements or rules (Gordon, 1988; Schön, 1983). Contextual patterns contribute to therapists' perceptions of the amount of control they have over their ability to carry out planned actions. These perceptions have a direct effect on their feelings of self-efficacy, self-confidence and autonomy (Ajzen and Madden, 1986; Bandura, 1997), all essential attributes for effective and creative reasoning. When therapists, because of organizational constraints, have a tenuous sense of self-efficacy and control, they have difficulty constructing images of how their actions can lead to a positive therapy outcome, and they will reason accordingly (Chapparo, 1997; Fidler, 1981).

The client and the client's life context

Knowledge of the client and the client's life context is fundamental to the clinical reasoning process. A core ethical tenet of occupational therapy is that intervention should be in concert with the client's needs, goals, lifestyle, and personal and cultural values (Chapparo and Ranka, 1997; Christiansen and Baum, 1997; Law, 1998). To this end, Mattingly and Fleming (1994) describe one of the primary goals of clinical reasoning as determining the meaning of disability from the client's perspective. At least five types of knowledge about the client are required to establish a picture of this meaning (Bridge and Twible, 1997; Crepeau, 1991; Dutton, 1996; Robertson, 1996). These are (a) knowledge of the client's

motivations, desires and tolerances; (b) knowledge of the environment and context within which client performance will occur; (c) knowledge of the client's abilities and deficits; (d) insight into the existing relationship with the client, its tacit rules and boundaries; and (e) a predictive knowledge of client potential in the long term. Knowledge from all these factors becomes a dynamic information flow during the process of assessment and intervention, demanding that therapists constantly update their understanding of how clients view themselves, how clients view therapy and the therapist and what clients think should be done.

Elements of this knowledge are used by therapists in the reasoning process to build a conceptual model of the client (Mattingly and Fleming, 1994; Rogers, 1983). Commonly, therapists use themselves as referents during this model creation (Chapparo, 1997), thereby ascribing meaning to the client's individual situation according to their own reality. Although this is viewed as a reasoning 'error' (Rogers, 1983), it is debatable to what extent therapists are able to uncouple their own values and perspectives to reach a full understanding of the client's situation. Rather, what is probable is that therapists develop an internal model of what they believe is the client's perspective, and work from that belief system.

Theory and science

Another source of motivation for clinical decision making is therapists' scientific knowledge about disease, human function and human occupation. Theory is purported to be useful because it gives direction for thinking, information about alternatives, and expectations of function and deficits (Mattingly and Fleming, 1994; Parham, 1987; Pelland, 1987). Professional knowledge has been described as applied theory whereby the process of 'naming' and 'framing' the problem occurs (Schön, 1983). This process requires identifying and classifying abstract constructs according to some theory base (such as depression, motor control, occupational role or cognitive ability). The identified construct becomes a cognitive mechanism that can facilitate the selection of strategies for assessment and treatment (Christiansen and Baum, 1997).

Theoretical knowledge alone, however, is an insufficient basis for effective clinical reasoning in occupational therapy. First, occupational therapy has a theory base that is incomplete and characterized by conflict. Second, therapists are required to make decisions in situations of uncertainty. Under these conditions, practical, intuitive knowledge is required. Such knowledge is tacit, founded in experience of clinical events (Gordon, 1988; Mattingly and Fleming, 1994; Rogers, 1983). Practical knowledge is integrated with theoretical knowledge to form a reasoning strategy that has been termed 'deliberative rationality' (Dreyfus and Dreyfus, 1986). When listening to therapists talk through their treatments this strategy can be observed as a personal theory of why events occur in therapy (Chapparo, 1997).

Therapists choose theories because of their potential to explain client problems. For instance, occupational therapists working with children are likely to choose developmentally based theories. However, therapists also choose one theory over another because of the congruence between the values implicit in the theory and the personal/professional values of the therapist, rather than because of any scientific merit. Many issues arising in conflicts between therapists and other professionals relate not to the logical soundness of the theoretical perspective but to the lines of thinking that arise from unspoken values embedded in the prescribed intervention approach (Parham, 1987).

Personal beliefs of the therapist

The fourth source of motivation is personal beliefs and values of the therapist. These are the fundamental beliefs and assumptions we have about ourselves, others and occupational therapy. Related to personal values, they can be internalized at several levels ranging from tentatively held beliefs to strong convictions. The strength with which a therapist adheres to a set of beliefs can differ from person to person as well as from situation to situation (Hundert, 1987). The place of these beliefs in clinical reasoning is to define the limits of acceptable behaviour for each individual therapist in any given clinical situation. Chapparo (1997), for example, in studying therapist thinking over a 3 year period was able to demonstrate that a set of 'personal norms' existed for each therapist studied. Moreover, there was a powerful causal relationship between these personal norms and clinical reasoning, as personal beliefs generated an expectation of personal behaviour during therapy and therefore expectations of personal satisfaction for the therapist.

Elements of each interpersonal interaction with a client are stored for use in future decision making. Knowledge that results from those personal experiences becomes personal knowledge and shapes what has been conceptualized as the architecture of self (Butt *et al.*, 1982; Fondiller *et al.*, 1990).

Attitude, behavioural expectancy and clinical reasoning

After defining clinical reasoning as a purposive social interaction, Chapparo (1997) used elements of attitude-behaviour theory (Ajzen and Madden, 1986) to demonstrate the effect of *attitude* on therapist thinking. In this model, actual therapy is found to be mediated through intention (what therapists choose to do) and expectancies (the perceived expectations of self and others). This mediation refers to the extent to which therapists believe that their therapy will meet the expectations of other people whose opinions they value. These other people may be clients or family members, or other professionals. *Attitude* (what therapists expect as outcomes of therapy) is derived from sets of beliefs derived from personal, theoretical and contextual knowledge outlined above. This conceptual model of reasoning is an explanation, not of the effects of general beliefs and attitudes on clinical reasoning, but of the effects of attitude towards a specific behaviour, in this instance, occupational therapy for a specific client. Attitudes therapists hold about their actions are the primary driving force in decision-making and are derived from salient beliefs, triggered by specific and changing events in therapy. Although a new area of study in the area of clinical reasoning, these tenets find support in attitude-behaviour research (Ajzen and Madden, 1986; Bandura, 1997).

Internal frame of reference

Clearly, clinical reasoning in occupational therapy is a phenomenon involving balancing of a number of personal, client-related, theoretical and organizational sets of knowledge. How therapists orchestrate their knowledge to determine which element receives precedence in reasoning is not yet clear. One emerging hypothesis is that knowledge used for clinical reasoning is housed within a highly individualized, complex internal framework structure, a personal internal frame of reference. Beliefs and attitudes are paramount sets of knowledge within this internal frame of reference and represent the therapist's internal reality of any clinical event (Chapparo, 1997). This knowledge is organized into facts about the therapist's everyday world of the clinic (external elements), the therapist's perceptions of what is real within the everyday world of the clinic (internal elements) and judgements about the everyday world of the clinic that can verified through action (attitude). Knowledge within this internal reality is viewed as a dynamic continuum of inquiry and is probably more correctly referred to as 'knowing' (Chapparo, 1997; Mattingly and Fleming, 1994). It is used during the clinical reasoning process to order, categorize and simplify complex data in order to develop a plan of action for intervention. In it resides the sum of cultural and personal biases of the therapist which serve to colour and interpret clinical reality and ultimately, clinical reasoning.

How do therapists think? The process of clinical reasoning

Considering the number of elements that impact on decisions therapists make, it is not surprising to find researchers proposing that multiple reasoning processes are used by occupational therapists. The third section of this chapter explores the ways in which the various elements of knowledge involved in clinical reasoning, as described previously, are processed to form pictures of client problems, client potential, therapy action and outcome.

Scientific reasoning

Occupational therapists use a logical process that parallels scientific inquiry when they try to understand the impact of illness and disease on the individual. Two forms of scientific reasoning identified by occupational therapy researchers are diagnostic reasoning (Rogers and Holm, 1991) and procedural reasoning (Mattingly and Fleming, 1994). These processes involve a progression from problem sensing to problem definition and problem resolution. Using information processing approaches put forward in medical models of clinical reasoning (Elstein and Bordage, 1979), Rogers and Holm (1991) outline a model of occupational therapy reasoning comprising cognitive operations identified as cue acquisition, hypothesis generation, cue interpretation and hypothesis evaluation.

As with earlier work (Rogers and Masagatani, 1982), Rogers and Holm's (1991) notion of diagnostic reasoning begins even before the therapist approaches a client. A 'problem sensing'

stage results in decisions being made concerning the information that is required to form an occupational diagnosis. It represents the therapist's interim, working and flexible identification of the general problem. It is probable that therapists have individual ideas about how well defined the problem should be before 'hypothesis generation' can begin.

Using procedural reasoning modes, therapists engage in a dual search for problem definition and treatment selection. Experienced therapists generate two to four hypotheses regarding the cause and nature of functional problems and several more concerning possible directions for treatment (Mattingly and Fleming, 1994). Hypotheses generated are then subjected to a process of critical reflection. Newer therapists generate fewer hypotheses, the tendency being to jump to conclusions about the nature and direction of therapy without weighing the grounds upon which the conclusion rests. The danger for experienced therapists is to place exclusive dependence on past experiences which have not been subjected to critical analysis through reflection. Without critical reflection, therapists forgo and cut short the act of inquiry that results in effective scientific reasoning.

Narrative reasoning

Implementing a therapy program that will potentially change life roles and functions for the client, occupational therapists are faced with profound problems of understanding. Specifically, they involve understanding the meaning of illness, disability and therapy outcome from the client's perspective. Understanding the meaning of a situation involves making an interpretation of it. This interpretation leads to subsequent understanding, appreciation and therapy action. What therapists perceive and fail to perceive and what they think and fail to think in the interpretive process is powerfully influenced by sets of beliefs, attitudes and assumptions that structure the way they interpret clinical experiences (Crepeau, 1991; Mezirow, 1991).

Two dimensions of making meaning are involved in narrative reasoning. Meaning schemes are sets of related and habitual expectations governing if/then relationships. Mattingly (Mattingly and Fleming, 1994) cites Bruner (1990) in linking these meaning schemes to a paradigmatic mode of thinking. For example, an occupational therapist with experience in stroke rehabilitation expects to see signs of left hemiplegia when referred a client with diagnosis of right cerebrovascular accident. Meaning schemes are habitual, implicit rules for interpreting and are strongly linked to knowledge.

Meaning perspectives are made up of higher-order schemata, theories and beliefs. They refer to the structure of assumptions and beliefs within which a new experience is interpreted. For example, occupational therapists make interpretations about clients based on values espoused by the notion of a 'helping profession', and their judgements are focused on client performance and satisfaction with occupational roles and tasks. Both meaning schemes and meaning perspectives selectively order and delimit clinical reasoning. They define therapists' expectations and therefore their intentions, and affect the activity of perceiving, comprehending and remembering meaning within the context of communicating with clients (Chapparo, 1997; Crepeau, 1991).

Mattingly (1994) describes how narrative thinking is central in providing therapists with a way to consider disability in phenomenological terms. She describes two types of narrative thinking. One is a 'mode of talk' that therapists use to shift disability from a physiological event to a personally meaningful one. The second involves the creation of images of the future for the client. The result of this type of thinking, as described by Mattingly, is purposeful occupational therapy that creates therapeutic activities which are meaningful to the client's life.

Ethical reasoning

Evidence suggests that personal values impact substantially on clinical reasoning processes in occupational therapy (Chapparo, 1997; Fondiller *et al.*, 1990; Haddad, 1988; Mattingly and Fleming 1994; Neuhaus, 1988; Rogers and Holm, 1991). A clinical problem becomes an ethical *dilemma* when it seems that an occupational therapy treatment decision will violate the therapist's values. In the process of choosing a therapeutic action using the reasoning processes outlined above, occupational therapists are often forced to balance one value against another. While this process is typically unconscious, it appears to drive decision making at various points throughout the treatment program.

Conditional reasoning

Fleming (1994) describes a third reasoning style, conditional reasoning. It involves projecting an imagined future for the client. Fleming uses the term 'conditional' in three different ways. First, problems are interpreted and solutions are realized in relation to people within their particular context. Second, therapists imagine how the present condition can be changed. Third, success or failure is determined by the level of client participation. It is a circular process, resulting in a flexible therapy program and is used by occupational therapists to assist clients to re-invent themselves through occupations. Chapparo (1997) extends the concept of conditional reasoning and describes a thinking process whereby therapists reconcile the actual (therapy) and the possible (intention) in terms of therapy outcome. It involves *reflection* (whereby the therapist's action turns in on itself), *conflict* (whereby therapists seek to reconcile choices made) and *judgement* (whereby therapists weight the soundness of decisions).

Pragmatic reasoning

Pragmatic reasoning goes beyond the therapist–client relationship and addresses the contexts in which therapy occurs (Schell and Cervero, 1993). Clinical reasoning focuses on practical action and therapists are compelled to think about what is achievable within their own or the client's world. As outlined above, these issues include organizational constraints, values and resources, practice trends, and reimbursement issues. Recent studies confirm that therapists' thinking is increasingly influenced by situations that occur in their practice world (Chapparo, 1997; Strong *et al.*, 1995).

Fleming (1994) created an image of an occupational therapist with a 'three-track mind'. The procedural track is used when therapists reason about the client's diagnosis. The interactive narrative track occurs when the therapist focuses on the client as a person. The conditional track creates an image of the client that is provisional, holistic and conditional on the client's participation. Alternatively, Chapparo (1997) used causal modelling to demonstrate that although therapists use multiple strategies (e.g. story telling, testing, questioning, imagining, feeling and moving) to acquire the multidimensional knowledge needed for reasoning, one mode of thinking is used to draw together very disparate areas of consideration (e.g. personal-emotional, contextual rules of operation, client needs, and science) into a coherent, integrated judgement about the course of action in therapy.

It is unclear from critical examination of the literature whether therapists use distinctly different types of reasoning that translate into mutually exclusive forms of thinking, or whether the different styles of reasoning which have been identified in each piece of research are images of thinking that have been constructed through the process of attempting to put words to a largely internal, tacit phenomenon. Descriptions of the different clinical reasoning processes that exist may actually be a reflection of the influence of the knowledge base of various researchers such as anthropology (Mattingly and Fleming, 1994), medicine (Dutton, 1996; Rogers and Holm, 1991), cognitive psychology (Bridge and Twible, 1997) and social psychology (Chapparo, 1997).

Conclusion

Clinical reasoning in occupational therapy, as in other health science professions, is a complex phenomenon that has only just begun to be described. It has been described as the use of multiple reasoning strategies throughout the various phases of client management. Procedural reasoning is used when therapists think about client problems in terms of the disease and within the context of occupational performance. Narrative reasoning (Mattingly and Fleming, 1994), using interactive processes, involves developing an understanding of the meaning of existing problems from the client's perspective. Conditional reasoning (Mattingly and Fleming, 1994) is a less definitive process by which occupational therapists imagine the client in the future, and, in so doing, imagine the therapy outcome and the therapeutic action required to achieve that outcome. Additionally, there is evidence of processes of ethical and pragmatic reasoning that further frame decision making personally and contextually.

There are many factors that act as motivating forces for clinical decisions. Among them are organizational structures and expectations, client needs and expectations, and theoretical and scientific knowledge about disease and human occupations. Within the therapist's internal frame of reference, perceptions of these external factors are integrated with personal beliefs about such things as perceived level of skill, personal knowledge, personal beliefs and perceived level of control. From this internal frame of reference, images of clients and their problems are created, as well as plans for therapeutic action, all of which serve to direct clinical-reasoning processes.

It is clear that current explanations and descriptions of clinical reasoning in occupational therapy are incomplete. Contemporary notions of clinical reasoning describe a highly individualistic mode of operation that is based in scientific knowledge and method, creative imagination, intuition, interpersonal skill, and artistry, operating within the frame of reference of the occupational therapy profession.

References

Ajzen, I. and Madden, T. J. (1986) Prediction of goal directed behaviour: Attitudes, intentions and perceived behavioural control. *Journal of Experimental Social Psychology*, **22**, 453–474.

Anderson, B. and Bell, J. (1988) *Occupational Therapy: Its Place in Australia's History*. Victoria: NSW Association of Occupational Therapists

Bandura, A. (1997) *Self Efficacy: The Exercise of Control*. New York: Freeman.

Barris, R. (1984) Toward an image of one's own: Sources of variation in the role of occupational therapists in psychosocial practice. *The Occupational Therapy Journal of Research*, **4**, 3–23.

Bissel, J. and Mailloux, Z. (1981) The use of crafts in occupational therapy for the physically disabled. *American Journal of Occupational Therapy*, **35**, 369–374.

Breines, E. (1990) Genesis of occupation: A philosophical model for therapy and theory. *Australian Occupational Therapy Journal*, **37**, 45–49.

Bridge, C. E. and Twible, R. L. (1997) Clinical reasoning: Informed decision making for practice. In *Occupational Therapy: Enabling Function and Well-being* (C. Christiansen and C. Baum, eds), pp. 158–179. Thorofare, NJ: Slack.

Bruner, J. (1990) *Acts of Meaning*. Chicago: University of Chicago Press.

Butt, R., Raymond, D. and Yamaguishi, L. (1982) Autobiographic praxis: Studying the formation of teacher's knowledge. *Journal of Curriculum Theorizing*, **7**, 87–164

Chapparo, C. (1997) Influences on clinical reasoning in occupational therapy. *PhD thesis*. Macquarie University, Australia.

Chapparo, C. and Ranka, J. (eds) (1997) *Occupational Performance Model (Australia)*. Monograph 1. School of Occupational Therapy, The University of Sydney, Australia.

Christiansen, C. (1990) The perils of plurality. *Occupational Therapy Journal of Research*, **11**, 259–265.

Christiansen, C. and Baum, C. (eds) (1997) *Occupational Therapy: Enabling Function and Well-being*. Thorofare, NJ: Slack.

Crepeau, E. B. (1991) Achieving intersubjective understanding: Examples from an occupational therapy treatment session. *American Journal of Occupational Therapy*, **45**, 1016–1025.

Day, D. J. (1973) A systems diagram for teaching treatment planning. *American Journal of Occupational Therapy*, **27**, 239–243.

Dewey, J. (1910) *How We Think*. Chicago: University of Chicago.

Dreyfus, H. and Dreyfus, S. (1986) *Mind over Machine: The Power of Human Intuition and Expertise in the Era of the Computer*. New York: Free Press.

Dutton, R. (1996) *Clinical Reasoning in Physical Disabilities*. Baltimore, MD: Williams & Wilkins.

Elstein, A. S. and Bordage, G. (1979) Psychology of clinical reasoning. In *Health Psychology: A Handbook* (G. Stone, F. Cohen and N. Adler, eds), pp. 109–129. San Francisco: Jossey-Bass.

Fidler, G. (1981) From crafts to competence. *American Journal of Occupational Therapy*, **35**, 567–573.

Fleming, M. H. (1994) Conditional reasoning: Creating meaningful experiences. In *Clinical Reasoning: Forms of Inquiry in a Therapeutic Practice* (C. Mattingly and M. H. Fleming, eds), pp. 197–235, Philadelphia, PA: F. A. Davis.

Fondiller, E. D., Rosage, L. J. and Neuhaus, B. E. (1990) Values influencing clinical reasoning in occupational therapy: An exploratory study. *Occupational Therapy Journal of Research*, **10**, 41–54.

Gordon, D. (1988) Clinical science and clinical expertise: Changing boundaries between art and science in medicine. In *Biomedicine Examined* (M. Lock and D. R. Gordon, eds), pp. 257–295. New York: Kluwer .

Haddad, A. M. (1988) Teaching ethical analysis in occupational therapy. *American Journal of Occupational Therapy*, **42**, 300–304.

Hagedorn, R. (1992) *Occupational Therapy: Foundations for Practice. Models, Frames of Reference and Core Skills*. London: Churchill Livingstone.

Harvey-Krefting, L. (1985) The concept of work in occupational therapy: A historical review. *American Journal of Occupational Therapy*, **39**, 301–307.

Hemphill, B. J. (1982) The evaluative process. In *The Evaluative Process in Psychiatric Occupational Therapy* (B. J. Hemphill, ed.), pp. 27–36. Thorofare, NJ: Slack.

Henderson, A. (1988) 1988 Eleanor Clarke Slagle Lecture. Occupational therapy knowledge: From practice to theory. *American Journal of Occupational Therapy*, **42**, 567–576.

Hopkins, H. L. and Tiffany, E. G. (1988) Occupational therapy – A problem-solving process. In *Willard and Spackman's Occupational Therapy*, 7th edn (H. L. Hopkins and H. D. Smith, eds), pp. 102–111. Philadelphia, PA: Lippincott.

Hundert, E. M. (1987) A model for ethical problem solving in medicine, with practical applications. *American Journal of Psychiatry*, **144**, 839–846.

Jacob, F. (1964) Occupational therapy in a psychiatric unit in a general hospital. *Australian Journal of Occupational Therapy*, **11**, 10–16.

Katz, N. (1985) Occupational therapy's domain of concern: Reconsidered. *American Journal of Occupational Therapy*, **39**, 518–524.

Kielhofner, G. (1992) *Conceptual Foundations of Occupational Therapy*. Philadelphia, PA: F. A. Davis.

Keilhofner, G. and Burke, J. (1977) Occupational therapy after 60 years: An account of changing identity and knowledge. *American Journal of Occupational Therapy*, **31**, 675–689.

Law, M. (ed.) (1998) *Client-Centered Occupational Therapy*. Thorofare, NJ: Slack

Licht, S. (1947) The objectives of occupational therapy. *Occupational Therapy Rehabilitation*, **28**, 17–22.

Line, J. (1969) Case method as a scientific form of clinical thinking. *American Journal of Occupational Therapy*, **23**, 308–313.

Llorens, L. (1972) Problem-solving the role of occupational therapy in a new environment. *American Journal of Occupational Therapy*, **26**, 234–238.

Mattingly, C. (1994) The narrative nature of clinical reasoning. In *Clinical Reasoning: Forms of Inquiry in a Therapeutic Practice* (C. Mattingly and M. H. Fleming, eds), pp. 239–269. Philadelphia, PA: F. A. Davis.

Mattingly, C. and Fleming, M. H. (1994) *Clinical Reasoning: Forms of Inquiry in a Therapeutic Practice*. Philadelphia, PA: F. A. Davis.

Meyer, A. (1922) The philosophy of occupational therapy. *Archives of Occupational Therapy*, **1**, 1–10.

Mezirow, J. (1991) How critical reflection triggers transformative learning. In *Fostering Critical Reflection in Adulthood* (J. Mezirow, ed.), pp. 82–95. San Francisco: Jossey-Bass.

Neistadt, M. and Crepeau, E. B. (eds) (1998) *Willard and Spackman's Occupational Therapy* 9th edn. Philadelphia, PA: Lippincott.

Neuhaus, B. E. (1988) Ethical considerations in clinical reasoning: The impact of technology and cost containment. *American Journal of Occupational Therapy*, **42**, 288–292.

Parham D. (1987) Toward professionalism: The reflective therapist. *American Journal of Occupational Therapy*, **41**, 555–561.

Pedretti, L. W. (1982) The compatibility of current treatment methods in physical disabilities with the philosophical case of occupational therapy. *Doctoral thesis*. San Jose University.

Pelland, M. J. (1987) A conceptual model for the instruction and supervision of treatment planning. *American Journal of Occupational Therapy*, **41**, 351–359.

Pinel, P. (1948) Medical philosophical treatise on mental alienation. In *Occupational Therapy Source Book* (S. Licht, ed.), p. 19. Baltimore, MD: Williams & Wilkins.

Reed, K. L. (1984) *Models of Practice in Occupational Therapy*. Baltimore, MD: Williams & Wilkins.

Reilly, M. (1960) Research potentiality of occupational therapy. *American Journal of Occupational Therapy*, **14**, 206–209.

Robertson, L. J. (1996) Clinical reasoning, part 1: The nature of problem solving, a literature review. *British Journal of Occupational Therapy*, **59**, 178–182.

Rogers, J. C. (1983) Eleanor Clarke Slagle Lectureship – 1983: Clinical reasoning: The ethics, science and art. *American Journal of Occupational Therapy*, **37**, 601–616.

Rogers, J. C. and Holm, M. (1991) Occupational therapy diagnostic reasoning: A component of clinical reasoning. *American Journal of Occupational Therapy*, **45**, 1045–1053.

Rogers, J. C. and Masagatani, G. (1982) Clinical reasoning of occupational therapists during the initial assessment of physically disabled patients. *Occupational Therapy Journal of Research*, **2**, 195–219.

Schell, B. R. (1998) Clinical reasoning: The basis of practice. In *Willard and Spackman's Occupational Therapy* (M. Neistadt and E. B. Crepeau, eds), pp. 90–99. Philadelphia, PA: Lippincott.

Schell, B. R. and Cervero, R. M. (1993) Clinical reasoning of occupational therapy: An integrative review. *The American Journal of Occupational Therapy*, **47**, 605–610.

Schkade, J. K. and Schultz, S. (1992) Occupational adaptations: Toward a holistic approach for contemporary practice, Part 1. *American Journal of Occupational Therapy*, **46**, 829–837.

Schön, D. A. (1983) *The Reflective Practitioner: How Professionals Think in Action*. New York: Basic Books.

Shannon, P. (1977) The derailment of occupational therapy. *American Journal of Occupational Therapy*, **31**, 229–234.

Slagle, A. C. (1922) Training aids for mental patients. *Occupational Therapy and Rehabilitation*, **1**, 11–14.

Spackman, C. (1968) A history of the practice of occupational therapy for restoration of physical function: 1917–1967. *American Journal of Occupational Therapy*, **22**, 67–76.

Stanage, S. M. (1987) *Adult Education and Phenomenological Research: New Directions for Theory, Practice and Research*. Miami, Florida: Kreiger

Strong, J., Gilbert, J., Cassidy, S. and Bennett, S. (1995) Expert clinicians' and students' views on clinical reasoning in occupational therapy. *British Journal of Occupational Therapy*, **58**, 119–123.

Van Deusen, J. (1991) The issue is: Can we delimit the discipline of occupational therapy? *American Journal of Occupational Therapy*, **44**, 175–176.

Yerxa, E. J. (1991) Seeking a relevant, ethical and realistic way of knowing for occupational therapy. *American Journal of Occupational Therapy*, **45**, 199–204.

Zemke, R. and Clarke, F. (eds) (1996) *Occupational Science: The Evolving Discipline*. Philadelphia, PA: F. A. Davis.

Section Three

Teaching clinical reasoning

14

Teaching clinical reasoning

Kathryn Refshauge and Joy Higgs

Teachers faced with the task of helping students in the health sciences develop their clinical reasoning skills need to understand the nature of clinical reasoning and how it develops, and need to develop strategies for teaching this complex skill to students. Earlier chapters in this book have addressed the nature of clinical reasoning. This chapter focuses on the task of teaching. The importance placed upon clinical reasoning by the health professions is evident in the increasing occurrence of explicit teaching of clinical reasoning in health science curricula (Elstein, 1981; Higgs and Jones, 1995; Neame *et al*., 1985; Rogers *et al*., 1991; Schwartz, 1991; Tanner, 1987).

Issues in teaching clinical reasoning

Deciding what to teach

The teaching of clinical reasoning should be based on 'an understanding of how competent individuals proceed in determining what observations to make, in identifying health problems from those observations, and in deciding on appropriate actions; and an understanding of the progression of such competence, from beginning level to the development of expertise' (Tanner, 1987, p. 155). Teachers are faced with the question, 'which model of clinical reasoning should I encourage my students to emulate?'. The choice could be hypothetico-deductive reasoning (Elstein *et al*., 1978), pattern recognition (Barrows and Feltovich, 1987), problem solving (Bashook, 1976), the phenomeno-

logical model adopted in occupational therapy (Mattingly, 1991), models of backward reasoning and forward reasoning (Patel and Groen, 1991), models as in nursing which emphasize intuition (Benner and Tanner, 1987) or a combined model (Higgs and Jones, 1995). A sound plan for teaching encompasses elements of clinical reasoning, including knowledge, reasoning ability and metacognition within the model. In addition, learners need to develop their own understanding of the clinical reasoning process and of how they reason, as well as how to critique their reasoning. For instance, students continue to incorporate into their understanding of clinical reasoning their unique and evolving knowledge bases (comprising theoretical, research, experiential and personal knowledge), their learning and thinking approaches, and the sets of values, beliefs and attitudes against which they compare new information and make decisions. Each of these factors influences students' clinical reasoning behaviour. For instance, if new knowledge or ideas are incongruent with their belief system, individuals may reject the new information. In addition, people lean towards a confirmatory bias, where they tend to accept information that supports their beliefs, and reject or ignore information that conflicts with their beliefs (Elstein *et al*., 1978). To enhance the reasoning processes of health professionals, it is incumbent upon both the teacher and the learner to explore the values or belief systems of the students, to ensure that they explore new ideas and process information in appropriate ways.

Curriculum framework and design

Clinical reasoning may be taught as a separate subject within a curriculum or as an integral aspect of all areas/subjects within the curriculum. The first option has the advantage of drawing attention to this skill rather than diffusing it among the various other learning goals of the curriculum. More time can be spent in refining individual students' clinical reasoning skills or in identifying and addressing deficiencies in their knowledge and reasoning abilities. However, the more general approach has the potential advantages of reinforcing both reasoning and the integration of knowledge in all areas of learning, and of promoting transfer of learning from classroom to clinical settings.

Shepard and Jensen (1990) refer to explicit and implicit curricula, the latter indicating the messages received by students as to the importance of many aspects of their learning program which are not clearly articulated in formal curriculum documents. Both these forms of curriculum reinforce and direct students' learning. These authors, with Everingham and Feletti (1999), emphasize the importance of using both explicit and implicit curricula to promote reflection in learning and the development of reflective knowledge and skills. Such abilities can help learners (and clinicians) to deal with what Schön (1987) labels 'the indeterminate zones of practice' or the uncertainty, uniqueness and value conflicts which characterize human situations. What is needed with these situations is a *reflective practitioner*, one who incorporates reflection into clinical reasoning practices.

Mismatches between implicit and explicit curricula cause confusion and less than optimal learning. It is important, therefore, for teachers to avoid what has been described as a discrepancy between 'espoused theory' and 'theory-in-use' (Bowden, 1988). In studying practice in a number of university programs, Bowden (1988, p. 257) found that teachers wanted students to possess qualities such as 'problem-solving ability in their profession, lateral thinking, insight, integrity, perspective, self-motivation, ability to 'self-learn', and an understanding of the structure of (relevant) knowledge'. (Such outcomes would be desirable in a clinical reasoning course.) However, when investigating why students did not achieve these outcomes, Bowden identified that a mismatch had occurred between espoused theory (and its intended outcomes) and the ways in which the students were actually taught and assessed. The

challenge for the educator, then, is to select an educational philosophy or conceptual framework which is appropriate for the subject to be taught and to authentically adopt this 'espoused theory' in practice.

We would argue that the ideal choice of educational philosophy and framework for clinical reasoning programs is adult learning. This is because both clinical reasoning and adult learning involve a complex, interactive set of characteristics and capabilities:

- A relevant and sound knowledge base.
- A willingness to take responsibility for decisions and actions.
- Cognitive (learning and reasoning) processes.
- Ability to seek information and knowledge as required (in order to learn or to make clinical decisions).
- Capacity to engage in self-monitoring and self-evaluation, and to take responsibility for self-development and for decisions made.

According to Finger (1990), adult learning provides a means of achieving transformation of learners and their situation, since this approach helps learners find a 'way out' of problem situations. Adoption of this approach, therefore, would enable students to learn through the experience of solving their learning problems while at the same time learning about clinical reasoning or the transformation of clinical problems into solutions. The notion of changing students' conceptions of aspects of the world around them is regarded by Ramsden as 'the core of education' (Ramsden, 1988a, p. vii). Education can be enhanced, argues Ramsden (1988b), by understanding how students are thinking and learning, by helping students learn to understand how subject experts see relevant phenomena and by enabling students to change their conceptions of these phenomena.

The principles and practice of adult learning come closest to this goal. In adult learning students need to take an active part in the learning process, the teacher and learner are engaged in interdependent learning (Griffith, 1987), and learning is directed towards growth of the learner. Table 14.1 (from Terry and Higgs, 1993) provides an overview of environmental conditions which promote adult learning, teaching decisions the educator and learner need to make to engage successfully in adult learning and the characteristic behaviours of effective adult learners. This overview provides a guide for teachers wishing to adopt the adult learning approach.

Table 14.1 Adult learning conditions and behaviours

Environmental conditions	Decision making/management factors	Adult learning behaviours
Motivation	Shared goals	Problem solving
Acceptance of learner as person	Shared management	Interacton with teacher and other
Freedom/autonomy	Mutual decision making/planning	learners
Individuality	Shared resource acquisition	Active participation in learning
Emphasis on abilities/experience	Learner involvement in learning needs,	Self-correction
Student-centred learning	diagnosis and evaluation	Interdependence
Resource-rich environment	Learner direction in posing questions/	Critical reflection
Mutual respect/trust	seeking answers	Progressive mastery
Teacher support/facilitation	Effective communication	Active seeking of meaning
Learning via experience relevant to	Choice in participation	Individual pacing
learner	Collaborative facilitation	Empowered self-direction
Praxis – integrating reflection, theory,	Ongoing review by teacher and learners	Internal drive/motivation
practice, experience	Learner identification of community	Reciprocal learning
Interaction between learners	goals and needs as part of own	Experiential learning
Effective/appropriate group dynamics	learning context	
Security/support	Learner acceptance of responsibility	

From Terry and Higgs (1993).

Teaching knowledge that is purposeful and requires deep learning

Health professionals today need to be capable of performing competently in an autonomous, professional capacity, of maintaining this competence, and of generating knowledge throughout their careers. They also need to be able to respond to the changing health care needs of the community (Cox, 1988). Effective reasoning and decision-making abilities can enhance the likelihood of an individual successfully achieving these outcomes. Success in the above behaviours requires the ability to acquire knowledge using a deep learning approach.

Research in the area of student learning (Entwistle and Ramsden, 1983) has identified that contexts and curricula which foster deep learning are characterized by freedom in learning, less formality, good teaching input, a good social climate and clear goals. Surface or rote learning approaches are more likely to occur where there are heavy workloads. Curriculum planning therefore needs to ensure that learning environments are created that will foster deep learning. Table 14.2 (from Ramsden, 1988b, p. 19) presents an overview of deep and surface approaches to learning.

The learning environment

The above discussion emphasizes the importance of the learning environment. According to Ramsden (1985) the effects of learning environments

Table 14.2 Deep and surface approaches to learning

Deep approach Intention to understand	Surface approach Intention to complete task requirements
Focus on 'what is signified' (e.g. the author's argument	Focus on the 'signs' (e.g. the text itself)
Relate and distinguish new ideas and previous knowledge	Focus on discrete elements
Relate concepts to everyday experience	Memorize information and procedures for assessments
Relate and distinguish evidence and argument	Unreflectively associate concepts and facts
Organize and structure content	Fail to distinguish principles from evidence, new information
Internal emphasis: 'A window through which aspects of	from old
reality become visible, and more intelligible' (Entwistle	Treat task as an external imposition
and Marton, 1984)	External emphasis: demands of assessments, knowledge but
	off from everyday reality

From Ramsden (1988b).

can be best understood if they are thought of as operating at the levels of the learning task, the teacher, the department or course and the institution. In planning a learning program the teacher needs to consider the environmental influences and constraints at each of these levels and also the opportunities which different learning environments provide. In problem-based learning curricula, many environmental levels may be well co-ordinated to reinforce the learning of clinical problem solving skills and knowledge throughout students' learning experiences.

More conventional curricula are frequently divided into a 'pre-clinical' component (or an on-campus program which is likely to include the teaching of clinical as well as pre-clinical skills and knowledge) and a subsequent 'clinical' or 'fieldwork' component. Clinical reasoning can be explored either in the classroom or in the clinic.

In the classroom students can learn from mistakes, explore alternative treatment decisions, change their minds and examine many detailed aspects of knowledge use and evaluation, in the absence of both time constraints and the potential negative effects on patients which can occur in the clinical context. The classroom setting also allows for discussion of students' thinking and the potential effects their decisions may have, and encourages feedback from both peers and teachers. However, attention must be devoted to transfer of these skills from the classroom to the clinical context. To enhance transfer into the clinical setting, it is essential that clinical educators develop a clear understanding of the process of teaching clinical reasoning that is consistent with classroom teaching. They need to create time to facilitate students' reasoning and use of knowledge, and to provide feedback on these areas as well as on technical skills.

On-campus pre-clinical teaching in health science curricula commonly addresses the basic and applied sciences (e.g. anatomy, physiology and biomechanics) and the medical sciences (e.g. pathology) which form an essential part of the clinician's knowledge base. In addition, students study specific health science subjects such as occupational performance, paediatric nursing, obstetrics and musculo-skeletal physiotherapy. In these clinical subjects structured learning activities can be implemented which are aimed at promoting the development of clinical reasoning skills and practice knowledge and the integration of knowledge students have gained from life

experiences, and developed throughout their curricula. Such learning activities can include small group learning tutorials, peer teaching, cognitive mapping, role play, verbalizing interpretation of patient data in simulated clinical settings and experts discussing their interpretation of a problem. Peer teaching is another useful method of fostering the development and evaluation of knowledge. Communicating thoughts, arguments and rationales requires students to understand and organize what they know and how they use knowledge. Experience in peer teaching (Higgs, 1990) has shown that when learners are attempting to create learning experiences for others, they learn a great deal about the nature of their own knowledge, the breadth of this knowledge, the cognitive links they make, and the value and validity of their knowledge.

As well as developing reasoning skills and knowledge in the classroom, students need to test the application of this knowledge in appropriate contexts. Clinical education provides this context. During clinical placements much of the daily activity of health science students relates to clinical problem solving, since students are continually seeking, absorbing, interpreting, evaluating and summarizing clinical information, and making clinical decisions on the basis of this information (Whelan, 1988). Experiences during clinical education promote an understanding of patients' conditions and needs as well as of the students' abilities in meeting these needs.

The reality of the clinical setting has many advantages for the exploration of clinical reasoning in action, even though it incorporates constraints such as time pressures and potential dangers to the patient. During clinical education, students can gain skills in many broad areas such as interpersonal communication, assisting patients with movements, team work and writing skills, as well as the technical skills of their discipline. The complex environment with its immediacy, variability, personality factors of patients and staff, and reality of consequences of actions, is an important context for learning. It has been found (Norman, 1990) that the context in which learning occurs has a profound effect on students' ability to recall learning, with recall occurring best in situations similar to that in which it was learned. Finally, the role of patients in teaching and providing feedback is a further advantage of clinical settings. It is necessary, therefore, that health science curricula actively utilize both classroom and clinical settings for this purpose.

Processing learning experiences

Regardless of the learning environment, the key factor to students' learning remains their experiences and the way they learn from them. Learning through experience is what people do throughout their lives. It has been described as 'simultaneously an educational philosophy, a range of methodologies, and a framework for being, seeing, thinking and acting, on individual and collective levels. It involves the active transformation and integration of different forms of experience. These processes lead to new understandings, and the development of a wide range of capabilities' (McGill and Weil, 1989, p. 245). Boud (1993, p. 35) describes the key contributing elements of experience as a basis for learning as follows:

- Experience is the foundation of, and stimulus for learning.
- The effects of prior experience influence all learning.
- Learners actively construct their own experience.
- Learning is a holistic process which has affective, cognitive and conative features.
- Learning is socially and culturally constructed.
- Learning occurs in a socio-emotional context.

Simply participating in learning activities is not enough to generate learning or new knowledge. Many learners are not fully aware of the interactions in which they are participating or of the potential of their social, psychological and material environment as a source of learning, and require reflection to fully utilize this experience for learning (Boud and Walker, 1991). They need to learn to be reflective practitioners (Schön, 1987).

Assessment and feedback

Teachers need to re-evaluate the purpose of assessment and to re-interpret assessment as a holistic process acknowledging the inseparable link between learning and assessment (Boud and Higgs, 1999). They need to consider the effects of assessment and the strategies used in order to promote optimal learning.

What and how students learn is also influenced by what they are assessed upon and how they are assessed (Elton, 1982; Newble and Jaeger, 1983; Ramsden, 1984). It has been demonstrated (Ramsden, 1984) that it is easier to encourage students to adopt a surface (or rote learning) approach than a deep (or meaningful) learning approach and that the learning approach can be strongly influenced by the choice of assessment methods. Deep learning is fostered through assessment which rewards understanding, such as essay writing, as opposed to examinations based on recall of information (Watkins, 1984).

As discussed earlier, students seek messages from the curriculum (e.g. from stated goals, learning activities and assessment) to guide their learning. Students' perceptions of these messages and of conflicts between them can result in their adopting learning behaviours contrary to those intended by the teachers. In particular, learning behaviour and outcomes are influenced by the learner's perception of the demands of assessment (Ramsden, 1984). In designing and conducting assessment procedures, therefore, the nature of the assessment process and how it is presented to and perceived by the learners is important. The method of assessment also needs to be reliable and valid for the behaviour being assessed, whether it be understanding, recall or evaluation.

There needs to be consistency between the goals of learning, the activities used, the feedback given and the assessment procedures implemented. If deep learning is desired to enhance the value as well as the breadth of the learner's knowledge, then learning activities, feedback and assessment procedures must all be consistently aimed at encouraging deep learning.

The role of the teacher and learner in adult learning programs

Health sciences education is a process of socialization into the professional role, which amplifies the parallel responsibilities of the learner and the autonomous clinician for their decisions and actions. In adult learning environments which seek to foster deep learning, there is a dual emphasis on the teacher creating a climate which Rogers (1983) labels 'responsible freedom' and on the learners accepting both the privileges and responsibilities such freedom entails. To succeed in this environment students need to develop higher learning skills including self-direction, critical self-appraisal and metacognition, to participate actively both in the learning activities provided and in the management of their learning, and to seek help, guidance and feedback when appropriate.

An important factor to remember in planning for this creative, interdependent and dual (teacher and learner) managed learning environment is that not all learners will enter the current learning program with these advanced learning skills. Matching the teaching strategy to 'learner task maturity' [i.e. the level of readiness and ability to the learner to deal with demands of a specific learning task at a given time (Higgs, 1993)] is an important consideration in promoting learner independence and responsibility.

Experiencing clinical reasoning as an interactive process

In addition to the process of reasoning itself, health science students need to learn to interact with others as part of the reasoning process. To do so they need to learn how to communicate their reasoning and how to involve their clients in the reasoning process.

The community and government-led demands for accountability which accompany the increased autonomy of health professionals and increased participation expectations of consumers require effective communication and justification of clinical decisions. In addition to behaving in a competent, ethical and professional manner, clinicians need to be able to explain, clearly and credibly, the scientific and therapeutic bases for their actions and the expected outcomes, within the context of the individual client's needs, wishes and situation. Students can learn to communicate and justify their decisions effectively through clinical reasoning learning activities such as verbalizing their interpretation of patient data, and justifying their choice of intervention.

Conclusion

Clinical reasoning teaching is widely regarded as an essential part of health science curricula. It provides a framework for integrating students' learning, for preparing them for their role as autonomous, responsible health care professionals and for helping them deal with the complex and variable elements of clinical practice. By making clinical reasoning a conscious and strategic part of their clinical practice, student and graduate clinicians are encouraged to examine and express their opinions and ideas and to develop a greater awareness of how they reason and how their knowledge, values and beliefs influence their clinical reasoning.

The challenge faced by health science educators of enhancing skills in clinical reasoning can be met by addressing four key elements: a comprehensive, valid and well-organized knowledge base; reasoning skills (i.e. cognitive, evaluative and metacognitive skills); a value and belief system; and clinical skills and clinical experience. This chapter has presented adult learning as an ideal framework for the development of these clinical reasoning skills and for fostering deep and lifelong learning. Learners' active participation in creating and managing their learning experiences and in deriving meaning from them is at the core of this learning approach.

References

Barrows, H. S. and Feltovich, P. J. (1987) The clinical reasoning process. *Medical Education*, **21**, 86–91.

Bashook, P. G. (1976) A conceptual framework for measuring clinical problem-solving. *Journal of Medical Education*, **51**, 109–114.

Benner, P. and Tanner, C. (1987) Clinical judgment: How expert nurses use intuition. *American Journal of Nursing*, January, 23–31.

Boud, D. (1993) Experience as the base for learning. *Higher Education Research and Development*, **12**, 33–44.

Boud, D. and Higgs, J. (1999) Assessment and learning. In *Educating Beginning Practitioners* (J. Higgs and H. Edwards, eds), pp. 221–227. Oxford: Butterworth-Heinemann.

Boud, D. and Walker, D. (1991) *Experience and Learning: Reflection at Work*. Geelong, Victoria: Deakin University Press.

Bowden, J. (1988) Achieving change in teaching practices. In *Improving Learning: New Perspectives* (P. Ramsden, ed.), pp. 255–267. London: Kogan Page.

Cox, K. (1988) Professional and educational context of medical education. In *The Medical Teacher* (K. Cox and C. E. Ewan, eds) (2nd edn), pp. 4–8. Edinburgh: Churchill Livingstone.

Elstein, A. S. (1981) Educational programs in medical decision making. *Medical Decision Making*, **1**, 70–73.

Elstein, A. S., Shulman, L. S. and Sprafka, S. A. (1978) *Medical Problem Solving: An Analysis of Clinical Reasoning*. Cambridge, MA: Harvard University Press.

Elton, L. R. B. (1982) Assessment for learning. In *Professionalism and Flexibility in Learning* (D. Bligh, ed.). Guildford: SRHE.

Entwistle, N. J. and Ramsden, P. (1983) *Understanding Student Learning*. London: Croom Helm.

Everingham, F. and Feletti, G. (1999) Curriculum management in a changing world: The new imperative. In *Educating Beginning Practitioners* (J. Higgs and H. Edwards, eds), pp. 79–87. Oxford: Butterworth Heinemann.

Finger, M. (1990) Does adult education need a philosophy? Reflections about the function of adult learning in today's society. *Studies in Higher Education*, **12**, 81–98.

Griffith, G. (1987) Images of interdependence: Authority and power in teaching/learning. In *Appreciating Adults Learning: From the Learners' Perspective* (D. Boud and V. Griffin, eds), pp. 51–63. London: Kogan Page.

Higgs, J. (1990) Fostering the acquisition of clinical reasoning skills. *New Zealand Journal of Physiotherapy*, **18**, 13–17.

Higgs, J. (1993) The teacher in self-directed learning: Manager or co-manager? In *Learner Managed Learning* (N. J. Graves, ed.), pp. 122–131. Leeds: World Education Fellowship.

Higgs, J. and Jones, M. (1995) Clinical reasoning. In *Clinical Reasoning in the Health Professions* (J. Higgs and M. Jones, eds), pp. 3–23. Oxford: Butterworth-Heinemann.

Mattingly, C. (1991) The narrative nature of clinical reasoning. *The American Journal of Occupational Therapy*, **45**, 998–1005.

McGill, I. and Weil, S. W. (1989) Continuing the dialogue: New possibilities for experiential learning. In *Making Sense of Experiential Learning: Diversity in Theory and Practice* (S. W. Weil and I. McGill, eds), pp. 245–272. Milton Keynes: The Society for Research into Higher Education and Open University Press.

Neame, R. L. B., Mitchell, K. R., Feletti, G. I. and McIntosh, J. (1985) Problem-solving in undergraduate medical students. *Medical Decision Making*, **5**, 312–324.

Newble, D. I. and Jaeger, K. (1983) The effect of assessments and examinations on the learning of medical students. *Medical Education*, **17**, 165–171.

Norman, G. R. (1990) Editorial: problem-solving skills and problem-based learning. *Physiotherapy Theory and Practice*, **6**, 53–54.

Patel, V. L. and Groen, G. J. (1991) The general and specific nature of medical expertise: A critical look. In *Toward A General Theory Of Expertise: Prospects and Limits* (A. Ericsson and J. Smith, eds), pp. 93–125. New York: Cambridge University Press.

Ramsden, P. (1984) The context of learning. In *The Experience of Learning* (F. Marton, D. Hounsell and N. Entwistle, eds), pp. 000–000. Edinburgh: Scottish Academic Press.

Ramsden, P. (1985) Student learning research: Retrospect and prospect. *Higher Education Research and Development*, **4**, 51–70.

Ramsden, P. (1988a) Preface. In *Improving Learning: New Perspectives* (P. Ramsden, ed.), pp. vii–ix. London: Kogan Page.

Ramsden, P. (1988b) Studying learning: Improving teaching. In *Improving Learning: New Perspectives* (P. Ramsden, ed.), pp. 13–31. London: Kogan Page.

Rogers, C. R. (1983) *Freedom to Learn for the 80s*. Columbus, OH: Charles E. Merrill.

Rogers, J. C., Swee, D. E. and Ullian, J. A. (1991) Teaching medical decision making and students' clinical problem solving skills. *Medical Teacher*, **13**, 157–164.

Schön, D. A. (1987) *Educating the Reflective Practitioner*. San Francisco: Jossey-Bass.

Schwartz, K. B. (1991) Clinical reasoning and new ideas on intelligence: Implications for teaching and learning. *The American Journal of Occupational Therapy*, **45**, 1033–1037.

Shepard, K. F. and Jensen, G. M. (1990) Physical therapist curricula for the 1990s: Educating the reflective practitioner. *Physical Therapy*, **70**, 566–573.

Tanner, C.A. (1987) Teaching clinical judgement. *Annual Review of Nursing Research*, **5**, 153–173.

Terry, W. and Higgs, J. (1993) Educational programmes to develop clinical reasoning skills. *Australian Journal of Physiotherapy*, **39**, 47–51.

Watkins, D. (1984) Student perceptions of factors influencing tertiary learning. *Higher Education Research and Development*, **3**, 33–50.

Whelan, G. (1988) Improving medical students' clinical-problem-solving. In *Improving Learning: New Perspectives* (P. Ramsden, ed.), pp. 199–214. London: Kogan Page.

15

The Internet and clinical reasoning

Allan Christie, Paul Worley and Mark Jones

Clinical reasoning is a cognitive process that is difficult to explain, demonstrate and assess. Therefore teaching clinical reasoning requires educational methods that make the internal process more accessible. Clinical reasoning is also closely associated with knowledge and practice. Thus learning clinical reasoning requires educational experiences which promote active integration of cognitive processes, clinical experiences and the associated knowledge into learners' existing knowledge structures. Clinical reasoning is becoming more cognitively demanding as the body of knowledge within respective health professions continues to grow.

Educational technology in the form of knowledge resources can assist clinicians in their reasoning by providing support systems for clinical decision making and by providing greater access to the collective knowledge of the profession and beyond. 'Technology' is an umbrella term that may be defined as the totality of the means employed to provide objects necessary for human support. Our approach to the use of technology in education is that it must be a tool to support the clinical education process and not direct it. It is not the technology that is important, but rather what it allows the clinician to achieve with respect to health outcomes, and what it allows the learner to achieve with respect to the attainment of knowledge and the development of problem-solving skills. Two important components which facilitate the learning of clinical reasoning are (a) ready access to information and (b) a system in which the learner is an active participant in the learning process. Computer-facilitated learning technologies and the Internet both have much to offer with

respect to these factors; in addition, they allow students to learn at their own pace, in their own time and place.

In the first edition of this book we discussed computer-facilitated learning and computer support systems and their role in clinical reasoning. The focus of this chapter is on the role of the Internet in facilitating clinical reasoning in both student learning and clinical practice. This chapter also provides a listing of Internet resources related to clinical reasoning, to assist readers in their ongoing research and practice in this field.

What is the Internet?

The Internet is an interconnection of a massive network of computers, all sharing information, using a simple protocol for this data exchange. Having began life in 1969, it celebrates its 30th birthday this year. The Internet is much more than simply the World Wide Web, although with 1.5 million new web pages being added daily it is not surprising that this particular application commands so much attention. A few other statistics will serve to underline the importance of the Internet as an essential tool of professional life. It is estimated that there are approximately 150 million people worldwide who use the Internet at least once a week. The USA has by the far the largest number of users with approximately 77 million, followed by Japan with 10 million and the UK with 8 million. Australia is sixth with 4.5 million, giving it one of the highest per capita rates in the world.

The Internet and learning clinical reasoning

Experiential learning is the traditional method of clinical instruction. It was Osler (1962) who led the call at the turn of this century to bring the student to the patient. In his day this meant bringing students to the bedside of patients in urban public hospitals, and the 'teaching hospital' was born. The Flexner Report on Physician Education (Flexner, 1910), released a decade later, articulated the importance to clinicians of a sound understanding of the biological sciences that underpin clinical reasoning.

These two elements of instruction, the clinical experience and the underlying scientific framework, along with the technological and scientific advances spawned by this coalescence, soon saw the community's academic clinical expertise become concentrated in large, research-oriented, university-affiliated tertiary teaching hospitals. Here students have been instructed in the art and techniques of inductive clinical reasoning by clinicians employed not for their teaching abilities but primarily for their clinical experience or research capability.

Recently, the teaching capacity of these institutions has come under a number of threats.

(a) *Information overload*. The partnership of basic scientist and clinician has had some remarkable results. The resultant knowledge explosion of the late 20th century has resulted in the situation where there are now over two million medically relevant research articles published every year. Thomas Edison claimed at the turn of the century that we do not know one-millionth of one per cent about anything. How many health science students feel the same today? How does a clinical student incorporate this constantly evolving knowledge into their clinical learning?

(b) *Research dominance*. Some have claimed that this research success in recent decades has come at the expense of clinical learning opportunities for clinicians in training. Bloom (1989) has even proposed that the only reason research-based institutions have retained a clinical teaching role is to give their research programs public credibility. The present reliance of most universities on external competitive grant funding has understandably focused the institutions' efforts on research. The money available for clinical

education pales into insignificance when placed alongside the funding for biomedical research. Are the resulting research-oriented clinicians best placed to instruct students in clinical reasoning?

(c) *Narrow patient profile*. The advances in investigative and therapeutic technology, and the escalating cost of these interventions, have caused a change in the patient profile of teaching hospitals. Increasingly, we have seen a concentration on selected major acute illnesses to the exclusion of less severe acute illnesses and many categories of chronic illness, which are the main burden on the health system. How then are students to find appropriate clinical material on which to cut their clinical reasoning teeth? Is there a paradoxical incongruity between the stated broad curricular goals of many health education institutions, which often emphasize an understanding of the common clinical problems facing their profession, and both the narrow patient base provided for student learning and the sub-specialized experience of available clinical tutors?

(d) *Student access*. The funding of clinical services in many western nations has been under close public scrutiny in recent years. In most countries there has been increasing external control on clinical practice, through either commercial insurance contracts or 'outcomes-based' and 'input-efficient' legislative initiatives. This external input has contributed to an increasingly 'efficient' tertiary hospital sector, with efficiency often measured in decreased 'occupied bed days' for hospital-based intervention. To meet new criteria, hospitals have naturally focused on areas (e.g. early discharge) where efficiencies are easiest to attain, resulting in a further skewing of the caseload available for clinical learning. How does an educational institution reconcile its financial need to have patients discharged as soon as possible with the obligation to allow clinicians and students time to interact 'at the bedside'? How do students find suitable and accessible clinical material for learning when the patient has often been discharged before the student was even aware of the admission? How do clinicians, under increasing pressure from health administrators to see more patients in less time, find the time to instruct their students in clinical reasoning?

These questions point to some of the problems faced by an increasingly complex and dis-articulated learning environment for clinical reasoning. Can a communication and networking tool such as the Internet assist us in this complex milieu?

The Internet is primarily an electronic communication tool that can link people to people or people to information in ways not previously possible. Considering that these two relationships are also the building blocks of learning clinical reasoning, it is not surprising that there are numerous examples of institutions using the Internet to overcome the disconnectivity that we have described above.

As access to appropriate patients is no longer predictably available in tertiary hospitals, many institutions are looking to community-based clinical learning. This focus enables students to find suitable clinical material to stimulate enquiry and hypothesis generation. As students in such sites often do not have proximate access to library facilities, the Internet as an information source can be invaluable in the learning process. The Internet can also be useful to students on the main campus, because no library can provide on-site access to all the information an inquisitive student will require.

There is an important role for academic institutions to provide guidance to students regarding the credibility of Internet sites. This accreditation process, along with training for students in critical appraisal, is an essential prerequisite if students are to know how to trust the information they access through the Internet.

Many clinical reasoning dilemmas lead naturally to a discussion with an expert in the field. With phone calls unanswered, appointment books full or the professor 'at an important meeting', access to these overworked experts can be difficult for students in the hospital, let alone students learning in the community. This is where *E-mail* can be useful. E-mail is an inexpensive asynchronous electronic communication medium. It enables people to communicate effectively and efficiently without having to negotiate common diary times to meet either physically or electronically. In this way, despite their time constraints, academics can be readily available to students. Students can ask their questions at the time of the clinical encounter and experts can answer at a time convenient to them, often while students are engaged in their next clinical learning activity. This facility provides opportunities for academics to plan their teaching activities in new ways. The increase in accessibility still takes significant time, which must be anticipated carefully.

E-mail access does not obviate the need for quality 'hands on' clinical supervision, but it does mean that the supervisor does not have to be an expert in every area. Students can also have more choice in the source from which or from whom they seek advice and this choice need not be bounded by institutional, state or even national boundaries. It is thus possible to create a clinical 'campus without walls' and encourage high-quality clinical learning in communities remote from the parent institution. This campus can incorporate group learning activities as well.

Tutorials can be held by means of Internet-based videoconferencing, utilizing a variety of commercially available software. E-mail-based formal tutorials can also be used, and chat groups or workgroups provide less formal methods of interacting in a 'classroom without walls'.

A rural example – The Parallel Rural Community Curriculum (PRCC)

One important application of Internet-facilitated learning of clinical reasoning is in the area of rural health. In many nations there is a maldistribution of health professionals resulting in inadequate numbers in rural areas (Strasser, 1995). Evidence has been available for decades to show that students who have positive learning experiences in rural communities are 2–5 times more likely to return to a rural area to practise compared to students who learn in an urban environment (Brazeau *et al.*, 1990). Concerned governments have therefore placed pressure on universities to increase the amount of clinical teaching that occurs in rural locations.

One of the difficulties that universities have faced in attempting to meet this challenge has been the apparent lack of appropriate educational resources in rural communities. There is an acknowledged wealth of clinical experience for students, but where are the health libraries, the experts or the peer interaction considered vital to the clinical learning process? Through the use of Internet resources, as documented above, the excellent clinical learning opportunities available in rural communities can be connected to the academic expertise and support available at the main city campus.

Experience in applying this model to undergraduate medical education[1] suggests that the

---

[1] Paul Worley

clinical reasoning capability of students trained in rural communities is equal to if not better than that of their tertiary hospital trained colleagues. The students with rural training have performed better than their colleagues in both objective structured clinical examinations and objective written clinical-reasoning tests. This program, known as the PRCC, has also encouraged students at the urban site to utilize information technology resources in their clinical learning. Clinical teachers at the tertiary hospital have likewise seen the time management benefits and have incorporated techniques developed for the PRCC in their hospital-based teaching.

It is important to note that students and staff have learned that simple technology is often more effective than the 'latest and greatest'. For instance, students often prefer to receive lectures by viewing videotapes rather than by video-conferencing. Once again, the issue of asynchronous communication is important here. The lecture times often conflict with other clinical learning opportunities. Videotapes can be viewed at a time that is convenient and sometimes more clinically relevant to the student, and the tape can be replayed for clarification. However, when interactivity is important, then Internet-based technologies such as E-mail, web-based messaging, electronic whiteboard and real-time chat come to the fore. It must also be said that whilst E-mail communication with supervising clinicians is cheaper and quicker than fax or phone, the E-mail is no use if it is not read! Our experience is that until all those involved in the enterprise are regular and effective users of the Internet, parallel communication with fax or phone is necessary. Although students are often great teachers of clinicians in using the Internet, adequate resources must be invested in staff training in Internet literacy.

While we have highlighted the academic uses of the Internet for these remote students, the Internet also provides an effective and inexpensive means of overcoming social isolation, especially isolation from peers and family. Learning to overcome this isolation is in itself an important skill for sustainable rural clinical practice. Although this is not at first glance a component of clinical reasoning, it could be argued that a lonely student will not learn as effectively as one with effective peer or family support.

Thus, through appropriate use of the Internet, universities are able to fulfil their social accountability by addressing the rural health workforce shortage whilst not compromising their academic accountability to students. By utilizing Internet communication resources, students can experience the best of all worlds: access to relevant clinical stimulation wherever that can be found, peer interaction and expert opinion from either validated references or experienced practitioners, wherever they may be found. If Osler was alive today, would he not be at the forefront of such transformation in learning clinical reasoning?

The Internet and clinical reasoning in professional practice

> To be conscious that you are ignorant is a great step to knowledge
> *Benjamin Disraeli (1835–1910), English statesman and writer*

The term 'evidence-based health care' has become almost a health care mantra during the last decade of the 20th century. But how can an individual practitioner know what the evidence says about every case seen? The proliferation of medical research, and its variable quality, make this a daunting task. Added to this is the increasing number of patients who wish to access such information themselves. The Cochrane Collaboration[2] is an international effort to prepare, maintain and promote the accessibility of systematic reviews of the effects of health care interventions. By accessing databases such as the Cochrane Database, both practitioner and patient can readily discover a quality-filtered synthesis of the world's research-based knowledge about their particular clinical problems. That is, if the information exists! The more health care practitioners strive to base their decisions on evidence, the more they find that relatively few areas of clinical practice have been subjected to randomized controlled trials (RCTs), the cornerstone of the Cochrane Collaboration. While RCTs should not be considered the only valid source of evidence or knowledge (see Chapter 36), information from all sources (e.g. RCTs, qualitative research, expert experience) can be made more accessible with the help of the Internet. Let us consider, then, how the Internet can assist in clinical reasoning in day to day practice.

Decision-support systems

Assistance with clinical reasoning in practice is available through expert systems that provide

---

[2] Australasian Cochrane Centre – see electronic address later in the text.

decision-support capabilities (Delitto *et al.*, 1989). Shortliffe (1987) defined a clinical decision-support system as any computer program that deals with clinical data or medical knowledge and which performs one or more of the following tasks: information management, attention focusing, and patient-specific consultation.

The *information management* category refers primarily to hospital information systems that permit the storage and retrieval of patient data but generally do not assist professionals in the use of the data to solve specific clinical problems. Interpretation is left to the individual.

Attention-focusing systems examine data for abnormal values or combinations of values, such as pharmaceutical applications that warn of adverse drug interactions. Focusing is the principle underlying the use of computer-generated reminders to increase compliance with predefined protocols of care.

The task of *patient-specific consultation* refers to what are commonly known as expert systems used in clinical diagnosis and therapy planning. Expert systems refer to knowledge-based structures that can contain protocols for eliciting input from the user and large databases with decision rules or algorithms to weigh the information obtained. That is, they use the knowledge provided by their creators to enter, organize and summarize data. The outputs from these systems are often patient classifications or diagnoses with suggested treatment strategies. However, making the final diagnosis for the patient's problems remains a uniquely human task. Such programs may be used in general medical practice, for instance.

A criticism of expert systems is that they tend to restrict thinking by fostering tunnel vision and over-reliance on the computer's as opposed to the clinician's knowledge and information processing. This is a reflection on the system's implementation and use rather than the capabilities of the tool itself. The elicitation of knowledge from experts, the engineering of that knowledge into the structure required by the specific expert system tool, and the integration of the final expert system into a total decision-support system are difficult, costly and time consuming tasks. It is easier to isolate a single area of concern and provide a tool to address that problem while holding all other factors constant. This forces users themselves to provide the breadth of vision so often lacking. If expert systems are regarded as aids to clinical decision making rather than as usurping that process, then the judgement of the clinician can be integrated

with the decision-enhancing responses of information-based systems. The feedback obtained from decision-support systems provides clear opportunity for the knowledge acquisition that is so integral to clinical reasoning.

Although decision-support systems have traditionally been confined to individual computers or networks at a particular site (often termed an 'Intranet'), as the speed of the Internet is increasing, the cost is decreasing, and security issues are being addressed, these systems will frequently be developed for Internet access.

Internet-based knowledge resources

Information processing theory assumes that human problem solvers are constrained by limitations of memory (Newell and Simon, 1972). A practitioner's clinical reasoning skills in a particular domain are closely related to the availability of knowledge in that domain as well as the practitioner's amount of case experience (Aegerter *et al.*, 1992; Cervero, 1988; Custers *et al.*, 1993; Elstein *et al.*, 1978).

Until recently, the use of information technology in providing access to a practical body of knowledge has been limited to resources (computer disks, peripheral devices such as CD-ROM players) that have a physical presence. With the burgeoning use of the Internet over the last 10 years, vast amounts of information and access to experts worldwide in related fields of interest are now readily available. Computer-mediated communication is now a common activity, with electronic mail, internet relay chat, electronic news groups and electronic discussion groups providing avenues for the discussion and dissemination of information on virtually any topic.

In an increasingly digital world, knowledge resources are proliferating at an incredible rate. Indeed, the amount of information available through computer networks can be overwhelming and information literacy skills need to be honed to take advantage of this resource. In addition, the commercial potential for successful Internet sites may raise questions of conflict of interest and bias as health care becomes increasingly market driven.

Examples of internet sites related to clinical reasoning

Given the phenomenal growth of the Internet which still continues to double every eight months or so what strategies can one use to manage the flow of data that all but threatens to swamp us with information?

Firstly, a decision needs to be made how widely the net should be cast. For 'clinical reasoning', do we also search for 'diagnostic reasoning', clinical decision making', 'clinical problem solving', 'evidence-based medicine' and so on. Using these keywords with a number of the popular Internet search engines soon returns more information than can be easily managed. For instance, searching for 'clinical reasoning' using the AltaVista search engine (http://www.altavista.com) returned nearly 1200 records. However, closer examination of these reveals very few providing relevant and useful information. More often these instances of 'clinical reasoning' relate either to course syllabi, research grant applications, book reviews, etc. The online resources that are available mainly pertain to conference papers and research reports with very few instances of teaching clinical reasoning via the online environment. Some useful resources are given below.

Groups, centres, associations, societies

- MIT Clinical Decision Making Group
  http://ga.org
- Artificial Intelligence Laboratory – University of Chicago CBR-MED Frequently Asked Questions
  http://www.cs.uchicago.edu/cbr-med/html/faq.html
- Laboratory for Computing, Cognition and Clinical Skills
  http://www.med.umich.edu/meded/lc3.html
- Australasian Cochrane Centre
  http://som.flinders.edu.au/FUSA/Cochrane/
- Centre for Evidence-based Medicine
  http://cebm.jr2.ox.ac.uk/
- American Medical Informatics Association
  http://www.amia.org/lkres.html
- Society for Medical Decision Making
  http://www.gwu.edu/~smdm/
- Society for Judgment and Decision Making
  http://www.sjdm.org/

Clinical reasoning information online

- Facilitating Clinical Reasoning Through Computer-based Learning and Feedback, Deborah A. Bryce, Nicholas J.C. King, Richmond W. Jeremy, and J. Hurley Myers
  (http://www.curtin.edu.au/conference/ASCILITE97/papers/Bryce/Bryce.html)

- Validated computer model for measuring clinical reasoning proficiency, strategy, thoroughness and efficiency, Dane M. Chapman, Judith G. Calhoun, Wayne K. Davis, Adrian P. VanMondfrans
  http://gema.library.ucsf.edu:8081/Originals/SAEMabs/SA179.html
- An Overview of Computer-assisted Instruction and a Qualitative Evaluation of a Program, Amy J. Clemens, RN, University of Maryland
  http://parsons.ab.umd.edu/~aclemens/text/article.html
- Medical Student Response to Computer Technology and Patient Simulation Software as a Way to Practice the Patient Encounter.
  http://www.odont.ku.dk/mhse/abstracts/54a.txt
- Bridging the Research-Practice Divide: Using General-Semantics in Physical Therapy Practice
  http://www.transmillennium.net/brucekodish/researchpractice.htm
- Clinical Reasoning, David Theige (PowerPoint presentation)
  http://osler.med.und.nodak.edu/presentations/clinReasoning/index.htm
- Introduction to Clinical Reasoning home page
  http://www.musc.edu/muscid/icrhomepage.html
- Evaluation of a Diagnostic Reasoning Program (DxR): Exploring Student Perceptions and Addressing Faculty Concerns, Deborah A. Bryce, Nicholas J. King, Celia F. Graebner and J. Hurley Myers
  http://www-jime.open.ac.uk/98/1/

Web-based education

- OT 620 (section A) – Winter, 1998 Clinical Reasoning III
  http://www3.gvsu.edu/wcb/schools/GV/pt/hooperb/4/
  A reasonable attempt at providing information and some interaction.
- MasterMed – a series of online cases to enhance clinical reasoning
  http://clinical.web.unsw.edu.au/mastermed/
  Appears to have potential but is password-protected – apparently undergoing evaluation.

General information sites

- Health One (Singapore)
  http://www.health1.nus.edu.sg/
- Medscape
  http://www.medscape.com

- Physiotherapy Global Links
  http://ptglobal.net
- American Educational Research Association Division I: Education in the Professions
  http://www.med.umich.edu/aera/literature.html
- RALE® (Respiratory Acoustics Laboratory Environment) Repository
  (http://www.RALE.ca/) presents digital recordings of respiratory sounds in health and disease.
- Many Journals are now available online. For example the *British Medical Journal* is available free of charge at http://www.bmj.com/

Non-Internet-based resources

The Internet is a very powerful tool for finding resources that are available but not necessarily in the online environment. Examples of non-internet-based resources include:
- Physiotherapy Global-Links
  Physical CD-ROM
  (http://www.netspot.unisa.edu.au/pt/physical.html)
- Health Uniserve in Australia
  List of electronic teaching materials
  http://health.uniserve.edu.au/scripts/dbml.exe?template=review.dbm
  Examples include:
- Clinical Decision Making
- Diagnostic Reasoning (DxR)
- Diagnostic Reasoning – Academic Series (Student Cases). Symptom-Based Case Studies on CD-ROM – A Problem-Based Learning Tool
  http://www.phoenix.net/~laser/img/DXR_ACAD.HTM
- University of Otago – School of Physiotherapy
  Interactive Clinical Reasoning in Manipulative Physiotherapy
  http://www.otago.ac.nz/ITS/etss/teachTechGrant/grants97.html

Clinical reasoning online

The authors of this chapter are developing an online resource for the teaching and learning of clinical reasoning. It is designed to take advantage of a number of key strengths of the Internet, i.e. access to up-to-date information, collaborative learning and timely access to both information and expertise. This learning module called 'Clinical Reasoning Online' will also make use of audio and video streaming to supplement text-based information. Specifically, this online learning module will include the following:

- Password access for registered users.
- Guest access for an overview purpose.
- Streaming audio using RealSystems player (http://www.real.com) providing weekly updates from key knowledge providers.
- Personalization of learning with ability to save study notes online, track progress through materials and filter information according to read/unread since last login/over a period of time/all, etc.
- Interactive web-based forums linked to E-mail lists.
- Real-time chat sessions for participants to share experiences and exchange ideas.
- Resources database for providing up-to-date information.

An example of this approach being used in another knowledge domain can be viewed at http://www.bba.unisa.edu.au

The online learning environment provides an excellent means of supplementing existing efforts to teach clinical reasoning and to facilitate the acquisition of knowledge. For example, when self-instructional interactive computer activities are designed to present real life clinical scenarios, students' cognitive processes such as hypothesis generation, hypothesis testing and problem formulation/re-formulation can be prompted. This form of active participation assists in activating students' existing knowledge while varying forms of feedback and resource direction enable integration of new information into the development of new knowledge structures. Experiential learning theory (Kolb, 1984) provides a useful basis on which interactive learning programs to facilitate the development of clinical reasoning and acquisition of knowledge can be created.

Clinical reasoning is becoming more cognitively demanding as the body of knowledge within respective health professions continues to grow. Educational technology in the form of knowledge resources can assist clinicians in their reasoning by providing support systems for clinical decision making and by providing greater access to the collective knowledge of the profession. Examples include comprehensive web sites such as Medscape (http://www.medscape.com), Physiotherapy Global-links, etc. These web sites provide 'one-stop shops' for information pertaining to a particular health-related discipline. For instance,

Medscape provides access to full-text articles, database searching of Medline, Toxline, Aidsline; medical dictionary; practice guidelines; clinical pearls; continuing medical education; quizzes and interactive cases.

Conclusion

Through this chapter the authors have sought to demonstrate the ways in which the Internet and its various applications (E-mail, World Wide Web, etc.) can assist in the teaching and learning of clinical reasoning and in clinical reasoning in practice. Access to up-to-date information and collaborative, interactive learning environments provides a powerful resource for both the student and clinician to acquire, maintain and enhance their clinical reasoning ability.

References

Aegerter, P., Auvert, B., Gilbos, V. *et al.* (1992) An intelligent computer-assisted instruction system designed for rural health workers in developing countries. *Methods of Information in Medicine*, **31**, 193–203.

Bloom, S. W. (1989) The medical school as a social organisation: The sources of resistance to change. *Medical Education*, **23**, 228–241.

Brazeau, N. K., Potts, M. J. and Hickner, J. M. (1990) The Upper Peninsula Program: A successful model for increasing the primary care physicians in rural areas. *Family Medicine*, **22**, 350–355.

Cervero, R. M. (1988) *Effective Continuing Education for Professionals*. San Francisco: Jossey-Bass.

Custers, E., Boshuizen, H. and Schmidt, H. (1993) The influence of typicality of case descriptions on subjective disease probability estimations. Paper presented at the *Annual Meeting of the American Educational Research Association, American Educational Research Association*, Atlanta, GA, April 12–16.

Delitto, A., Shulman, A. D. and Rose, S. J. (1989) On developing expert-based decision-support systems in physical therapy: The NIOSH low back atlas. *Physical Therapy*, **69**, 554–558.

Elstein, A. S., Shulman, L. S. and Sprafka, S. S. (1978) *Medical Problem Solving: An Analysis of Clinical Reasoning*. Cambridge, MA: Harvard University Press.

Flexner, A. (1910) *Medical Education in the United States and Canada: A Report to the Carnegie Foundation for the Advancement of Teaching*. Bulletin 4. Boston, MA: Updyke.

Kolb, D. A. (1984) *Experiential Learning: Experience as the Source of Learning and Development*. Englewood Cliffs, NJ: Prentice-Hall.

Osler, W. (1962) William Osler's farewell address to American and Canadian medical students. *Canadian Medical Association Journal*, **67**, 762–764.

Newell, A. and Simon, H. (1972) *Human Problem Solving*. Englewood Cliffs, NJ: Prentice-Hall.

Shortliffe, E. H. (1987) Computer programs to support clinical decision-making. *Journal of the American Medical Association*, **258**, 61–66.

Strasser, R. P. (1995) Policy on training for rural practice. *WONCA World Council Meeting*, June 1995.

16

Assessing clinical reasoning

David Newble, Geoffrey Norman and Cees van der Vleuten

The term *clinical reasoning* is used in varying ways. In this chapter we use it as a component of clinical competence which might elsewhere be referred to as 'clinical problem solving'. Our interest in its assessment reflects a wider concern with methods of assessment of both clinical competence and on-the-job clinical performance.

Clinical reasoning can be viewed as one of three components which comprise clinical competence, the others being relevant knowledge and relevant skills (see Figure 16.1). The latter includes interpersonal, clinical and technical skills. Clinical reasoning can broadly be considered to be the intellectual activity which synthesizes information obtained from the clinical situation, integrates it with previous knowledge and experience, and uses it for making diagnostic and management decisions. Each component of competence is influenced by a range of attitudinal aspects which are difficult to define and even more difficult to consider in any assessment procedure.

For assessment and test development purposes, the three components are often considered separately, so that specific tests are devised to assess relevant knowledge (e.g. multiple choice tests), relevant skills (e.g. an objective structured clinical examination) and clinical reasoning (e.g. patient management problems). In fact, these components are likely to be highly inter-related (Norman *et al.*, 1985).

Historical perspective

In the 1960s and 1970s there was considerable interest in the development of methods which assessed 'clinical problem-solving skills'. The interest arose partly from a concern to test at a greater depth than could be achieved with objective Multiple Choice Question (MCQ)-type tests and partly from an interest in the research being done at this time on the clinical reasoning process. The main thrust was to simulate on paper, and later by computer, the process by which a doctor took a history, obtained information from the physical examination and made diagnostic, investigational and management decisions.

Pioneering work in this field was done by Rimoldi (1961), who devised a card deck-based method to investigate the diagnostic ability of medical students. He showed differences in the performance of students of varying degrees of seniority compared to practising clinicians. He concluded that such a method could be used to measure objectively students' diagnostic skills and to train them in clinical reasoning. This technique was adapted by Helfer and Slater (1971) and called the *Diagnostic Management Problem*.

A slightly more sophisticated method was developed at the University of Illinois and called the *Patient Management Problem* (PMP) (McGuire and Babbott, 1967). A typical PMP begins with a variable amount of information about the patient. The student is then requested to collect

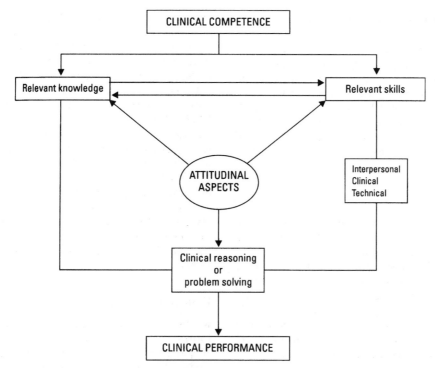

Figure 16.1 Components of clinical competence

further data sequentially in either a linear or branching fashion. A variety of technical devices are available to obscure the data until selected. After collecting history and examination data, ostensibly in the manner and order that would have pertained in the live patient situation, the student may be allowed to select investigations and/or make diagnostic and management decisions. The pathway of the student is compared to that of an expert or criterion group, and composite scores are determined for such aspects as thoroughness, efficiency and proficiency.

By 1974, 18 varieties of PMP could be identified (Galofre, 1974). PMPs became widely used for certification purposes, being accepted more on the basis of their perceived fidelity than their psychometric properties. They were perceived as a more valid measure of problem solving ability than other paper-and-pencil tests, with the advantage of being objectively scored.

Alternative approaches were also explored at this time. These included the *Sequential Management Problem* (SMP) (Berner *et al.*, 1974) and the *Modified Essay Question* (MEQ) (Hodgkin and Knox, 1975). Each of these introduces into the simulation varying amounts of sequential data and feedback. Student answers are written in, rather than selected from a fixed list of options, overcoming to some extent the cueing problem associated with most PMP formats (see below).

The SMP has not been used widely, probably because of the practical difficulties involved in collecting each section before the next is made available. Because of this, little information has been published on its reliability and validity (Neufeld and Norman, 1985). The MEQ, on the other hand, has been used quite extensively by the medical profession in some parts of the world, both for in-course assessments and for the certification of competence. This reflects, in part, the relative ease of construction of MEQs as compared to PMPs (Feletti, 1980). A typical MEQ once again begins with a case vignette. Students are asked to respond to questions in a short essay format. New information is provided sequentially which relates to differing and evolving circumstances of the same case. Some skill is required to avoid providing cues to earlier or subsequent sections of the MEQ. Few studies are available of the reliability and validity of this method but it has face validity, appears to be acceptable and is practicable (Feletti, 1980; Neufeld and Norman, 1985).

Patient management problems

Despite initial enthusiasm and widespread use there have been growing concerns about the credibility of PMPs, whether presented in written or computer-based format. These concerns relate partly to some technical and psychometric limitations and partly to research which raises doubt as to whether they are truly measures of problem solving. Some of these concerns are discussed below.

Cueing

One technical problem with PMPs is that of cueing. For scoring purposes, PMPs provide a predetermined and usually limited selection of responses. The presence of these lists acts as a prompt to the examinee which improves performance and distorts clinical problem-solving behaviour (Norman and Feightner, 1981; Goran *et al.*, 1973; McCarthy, 1966; Newble *et al.*, 1982). Great ingenuity has been shown in trying to minimize this effect, but it remains a significant problem.

Scoring

Scoring has been the major difficulty associated with PMPs. The development of a scoring system usually involves a panel of experts who decide, by consensus, on the acceptable pathways through the problem and on the weight (positive and negative) which should be given to the options in each section of the simulation. Students' scores are compared to those of the expert panel, and are used to calculate composite scores such as proficiency, efficiency, thoroughness and overall competence. Many forms of this weighted scoring system of varying complexity have been developed. However, correlations between methods are high (Bligh, 1980; Norcini *et al.*, 1983; Norman and Feightner, 1981).

In fact, this high correlation could have been anticipated. Numerous studies in a wide number of domains have shown that virtually all weighting schemes, regardless of complexity, have high correlations with simple counts of items (Wainer, 1976). Since most PMPs consist of large numbers of history-based items, physical examination findings and routine laboratory tests, nearly all scores reduce to a measure of thoroughness of data gathering, a measure which has been shown to be unrelated to diagnostic accuracy (Norman *et al.*, 1985). It is apparent that experts may follow many pathways through a problem and, moreover, experts take many shortcuts since they can use information more optimally than novices. The net result is that true expert performance on a PMP is frequently penalized (Marshall, 1977).

Confidence in PMPs has been further undermined by research comparing performance on PMPs of experienced clinicians with that of less experienced clinicians or students. In some studies, students have been shown to score higher than qualified doctors (Newble *et al.*, 1982). Conventional scoring systems may over-reward thoroughness, again leading to higher scores for less competent and less efficient problem solvers (Marshall, 1977). Despite efforts to deal with the problems associated with scoring, no satisfactory solution has been achieved (Swanson *et al.*, 1987).

Content or case specificity

Research has demonstrated consistently that performance on one PMP is a poor predictor of performance on another PMP. From a number of studies the correlation across problems was of the order of 0.1–0.3 (Norman *et al.*, 1985). This observation appears to undermine one of the original hypotheses underlying the development of problem-solving simulations, i.e. that they measure problem solving ability. If that was so, correlations between PMPs ought to be high, since those who are better problem solvers, either as a result of native ability or learned skills, should exhibit superior performance across a wide range of problems, independent of specific content knowledge. The explanation of this phenomenon is referred to variously as 'content specificity' or 'case specificity'. Interestingly, the finding is not peculiar to PMPs but is also seen for other methods which assess aspects of clinical competence and performance, including oral examinations (Swanson, 1987), vignette-based written tests (De Graaf *et al.*, 1987; Page *et al.*, 1995), chart audits (Erviti *et al.*, 1980), performance-based tests (Van der Vleuten and Swanson, 1990) and computer-based simulations (Swanson *et al.*, 1987).

Given these limitations, doubt has been cast on the value of the PMP and, indeed, for any format which involves extensive and lengthy testing with relatively few cases. Some authors have suggested they should not be used for decision making purposes until their validity has been more clearly established (Swanson *et al.*, 1987). However, the experience with PMPs has alerted us to our limited understanding of the nature of clinical reasoning. Among other things, it has stimulated research of a more fundamental nature into the cognitive functioning of medical students and doctors.

New concepts of clinical reasoning

In the 1970s and 1980s several studies showed that expert clinicians performed little better than less experienced doctors on a variety of simulations of clinical problem solving (Neufeld and Norman, 1985). This phenomenon occurred not only with PMPs but also with problems presented by real and standardized patients (Schmidt *et al.*, 1990). Such studies challenged the paradigms underlying previous test development. Knowledge gained from cognitive psychological research into the nature of clinical reasoning and the differences between experts and novices is now providing new insights which promise to redirect test development (Norman *et al.*, 1989; Regehr and Norman, 1996; Schmidt *et al.*, 1990). (See also Chapters 2, 4, 5 and 10.)

Current understanding would suggest that problem-solving ability is not a separate skill or entity which grows with training and experience and that it cannot be measured independent of relevant content knowledge. In other words, it has not generally been possible to establish that a person who is good at solving problems in one type of situation is predictably superior at solving problems in other types of situation. Chess grandmasters are exceptional only at solving chess problems (Chase and Simon, 1973; De Groot, 1965). Problem-solving ability appears to be highly dependent on knowledge, not just the amount of knowledge but also its specificity and the way it is structured, stored, accessed and retrieved. This is not to say that knowledge alone is sufficient for efficient and effective clinical reasoning. Higher-order control processes also play an integral role (Bransford *et al.*, 1986). These two components have been studied in great depth and from several different disciplinary perspectives, making generalization difficult and the terminology confusing for the uninitiated (Bransford *et al.*, 1986; Elstein *et al.*, 1990; Schmidt *et al.*, 1990). A simplified model is presented in Figure 16.2. We have chosen *higher order control processes* as a relatively neutral term to include a wide range of intellectual strategies which may be brought to bear as problems are being solved. A flavour of the other terms used by writers in this aspect of problem solving can be gained from this list: metacognition; executive thinking; categorization; rehearsal, organization and re-organization; chunking; debugging; the deep approach; hypothetico-deductive thinking.

Organized knowledge is held by some to be the key to successful problem solving. It is the specificity of the knowledge and how it is structured and retrieved in relation to the problem that determines success and expertise (Norman *et al.*, 1989). One such theory proposes that knowledge is structured in various ways or levels (Bordage and Lemieux, 1991). Novices tend to have low or dispersed levels of knowledge. As experience grows knowledge is elaborated and compiled into complex structures and schemata. The organization is heavily influenced by the context in which the experience was attained.

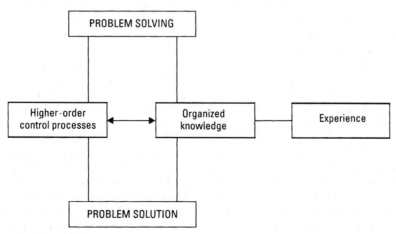

Figure 16.2 Aspects of problem solving

An alternative theory of knowledge organization proposes three different kinds of information relevant to solving clinical problems. The most elementary is knowledge of disease processes and causal relationships, the basic science of medicine. At a later level, students acquire 'illness scripts' which are quite literal list-like structures relating signs and symptoms to disease prototypes (Felto-vich and Barrows, 1984). At the highest level of functioning, the expert uses a sophisticated form of pattern recognition characterized by speed and efficient use of information (Brooks *et al*., 1991; Schmidt *et al*., 1990). It is theorized that this latter representation is drawn to a large degree from direct experience with patients, and that pattern recognition is, in fact, recognition at a holistic level of the similarity between the present patient and previous patients. Some studies have experimentally demonstrated some features of this process. For example, recent experience has demonstrated that similar appearing dermatologic lesions can influence diagnostic accuracy and expert radiologists have been shown to recognize chest lesions using a process which is apparently only loosely related to the presence or absence of specific signs (Brooks *et al*., 1991). In fact, in the latter case, a biasing history can change not only the likelihood of diagnosis but also the judgement of the presence or absence of specific signs (Norman *et al*., 1992). Seeing a vivid example of a clinical problem as much as several weeks earlier can change diagnostic judgements of other cases which match only on age, sex and chief complaint (Van Rossum *et al*., 1989).

This is not to indicate that all expert clinical reasoning occurs by pattern recognition. It is hypothesized that when experts find themselves in a position where clear analogies are not present and the problem is difficult, they may revert to more analytical methods and, in rare circumstances, may analyse the problem with basic principles available to the beginning medical student.

It is evident, therefore, that effective clinical reasoning may follow one of several routes. If the problem is one with which the person has had considerable previous experience, then the problem is probably recognized very early by a pattern recognition process. Little active thinking is required and there is a rapid resolution of the problem. In fact, the problem is not really a problem any more for that person. On the other hand, if the situation does present a problem for that person, more systematic intellectual activities must be brought into play, either formal testing of hypoth-

eses through accumulation and weighting of specific data, or causal reasoning at the level of basic disease mechanisms. An individual will demonstrate a range of approaches, both within and across problems, depending on previous experience and exposure to problems of a similar nature.

To the extent that this view is correct, it is evident that early attempts to assess clinical reasoning were doomed. We cannot consider it a generic process. Instead, we must contemplate the evaluation of several qualitatively different strategies. Some, like pattern recognition, are efficient and indeed may be over in seconds. These strategies will defy any attempt at measurement of the process. Some, like causal reasoning, are focused on detailed reasoning about mechanisms and are little concerned with data acquisition. As a result, they are inadequately captured by a focus on observable behaviours like history taking and physical examination. These issues have serious implications for assessment.

New developments

It is not very encouraging, but probably close to the truth, to say that we have no method of assessing clinical reasoning which stands up to critical scrutiny. On the other hand, we are at the cutting edge of test development.

The research referred to in the previous section is likely to form the basis for much of this new development. Preliminary attempts are being made to transpose the experimental laboratory instruments of psychologists into practical methods of testing competence (Norman, 1989). Others are attempting to modify current test methods to take into account the new concepts (Case *et al*., 1991).

Taking the model of problem solving (Figure 16.2) as a guide we could approach assessment in one of several ways. We could ignore the reasoning process entirely and focus assessment on the problem solution or 'outcome'. This would entail presenting the student with an appropriate range of problems in a high fidelity format and concentrating on the quality of the problem solution in terms of diagnosis or management plan. That might be a logical and even desirable approach in the postgraduate sphere, but has less attraction in the undergraduate phase where information on the intermediate stages of problem-solving would be of interest from a teaching as well as from an assessment point-of-view. Such a 'process' approach would attempt to measure aspects of higher order control processes and aspects of the organized knowledge/experience, i.e. both its presence and its utilization.

Some progress is being made in developing measures for some aspects of the clinical reasoning process, though most must still be regarded as experimental. For example, several workers have explored methods similar to those used in the classic studies of chess grand masters (Chase and Simon, 1973; De Groot, 1965) with chess scenarios replaced by clinical case protocols. In one exploratory study, Newble and Raymond (1992) showed a rising trend in the ability to recall medical case-based material associated with increasing medical expertise. This trend was not evident for the recall of non-medical material. In another study, Schmidt and Boshuizen (1993) showed that severely restricting the reading time of exposure to clinical material allowed differences in recall relating to expertise to emerge. The demands on memory can also be altered by adjusting the complexity of the task. For instance, Norman *et al.* (1989) showed that the use of fluid and electrolyte problems, combined with instructions to solve the problem and then recall the data, led to large differences in recall related to expertise. While such studies provide some support for the validity of the previously described concepts as a basis for understanding the clinical reasoning processes of medical practitioners they are unlikely to be of great value as forms of assessment. Speeded 'recall of data' tests might well be good discriminators but it is hard to imagine them being acceptable for routine use.

Other workers have been seeking more practical ways of exploiting the relationship of expertise to the organized knowledge base and clinical experience. Case *et al.* (1988) have devised a 'pattern recognition test' in which students are presented with a series of brief case scenarios based on a single chief complaint (e.g. shortness of breath) and must select the most appropriate diagnosis from a long menu of potential diagnoses (see Table 16.1). Such a format, if proved to be valid, would be attractive because of its adaptability for machine scoring and computer analysis.

An alternative approach is to present students with less familiar and more complex scenarios which might require some deductive reasoning as well as pattern recognition. That such an approach may have merit has been demonstrated by Norman *et al.* (1994). They showed that complex written clinical situations containing a minimum of clinical information and laboratory data could clearly differentiate between first-year residents, second-year residents and specialists. They also showed that the experts were more likely to use physiological concepts to explain abnormal patterns of laboratory data, and were less likely to rely on pattern recognition in these complex and atypical situations.

It is a little more difficult to conjecture how one might measure higher order control processes. The research methods used by Patel and Groen (1991), with propositional networks and characterization of forward and backward reasoning, are an attempt in this direction. Another similar approach has been to concentrate on the underlying reasoning

Table 16.1 Example of long menu extended-matching question

Theme:	*Shortness of breath*		
Options:	A. Anaemia	K.	Lung cancer
	B. Aortic stenosis	L.	Metabolic acidosis
	C. Aspiration pneumonia	M.	Mitral insufficiency
	D. Asthma	N.	Mitral stenosis
	E. Bacterial pneumonia	O.	Myocardial infarction
	F. Chronic obstructive pulmonary disease	P.	Pneumocystis carinii
	G. Congestive heart failure	Q.	Pneumothorax
	H. Hypertrophic outlet obstructive cardiomyopathy	R.	Primary pulmonary hypertension
	I. Hyperventilation	S.	Pulmonary embolism
	J. Laryngeal spasm	T.	Pulmonary fibrosis–silicosis

Lead in: For each patient with shortness of breath, select the most likely diagnosis.

1. A 55-year-old woman who smokes has had a chronically productive cough and progressive shortness of breath for 5 years
2. A 64-year-old woman has had shortness of breath, a temperature to 101.5°F, purulent sputum and pleuritic chest pain on the left for 3 days
3. A. . . . .
4. A. . . . .
etc.

process as the student tries to understand the pathophysiological mechanisms involved in the problem (Des Marchais *et al.*, 1993; Jean *et al.*, 1993). However, such methods are too labour intensive as yet for routine applications.

Regardless of the approaches and methods that will eventuate from these research efforts, several things have become clear. The first is that the assessment must be anchored in case-based material presented in a way that will induce and sample clinical-reasoning activities. Simply testing the recall of factual material is no longer tenable. The second is that laboriously taking a student through the full data gathering and investigational phase of a real or simulated clinical case is an inefficient approach when the concern is to evaluate clinical-reasoning skills. This is because of the content specificity problem and the consequent need to present students with large numbers of cases before satisfactory levels of test reliability can be achieved. For example, it has been shown that up to 8 hours of testing time may be required to achieve reliable assessments with PMPs because of this problem (Norcini *et al.*, 1985).

Such studies have triggered a search for more cost-effective methods. One possible approach emerged from the first Cambridge Conference (Norman *et al.*, 1985). The idea was based on the premise that any single case contained much 'dead wood' from a clinical-reasoning perspective. For example, in one case the critical challenge might be to elicit and interpret elements within the history, with little further being added by the physical examination and laboratory investigations. In another case the challenge might be the appropriate selection and interpretation of laboratory results. In other words, it may be possible to focus the problem-solving stimulus.

The concept of the 'Cambridge Case' has not been fully explored. However, one concrete outcome has been the *key feature* approach developed for the Medical Council of Canada certification examinations as an alternative to PMPs (Page and Bordage, 1995). In this procedure, clinical situations, as presenting in actual practice, are produced as a written case scenario. The 'key features' are identified on the basis of those elements critical to the resolution of the problem. Questions relating to the key features are then devised and may be posed in a variety of formats (e.g. short answer, MCQ or selection from longer menus of options). Such an approach allows a sample of 40–50 cases to be administered in the same time as that required to administer 12–15 PMPs. It should considerably enhance reliability (by sampling case situations more widely). Its validity as a test of clinical reasoning has yet to be proved but some recent research has produced encouraging results (Schuwirth *et al.*, personal communication).

Implications and advice for the teacher

As has become evident from this review, our success in developing valid measures of clinical reasoning for student assessment and research has been limited. If this is the disheartening reality, what should we as educators do in day-to-day practice? Should we discard whatever we are currently using and wait for better times? Or are there some guidelines that could be developed from the findings so far, which would allow us to proceed with some forms of assessment of clinical reasoning, albeit with caution.

Unfortunately there are no fixed answers to these questions. For instance, the answer may be quite different for tests which are to be used in undergraduate courses largely for formative purposes, compared to those which are to be used for major postgraduate certifying examinations where high levels of reliability are demanded.

There are several key points we would wish to make. First, it is hard to imagine a credible assessment of clinical competence which does not attempt to evaluate clinical reasoning skills. An assessment using less-than-perfect instruments is preferable to no assessment at all of this component. This is an issue of validity which must apply to the whole assessment procedure.

A second compelling argument not to discard our imperfect instruments is the very direct and powerful relationship between assessment and student learning. Academic success is largely defined by examination performance and academic success is what students are seeking. Thus, students will devote much of their energy to identifying and studying for what they believe will be in their examination (Newble and Entwistle, 1986). This impact of examinations on student learning will often be greater than that of the training program and is sometimes referred to as 'consequential validity'. Students may, in reality, be pursuing a program which is quite different to that which the teacher believes they are following – an effect called the 'hidden curriculum'. The implication is that such effects must be seen as inevitable, if not desirable. The only answer is to ensure a good match, at least in the student's mind, between the assessment procedures and the expected outcomes of the course. A failure to do so may have serious consequences (Newble and Jaeger, 1983). The bottom line is that if the imperfect instruments of clinical reasoning which are currently available are the best we have we should probably continue to use them until better ones have been developed.

If this is to be our recommendation we must, as a third point, emphasize that every effort should be made to reduce the known problems associated with our current test methods. A few suggestions are:

- Develop assessment tasks around appropriate real-life clinical scenarios. Such tasks may be presented in simple written form (e.g. MCQ, short answer), in more complex written form (e.g. MEQ, 'key features' approach), as written or computer-based simulations, in structured oral form, or by appropriate questioning of real or simulated patients. For assessing clinical reasoning, the method may actually be of less importance than we are intuitively inclined to believe.
- Concentrate on the content within the tasks. It must be of a complexity which ensures that the problem-solving process is induced. It should require the student to retrieve relevant information and apply it to make a diagnosis or make decisions about management. It should not be possible to answer the question by simple recall of knowledge.
- Focus the assessment on the expected level of expertise of the students. At lower levels (e.g. junior undergraduate) the focus should be more on the process of clinical reasoning and should reward thoroughness. At higher levels of expertise outcome and efficiency should be rewarded.
- Cueing effects should be avoided or minimized. This can be done simply by using open-ended questions and accepting the burden of marking. This process should not overstrain resources for the assessment of relatively small numbers of candidates (e.g. in medical schools) but can be a major difficulty for large national examinations with a cast of thousands. An alternative becomes the more innovative objective test formats such as those using long menus of options or pattern recognition items.
- Where direct observational methods are used it is important to find out what is going on in students' minds as they tackle the problem-solving task. This can be accomplished by asking students to verbalize thought processes during or after the patient encounter, by the use of probing questions by the assessor or via a post-encounter written assessment. These procedures should focus on hypothesis generation, diagnosis and decision making.
- Scoring systems should be kept simple. Most systems which have attempted to weight components differentially produce similar outcomes. Simple counts, limited pathways, simple decision rules for aggregating scores and avoidance of lengthy answers are all strategies to be recommended.
- Deal with the content-specificity problem. This requires sampling widely from as many problems or cases as possible. It is wiser to sample less within a single problem in favour of sampling more problems. If this process can be combined with the 'Cambridge Case' or 'key features' concept so much the better. It will maximize both efficiency and the clinical-reasoning value per problem or case.
- Avoid long unfolding cases with multiple pathways. While conceptually attractive and perhaps very valuable in a teaching situation, they are difficult to construct and administer, and a nightmare to score.
- Control other known sources of error such as those associated with marking and rating. Training of examiners for their roles and introducing structure into any rating or marking task can considerably improve reliability. As a general principle, more is to be gained by examiners scoring a single task or question for all candidates than scoring across a range of tasks or questions for a subset of candidates. This procedure effectively allows the effect of hawks and doves to even out. In an oral or viva situation, greater gains and reliability will be achieved by having single examiners assess students on two separate tasks rather than a pair of examiners assess students on only one task.

As a final comment, we would encourage experimentation. There is no one single best method of assessing clinical reasoning. Opportunities abound for creative activity and for teachers to contribute to the development of more valid and reliable test procedures.

References

Berner, E. S., Hamilton, L. A. and Best, W. R. (1974) A new approach to evaluating problem solving in medical students. *Journal of Medical Education*, **49**, 666–672.

Bligh, T. J. (1980) Written simulation scoring: A comparison of nine systems. Paper presented at the *American Educational Research Association Annual Meeting, American Educational Research Association*, New York.

Bordage, G. and Lemieux, M. (1991) Semantic structures and diagnostic thinking of experts and novices. *Academic Medicine*, **66**, S70–S72.

Bransford, J., Sherwood, R., Vye, N. and Rieser, J. (1986) Teaching thinking and problem solving. *American Psychologist*, **41**, 1078–1089.

Brooks, L. R., Norman, G. R. and Allen, S. W. (1991) The role of specific similarity in a medical diagnostic task. *Journal of Experimental Psychology: General*, **120**, 278–287.

Case, S. M., Swanson, D. B. and Stillman, P. S. (1988) Evaluating diagnostic pattern recognition: The psychometric characteristics of a new item format. In *Proceedings of the 27th Conference on Research in Medical Education*, pp. 3–8. Washington, DC: Association of American Medical Colleges.

Case, S., Swanson, D. B. and Van der Vleuten, C. (1991) Strategies for student assessment. In *The Challenge of Problem-Based Learning* (D. Boud and G. Feletti, eds), pp. 260–273, London: Kogan Page.

Chase, W. G. and Simon, H. A. (1973) Perception in chess. *Cognitive Psychology*, **4**, 55–81.

De Graaf, E., Post, G. and Drop, M. (1987) Validation of a new measure of clinical problem-solving. *Medical Education*, **21**, 213–218.

De Groot, A. (1965) *Thought and Choice in Chess*. The Hague: Mouton.

Des Marchais, J. E., Dumais, B. and Vu, N. V. (1993) An attempt at measuring ability to analyze problems in the Sherbrooke problem-based curriculum: A preliminary study. In *Problem-Based Learning as an Educational Strategy* (P. Bouhuijs, H. Schmidt, and R. Berkel, eds), pp. 239–248. Maastricht: Network Publications.

Elstein, A. S., Shulman, L. S. and Sprafka, S. A. (1990) Medical problem solving: A ten year retrospective. *Evaluation and the Health Professions*, **13**, 5–36.

Erviti, V., Templeton, B., Bunce, J. and Burg, F. (1980) The relationship of pediatric resident recording behaviour across medical conditions. *Medical Care*, **18**, 1020–1031.

Feletti, G. I. (1980) Reliability and validity studies on modified essay questions. *Journal of Medical Education*, **55**, 933–941.

Feltovich, P. J. and Barrows, H. S. (1984) Issues of generality in medical problem solving. In *Tutorials in Problem Based Learning: A New Direction in Teaching the Health Professions* (H. G. Schmidt and M. L. de Volder, eds), pp. 128–142. Assen: Van Gorcum.

Galofre, A. (1974) *A Review of Written Paper Management Simulations*. Chicago: Center for Educational Development, University of Illinois.

Goran, M. J., Williamson, J. W. and Gonnella, J. S. (1973) The validity of patient management problems. *Journal of Medical Education*, **48**, 171–177.

Helfer, R. E. and Slater, C. H. (1971) Measuring the process of solving clinical diagnostic problems. *British Journal of Medical Education*, **5**, 48–52.

Hodgkin, K. and Knox, J. D. E. (1975) *Problem Centred Learning: The Modified Essay Question in Medical Education*. Edinburgh: Churchill Livingstone.

Jean, P., des Marchais, J. E. and Delorne, P. (1993) *Apprendre a Enseigner Les Sciences de Sante*. Internal report. Montreal: University of Montreal.

Marshall, J. (1977) Assessment of problem-solving ability. *Medical Education*, **11**, 329–334.

McCarthy, W. H. (1966) An assessment of the effect of cueing items in objective examinations. *Journal of Medical Education*, **41**, 263–266.

McGuire, C. H. and Babbott, D. (1967) Simulation technique in the measurement of problem solving skills. *Journal of Educational Measurement*, **4**, 1–10.

Neufeld, V. R. and Norman, G. R. (1985) *Assessing Clinical Competence*. New York: Springer.

Newble, D. I. and Entwistle, N. J. (1986) Learning styles and approaches: Implications for medical education. *Medical Education*, **20**, 162–175.

Newble, D. I., Hoare, J. and Baxter, A. (1982) Patient management problems: Issues of validity. *Medical Education*, **16**, 137–142.

Newble, D. I. and Jaeger, K. (1983) The effect of assessments and examinations on the learning of medical students. *Medical Education*, **17**, 165–171.

Newble, D. I. and Raymond, G. A. (1992) Clinical memory as a potential measure of clinical problem solving ability. In *Approaches to the Assessment of Clinical Competence, Part 1*. (R. M. Harden, I. R. Hart and H. Mulholland, eds), pp. 347–351, Dundee: Centre for Medical Education.

Norcini, J. J., Swanson, D. B., Grosso, L. J., Shea, J. and Webster, G. D. (1985) Reliability, validity and efficiency of multiple choice questions and patient management item formats in the assessment of physician competence. *Medical Education*, **19**, 238–247.

Norcini, J. J., Swanson, D .B., Webster, G. D. and Grosso, L. J. (1983) A comparison of several methods of scoring patient management problems. In *Proceedings of the 22nd Annual Conference on Research in Medical Education* pp. 41–46. Washington, DC: Association of American Medical Colleges.

Norman, G. R. (1989) Reliability and construct validity of some cognitive methods of clinical reasoning. *Teaching and Learning in Medicine*, **1**, 194–199.

Norman, G., Allery, L., Berkson, L., Bordage, G., Cohen, R., Davis, W., Friedman, C., Grant, J., Lear, P., Morris, P. and Van der Vleuten, C. (1985) The psychology of clinical reasoning: Implications for assessment. Paper presented at the *Fourth Cambridge Conference*. Cambridge: Cambridge University School of Clinical Medicine.

Norman, G., Bordage, G., Curry, L., Dauphinee, D., Jolly, B., Newble, D., Rothman, A., Stalenhoef, B., Stillman, P., Swanson, D. and Tonesk, X. (1985) A review of recent innovations in assessment. In *Directions in Clinical Assessment: Report of the First Cambridge Conference* (R. E. Wakeford, ed.), pp. 9–27. Cambridge: Cambridge University School of Clinical Medicine.

Norman, G. R., Brooks, L. R. and Allen, S. W. (1989) Recall by experts and novices as a record of processing attention.

Journal of Experimental Psychology: Learning, Memory and Cognition, **5**, 1166–1174.

Norman, G. R., Brooks, L. R., Coblentz, C. K. and Babcock, C. J. (1992) The correlation of feature identification and category judgments on diagnostic radiology. *Memory and Cognition*, **20**, 344–355.

Norman, G. R. and Feightner, J. W. (1981) A comparison of behaviour on simulated patients and patient management problems. *Journal of Medical Education*, **55**, 529–537.

Norman, G. R., Trott, A. D., Brooks, L. P. and Smith, E. R. M. (1994) Cognitive differences in clinical reasoning related to postgraduate training. *Teaching and Learning in Medicine*, **6**, 114–120.

Page, G. G., Bordage, G. E. and Allen, T. (1995) Developing key features problems and examinations to assess clinical decision-making skills. *Academic Medicine*, **70**, 194–201.

Page, G. G. and Bordage G. E. (1995) The Medical Council of Canada's key features project: A more valid written examination of clinical decision-making. *Academic Medicine*, **70**, 104–110.

Patel, V. L. and Groen, G. J. (1991) The general and specific nature of medical expertise: A critical look. In *Toward a General Theory of Expertise: Prospects and Limits* (A. Ericsson and J. Smith, eds), pp. 93–125. Cambridge: Cambridge University Press.

Regehr, G. and Norman G. R. (1996) Issues of cognitive psychology: Implications for professional education. *Academic Medicine*, **71**, 988–1001.

Rimoldi, H. J. A. (1961) The test of diagnostic skills. *Journal of Medical Education*, **36**, 73–79.

Schmidt, H. G. and Boshuizen H. P. A. (1993) On the origin of 'intermediate effects' in clinical case recall. *Memory and Cognition*, **22**, 338–351.

Schmidt, H. G., Norman, G. R. and Boshuizen, H. P. A. (1990) A cognitive perspective on medical expertise: Theory and implications. *Academic Medicine*, **65**, 611–621.

Swanson, D. B. (1987) A measurement framework for performance-based tests. In *Further Developments in Assessing Clinical Competence* (I. R. Hart and R. M. Harden, eds), pp. 13–45. Montreal: Can-Heal Publications.

Swanson, D. B., Norcini, J. J. and Grosso, L. J. (1987) Assessment of clinical competence: Written and computer-based simulations. *Assessment and Evaluation in Higher Education*, **12**, 220–246.

Van der Vleuten, C. and Swanson, D. B. (1990) Assessment of clinical skills with standardized patients: State of the art. *Teaching and Learning in Medicine*, **2**, 58–76.

Van Rossum, H. J. M., Briet, E., Bender, W. and Meinders, A. E. (1989) The transfer effect of one single patient demonstration on diagnostic judgement of medical students: Both better and worse. In *Teaching and Assessing Clinical Competence* (W. Bender, R. J. Hiemstra, A. J. J. Scherpbier and R. P. Zwierstra, eds), pp. 435–440. Groningen: BoekWerk Publications.

Wainer, H. (1976) Estimating coefficients in linear models: It don't make no nevermind. *Psychological Bulletin*, **83**, 213–217.

17

Self-monitoring of clinical reasoning

Doris L. Carnevali

Clinical reasoning is a complex set of cognitive skills involving the use of existing knowledge, and the acquisition and processing of information. It is used to make accurate, specific judgements, diagnoses and prognoses about a person's or family's health status and situation, and to plan for rational, appropriate and individualized treatment or care. Achievement of expertise in clinical reasoning is a personal process. Others can offer knowledge, guidance and role models, but the accuracy, precision and efficiency associated with expertise in clinical reasoning must be developed by the individual clinician. Thus, it becomes a personal responsibility to consistently:

- Gain and systematically store discipline-specific knowledge and clinical experience on an ongoing basis.
- Achieve a working knowledge of the processes involved in clinical reasoning and critically practise those skills in varying clinical situations.
- Engage in self-evaluation and reflection on evaluation sought from others as a means of maintaining excellence and ongoing professional growth.

Ongoing self-evaluation of one's clinical reasoning tends to become an increasingly difficult professional task. As the clinician continues to make clinical judgements many times each day, over time the process becomes an automatic, unconscious activity (Benner, 1984; Schmidt *et al.*, 1990; Squire *et al.*, 1992). In the busy, demanding world of health care this is a normal and necessary evolution. Automaticity, however, can have advantages and disadvantages. Early, accurate sensing of the existence of a clinical problem and being able to take action without having laboriously and consciously to engage in the clinical reasoning process can be life saving. On the other hand, patterns of thinking and observing can become so habituated that flexibility and innovative approaches are no longer used and clinical judgements can become less accurate (Dawson and Arkes, 1987).

This latter possibility points up the need to periodically examine one's clinical reasoning behaviour. It is possible to seek awareness of one's cognitive activities and then to engage in self-analysis (Carnevali and Thomas, 1993). It is also possible to ask colleagues to critique one's judgements and the reported clinical reasoning that supports them, to gain fresh eyes with which to view one's practice. However, this will happen only if the clinician recognizes and values the need for recurring evaluation of clinical reasoning as a professional responsibility.

Attaining command of the complex mental and physical skills associated with expert clinical reasoning tends to be a slow, ongoing process resulting from integration of a growing body of theoretical and clinical knowledge and experience (Schmidt *et al.*, 1990). Having a knowledge base related to the clinical reasoning process itself is a basic foundation. Artistry and expertise is gained by repeated use of the skills in varying situations, and by systematically storing new experiences and knowledge for ease of retrieval.

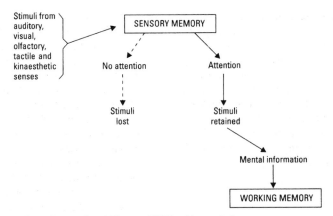

Figure 17.1 Sensory memory. From Carnevali and Thomas (1993) with permission

Expertise in the clinical reasoning process involves several components, including:

- Understanding what is known of memory systems and diagnostic reasoning processes.
- Systematically storing one's theoretical and clinical knowledge base in long-term memory, to facilitate its access for clinical judgement and decision making activities.
- Building a growing body of clinical experiences involving a variety of clinical phenomena, situations and treatments, and storing them for ease of retrieval.
- Gaining expertise in discipline-specific data acquisition and the use of one's cognitive processes in varying clinical situations and care settings.

This chapter offers some guidelines, cases and clinical exercises that can be used to improve clinical reasoning. The aspects to be addressed are: gaining working knowledge associated with memory as it is used in clinical reasoning and in the organization of knowledge for use in making clinical judgements and treatment decisions, and developing skills in information processing as it is used in making clinical judgements.[1]

Use of memory in clinical reasoning

Three forms of memory are currently thought to be involved in clinical reasoning. These are sensory, working (or short-term) and long-term memory (Ashcraft, 1989; Baddeley, 1990). Each form of memory serves particular functions in clinical

reasoning and has particular capacities and limitations. The clinician's knowledge and clinical experience need to be stored with these capacities and limitations in mind so that each type of memory can be used most effectively (Carnevali and Thomas, 1993). In addition, the clinical reasoning process itself must utilize strategies that acknowledge and accommodate both the richness and constraints of memory.

Sensory memory

Sensory memory is the entry point to the memory system and holds incoming stimuli for 0.5–3.0 seconds (Ashcraft, 1989). It is here that incoming stimuli from the clinical situation are either translated into mental representations for transmission to working memory; or they are lost (Coltheart, 1983) (refer to Figure 17.1). Effective use of sensory memory for clinical reasoning depends upon having working knowledge of:

- Significant cues associated with clinical phenomena within one's discipline-specific domain. These include not only the clear, obvious stimuli, but also those that are subtle or ambiguous as well as those that are extraneous or should not be present.
- The discipline-specific language used to transform stimuli into mental information. This is the initial identification or interpretation of sensory stimuli. In the cognitive science literature, this assignment of descriptors to incoming stimuli is called encoding (Ashcraft, 1989; Baddeley, 1990).

Students in any health care field learn from lectures, reading and clinical experiences about

---

[1] For further exercises see Chapter 3 in Carnevali and Thomas (1993) and Carnevali (1995).

salient risk factors and recognition features (or cues) associated with specific phenomena. They also learn the language or images used to describe them. This knowledge can be stored in such a way as to affect the initial cognitive processes of seeking, giving attention to and labelling stimuli coming into sensory memory. With ongoing patient (and family) encounters, thoughtful clinicians can modify, sharpen and refine their skills in initially noticing and encoding significant stimuli entering sensory memory.

Sensory memory exercises

(a) As you listen to lectures and read about clinical phenomena in your health care field, identify specifically the associated risk factors and manifestations you should seek, notice and label. Make note of cues that should not be present. Identify words or images that are used to represent the norms and variations in these stimuli. Identify the range of clinical situations and settings in which these phenomena and stimuli might be encountered and the variety of ways such data might be sought or present themselves.

(b) Engage in a patient encounter. Try to be aware of the incoming stimuli you notice and the initial words or images you use to transform stimuli into mental representations.

(c) Ask a colleague or mentor to join you in engaging in a clinical encounter and repeat Exercise (b). Compare what each of you noticed and the initial descriptors you used. Analyse the differences in clinical reasoning and judgements that could arise from these differences. Accept the differences without trying to modify them.

(d) Recall clinical situations in which you failed to notice significant stimuli or used incorrect or too general words or images to represent them. Consider the kinds of clinical judgement that could result from failing to attend to incoming stimuli or ineffectively labelling them.

Working memory

Incoming stimuli that have been transformed into mental information move from sensory memory to working memory, the next component of the memory system used in clinical reasoning. Working memory can be likened to a processing centre or workroom of the memory system that temporarily takes in and uses mental information from both sensory memory and long-term memory (Ashcraft, 1989; Salame and Baddeley, 1982; Waldorp, 1987) (refer to Figure 17.2). Working memory is required to accomplish a tremendous workload during

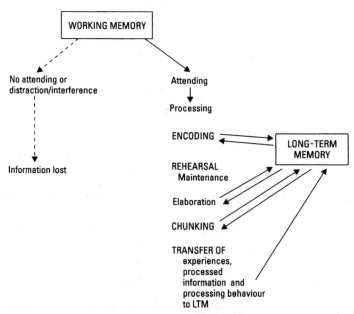

Figure 17.2 Working memory. From Carnevali and Thomas (1993) with permission

clinical reasoning. Despite this extensive work-load, working memory has major limitations and constraints including:

- Restricted duration (i.e. 15–20 seconds unless mental rehearsal takes place).
- A capacity of only five to nine chunks of information at any time (Miller, 1956). A chunk is a cluster made up of one or more units of related information that has become a familiar pattern and thus can be recognized as a single item (Larkin *et al.*, 1980).
- Easy loss of information through distraction.

These constraints shape strategies involved in effective clinical reasoning (Carnevali and Thomas, 1993; Elstein *et al.*, 1978). Such strategies include:

- Assigning more specific descriptors and interpretation to mental information received from sensory memory.
- Rehearsal for maintaining or elaborating on information received.
- Clustering information into related chunks to permit more effective judgements and to save space in working memory.
- Transferring information to and from long-term memory (Ashcraft, 1989; Baddeley, 1990; Craik and Lockhart, 1972).

Assigning more specific meaning

The initial encoding of stimuli in sensory memory tends to be a general tag or label. For example, a pulse may be identified as to location (e.g. radial, pedal, carotid), strength (e.g. full, weak), rate (e.g. rapid, slow) and pattern (e.g. rhythmic, arrhythmic). However, it can be more precisely encoded in terms of an actual numerical rate, a 0 to 4+ volume and the specific rhythmic pattern (Wild *et al.*, 1991). Richness and precision in encoding information in working memory have been found to be useful in subsequent cognitive tasks such as discrimination and differential diagnosis (Baddeley, 1990; Moscovitch and Craik, 1976). Professional growth requires clinicians to continually evolve qualitative and quantitative language or imagery to accurately describe and interpret clinical information received in working memory.

Maintenance rehearsal

Information is readily forgotten in working memory. Therefore, if one is collecting patient data and does not have access to paper and pen to record these data when they are obtained, one can mentally rehearse or repeat the information several times so as to fix it more firmly into memory until it can be recorded.

Elaborative rehearsal

Elaborative processing of information is both a more effective and more demanding means of retaining information needed for clinical reasoning in one's working memory, and it is thought to result in greater long-term learning and more effective recall. It involves semantics, previously stored knowledge and clinical experience as a basis for processing current data. It involves drawing relationships between what is already known and the information currently being processed.

The following case illustrates elaborative rehearsal. A nurse is caring for a dying patient who is managing the experience by use of hope and denial. Today, for the first time she hears the patient speak of his impending death. The nurse links this to her knowledge of the stages of grief. Later in the day, the patient reverts to speaking about feeling better and expecting a cure. Throughout the next day the patient vacillates between hope of cure and awareness of the reality of impending death. Prior to this clinical experience the nurse's concept of grieving had not included repeated vacillation between the elements. In future encounters with dying patients her knowledge would incorporate this possibility (Carnevali and Reiner, 1990; Carnevali and Thomas, 1993).

Clustering/chunking information

An important cognitive skill involved in using working memory for clinical reasoning is clustering incoming information into meaningfully related clusters or chunks (Larkin *et al.*, 1980). Most clinical judgements are based upon conscious or unconscious recognition of cue patterns. This pattern recognition emerges from knowledge or clinical experience previously stored in long-term memory.

Chunking conserves space in working memory. An entire chunk is *tagged* and used as one unit. Clinicians who are expert in working with particular phenomena tend to integrate more pieces of information into each chunk and to assign useful tags. A clinician viewing a patient with apparently normal respirations might cluster all of the sights and sounds into a chunk and tag it 'respiration'. On the other hand, a clinician seeing a patient with abnormal breathing might group 10 cues into one chunk and tag them 'emphysema'.

Chunking is learned from both theory and clinical experience. Lectures, books, and encounters with health care professionals provide knowledge about a discipline's usual and variant clustering of information relating to risk factors, the manifestations of clinical phenomena and the underlying dynamics that produce clinical findings. However, clinicians need personal experiences with commonalities and variations in conditions, situations, and responses in order to store living, working knowledge of patterns and chunks of related findings (Schmidt *et al.*, 1990). Novices will tend to have fewer items in each chunk, not having had the clinical experiences needed to 'put things together' effectively (Tanner, 1984; Tanner *et al.*, 1987). Clinicians who have sound theoretical foundations and multiple experiences with particular phenomena will unconsciously chunk more items and integrate them at more sophisticated levels within their area of expertise (Corcoran, 1986a,b).

Exercises in chunking

(a) Think about a diagnosis, situation or response in your discipline that you know well; one where you believe you can 'chunk' clinical information easily and effectively. Identify and 'tag' the different chunks or patterns of information associated with that phenomenon. Under each chunk heading list the kinds of data you would incorporate. Then, repeat this exercise with a phenomenon with which you are less theoretically and clinically familiar. Compare the familiar with the unfamiliar exercise. Think about how your chunks in each instance would fit the five to nine chunk limitation of working memory and how they could affect your clinical reasoning expertise.

(b) Encounter a patient. Gather data and group them in chunks. 'Tag' the chunks. Ask a health care professional from a different field or subspecialty (e.g. a medical-surgical nurse and a psychiatric nurse) to see the patient or listen to your full, unchunked description of the patient. Ask that person how she or he would cluster the data. Compare it with your own. Would you chunk any differently the next time based on this experience? Why?

Transfer of information to and from long-term memory

As can be seen from the discussion of the activities taking place in working memory, movement of information between working memory and long-term memory is almost constant. New information and experiences taken into working memory move on to long-term memory. These include:

- Experiences stored in episodic memory.
- Knowledge (new or revised) stored in semantic memory.
- The activities of processing, retrieval and transfer thought to be stored both in episodic memory, and an area identified sometimes as production memory (Anderson, 1985).

Repeated practice and building of efficient, often complicated organizational systems for storing information in long-term memory eventually allows clinicians to move between working memory and long-term memory so quickly that the boundaries between the two components of memory become blurred. At this stage the clinician is said to have developed skilled memory (Ericsson *et al.*, 1980; Waldorp, 1987). In addition, repeated experiences of making clinical judgements and treatment decisions about specific phenomena tend to build the connections (Squire *et al.*, 1992).

Long-term memory in clinical reasoning

Long-term memory acts like a library of knowledge and experience that a clinician consults to identify and interpret information in working memory. Long-term memory appears to have unlimited capacity and little forgetting. However, problems can occur in gaining access to and retrieving knowledge and experience when they are needed.

The two major divisions of long-term memory are semantic memory, containing knowledge, and episodic memory, containing experiences. These are highly interactive in clinical reasoning. Schmidt *et al.* (1990) hypothesize that novices in clinical reasoning primarily use theoretical knowledge from semantic memory, gradually adding clinical knowledge, called 'problem scripts'. Expert clinicians rely more on 'patient instance scripts' drawn from episodic memory for comparison with findings in the current situation as a basis for making clinical judgements. Access is gained to both semantic and episodic memory by transmission of a unit or chunk of information from working memory to long-term memory. This accessing information from the current situation tends to communicate common, essential properties associated with the phenomenon to be recognized and understood. Gaining access to the needed diagnostic concepts in long-term memory is thought to begin with one concept and then to spread along connecting pathways to other related concepts as shown in Figure 17.3. This suggests that clinicians need to store theoretical knowledge by 'cross filing' it in terms of other potential diagnostic explanations as well as clinical ramifications.

Findings in the current patient situation that confirm previous knowledge can be processed to strengthen that part of the semantic diagnostic concept or linkages between concepts. Those which extend or are at variance with one's currently held knowledge can be used to modify the stored concept, as should disconfirming findings. In this way clinical practice and new knowledge are used in an ongoing way to sharpen one's diagnostic concepts and linkages in long-term memory.

Organisation of knowledge for clinical reasoning

Diagnostic concepts (i.e. knowledge about any discipline-specific phenomenon or situation) which are stored with a consistent structure can offer greater ease of access for future clinical reasoning and ongoing storage of new knowledge.

In the medical field, knowledge about pathology is usually organized to highlight the nature of the phenomenon, recognition features, prognostic variables, complications and treatment options. Other disciplines can use a comparable organizational structure to advantage [refer to Carnevali and Reiner (1990) for examples of organizational structures in nursing].

Since professional expertise in clinical reasoning is based upon access to correct, up-to-date knowledge and appropriate use of earlier clinical experiences, efficient storage and updating of one's clinical knowledge files is an ongoing professional responsibility. There is no question that new knowledge and experience regularly move from working memory to long-term memory without awareness. On the other hand, thinking about future uses of new information and about patient instances in relation to clinical reasoning can provide a useful basis for the effective storage of such information in long-term memory and can make it more accessible for future clinical reasoning (Baddeley, 1990; Moscovitch and Craik, 1976).

Exercises in the use of an organizational system for storing knowledge

(a) Set up a structural outline for storing knowledge in your discipline, preferably one that highlights recognition features such as risk factors and manifestations, underlying mechanisms

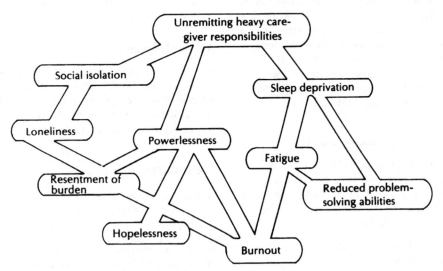

Figure 17.3 Example of linkages between diagnostic concepts in long-term semantic memory. From Carnevali and Thomas (1993) with permission

differential diagnoses or problem categories, prognostic variables, complications of untreated problems and iatrogenic complications, treatment or management options and evaluation criteria. After each heading, identify relevant content in each category based on the knowledge and perspectives of your discipline.

(b) Select a diagnostic concept or problem area commonly occurring in your discipline with which you are personally familiar. Using the theoretical and clinical knowledge and experience you already possess, organize your knowledge using the structural guidelines developed in Exercise (a). Refine your diagnostic concept by consulting the literature as needed and by testing it in your encounters with patients who have problems within this diagnostic concept. Repeat this exercise with additional concepts until your concept library attains consistent structure.

Using patient instances

As clinicians develop professional practice expertise a transition is made in the clinical reasoning process they adopt. Initially their reasoning relies heavily on the use of theoretical knowledge. Increasingly, however, their reasoning relies more on the recall and use of patient instances as the basis for recognizing and understanding the presenting situation (Schmidt *et al.*, 1990). This suggests that patient instances, like new knowledge, need to be 'filed' in some systematic way. Each patient instance offers either confirmation of, or variation from, earlier patterns of risk factors, etiology and manifestations. It can also offer a strengthening of previously encountered linkages with related problem areas or new areas. Some degree of awareness of the need to update one's patient instance file with new patient encounters is important for professional growth.

Using the clinical reasoning process

Activities actually undertaken in the processing of information involved in clinical reasoning are certainly not linear, even though diagrammed steps and logic would make them seem to be so. However, it is possible to:

- Identify components of the reasoning process and delete the table.
- Achieve a working understanding of them.
- Develop skill in the use of each of them.

Conclusion

The clinical reasoning process can be used with or without awareness. Therefore it seems wise to initially and periodically check on one's current practices in the clinical reasoning process to determine whether unwanted or ineffective strategies are being used. The people who depend upon professionals for care in health and illness bring with them the complexities inherent in all human beings. Their presenting problems in health promotion, risk reduction, or in living with pathology and its treatment are rarely simple. Therefore, real challenges face health care professionals in any discipline who seek to provide care that is tailored to the individual's situation and is also rational, therapeutic and cost-effective.

Clinical reasoning is the critical foundation to problem identification and resultant treatment decisions. Individuals in some disciplines have thought that the process should be made simple. Unfortunately this is not possible, given the complexity of human beings and their health problems. The only solution is to accept the difficulty as given and then to strive to master the knowledge base, the data collection skills and the cognitive processes needed to adequately address the requirements in the situation. Achieving and maintaining excellence in clinical reasoning in any health care field is a lifelong pursuit. Only by acknowledging its difficulties and regularly engaging in critical practice is it possible to gain the consistent competence required to effectively and predictably meet patients' and their families' health care needs.

Acknowledgement

This is a condensed version of the chapter by the same title and author, which appeared in the first edition of this text. Our thanks to Joan Rosenthal who assisted in the revision of this chapter. Figures are derived from the first edition.

References

Anderson, J. F. (1985) *Cognitive Psychology and its Implications*, 2nd edn. New York: Freeman.

Ashcraft, M. (1989) *Human Memory and Cognition*. Glenview, IL: Scott Foresman.

Baddeley, A. (1990) *Human Memory*. Boston: Allyn & Bacon.

Benner, P. (1984) *From Novice to Expert: Excellence and Power in Clinical Nursing Practice*. Menlo Park, CA: Addison-Wesley.

Carnevali, D. (1986) Loneliness. In *Nursing Management for the Elderly*, 2nd edn (D. Carnevali and M. Patrick, eds), pp. 287–298. Philadelphia, PA: Lippincott.

Carnevali, D. (1995) Self-monitoring of clinical reasoning. In *Clinical Reasoning in the Health Professions* (J. Higgs and M. Jones, eds), pp. 179–190. Oxford: Butterworth-Heinemann.

Carnevali, D. and Reiner, A. (1990) *The Cancer Experience: Nursing Diagnosis and Management*. Philadelphia, PA: Lippincott.

Carnevali, D. and Thomas, M. (1993) *Diagnostic Reasoning and Treatment Decision Making in Nursing*. Philadelphia, PA: Lippincott.

Coltheart, M. (1983) Iconic memory. *Philosophical Transactions of the Royal Society of London*, **302**, 283–294.

Corcoran, S. (1986a) Task complexity and nursing expertise as factors in decision making. *Nursing Research*, **35**, 107–112.

Corcoran, S. (1986b) Expert and novice nurses' use of knowledge to plan for pain control: How clinicians make their decisions. *The American Journal of Hospice Care*, **3**, 37–41.

Craik, F. and Lockhart, R. (1972) Levels of processing: A framework for memory research. *Journal of Verbal Learning and Verbal Behavior*, **11**, 671–684.

Dawson, N. and Arkes, H. (1987) Systematic errors in medical decision making. *Journal of General Internal Medicine*, **2**, 183–187.

Elstein, A. S., Shulman, L. S. and Sprafka, S. A. (1978) *Medical Problem Solving: An Analysis of Clinical Reasoning*. Cambridge, MA: Harvard University Press.

Ericsson, K., Chase, W. and Faloon, S. (1980) Acquisition of a memory skill. *Science,* **208**, 1181–1182.

Larkin, J., McDermott, J., Simon, D. and Simon, H. (1980) Expert and novice performance in solving physics problems. *Science,* **208**, 1135–1142.

Miller, G. (1956) The magical number seven, plus or minus two: Some limitations on our capacity for processing information. *Psychological Review*, **63**, 81–97.

Moscovitch, M. and Craik, F. (1976) Depth of processing, retrieval cues and uniqueness of encoding as factors in recall. *Journal of Verbal Learning and Verbal Behavior*, **15**, 447–458.

Salame, P. and Baddeley, A. (1982) Disruption of short-term memory by unattended speech: Implications for the structure of working memory. *Journal of Verbal Learning and Verbal Behavior*, **21**, 150–164.

Schmidt, H., Norman, G. and Boshuizen, H. (1990) A cognitive perspective on medical expertise: Theory and implications. *Academic Medicine*, **65**, 611–621.

Squire, L., Ojemann, J., Mielin, F., Peterson, S., Videen, T. and Raichle, M. (1992) Activation of the hippocampus in normal humans: A functional anatomical study of memory. *Proceedings of the National Academy of Sciences*, **89**, 1837–1841.

Tanner, C. A. (1984) Toward development of diagnostic reasoning skills. In *Diagnostic Reasoning in Nursing* (D. Carnevali, P. Mitchell, N. Woods and C. Tanner, eds), pp. 57–104. Philadelphia, PA: Lippincott.

Tanner, C. A., Padrick, K. P., Westfall, U. and Putzier, D. (1987) Diagnostic reasoning strategies of nursing and nursing students. *Nursing Research*, **36**, 358–363.

Waldrop, M. (1987) The workings of working memory. *Science*, **237**, 1564–1567.

Wild, L., Craven, R. and Cunningham, S. (1991) Assessment of vascular function. In *Medical Surgical Nursing: Pathophysiological Concepts*, 2nd edn (M. Patrick, S. Woods, R. Craven, J. Rokosky and P. Bruno, eds), pp. 802–811. Philadelphia, PA: Lippincott.

18

The case study as an instructional method to teach clinical reasoning

Susan Prion

Health care has changed dramatically in the past 10 years. New nursing graduates are expected to demonstrate proficiency with medical and nursing procedures, interpersonal competence, a comprehensive grasp of complex theory, effective diagnostic abilities, a mastery of cost-saving techniques and strategies, to work effectively in diverse teams, and to manage complex technology, all while remaining consumer oriented and community based (Watson and West, 1996). Schools of Nursing are becoming increasingly creative in their attempts to teach students the knowledge, skills and clinical reasoning proficiency that they will need to be successful as practising nurses. Studies of the clinical reasoning of experienced nurses have helped provide some understanding into the processes that these experts use in day-to-day problem solving regarding patient care (e.g., see Carnevali et al., 1984; Corcoran, 1986; Fonteyn, 1991; Radwin, 1990; Tanner et al., 1987) and those insights have guided nursing instructors in their selection of pedagogical strategies for the classroom.

This chapter describes one attempt to meet the challenge of teaching clinical reasoning to novice nurses. It is based on a model suggested by a survey of research on clinical reasoning by Radwin (1990) and uses case studies to simulate the reality of patient care situations. This case study approach aids creation of knowledge, promotes a realistic analysis of patient condition, demonstrates a holistic application of the clinical reasoning process and provides an opportunity to apply information from the entire nursing curriculum.

Case studies as an instructional method are particularly useful to provide a model of the clinical-reasoning process for students. The opportunity for questions to an expert instructor about specific content, inferences that were made, cue groupings, decision making about relevant and irrelevant cues, and the types of additional information that would be needed are all helpful for the beginning student to start to approximate the clinical reasoning processes of competent nurses.

Much has been written in the health care literature about problem-based learning (PBL) (Albanese and Mitchell, 1993; Frost, 1996; Heliker, 1994; Norman, 1988; Norman and Schmidt, 1992; Vernon and Blake, 1993; Walton and Matthews, 1989). The case study approach described in this chapter is a type of PBL, but intentionally limited in its scope. PBL can be defined as a method of learning that has the following characteristics: (a) use of clinical case studies, either real or hypothetical, (b) small group discussions, (c) collaborative yet independent student work, (d) hypothetico-deductive reasoning, and (e) faculty guidance and direction of the group process rather than imparting of information (Vernon and Blake, 1993). PBL is most effective when students can work through problem situations and generate plausible solutions by drawing on relevant literature and prior knowledge and experience (Andrews and Jones, 1996). Most undergraduate nursing students, especially beginning ones, have limited prior nursing/medical knowledge or experience on which to build. Therefore, the case study method described here fulfils two educational goals: to create knowledge and to practise effective clinical reasoning within a safe and well-controlled learning environment.

The clinical reasoning model

The clinical-reasoning process model (see Figure 18.1) used by the author at the University of San Francisco is loosely based on the work of Radwin (1990) and Tichenor *et al.* (1995). It is further informed by the work on *cognitive elaboration* by Craik and Tulving (1975), and related research about *cognitive schemata* by Rumelhart and Ortony (1977), Mayer (1992), and Chi *et al.* (1988). These studies describe the components and stages of understanding that are common to most models of the diagnostic reasoning process, and the mental representation that enables reasoning to progress. The stages of Radwin's model are the basis for educational strategies that evoke the desired knowledge acquisition and clinical-reasoning behaviours in students.

In any clinical situation, the nurse is initially confronted with a set of presenting cues that can be designated as the *situation prime*. These cues may consist of the patient's medical diagnosis, the topic of the practice case study or the hypothetical patient's chief complaint. The situation prime acts as a crude sifting mechanism that immediately narrows the field of possible diagnostic hypotheses. If the situation prime seems to suggest that it is a cardiac patient, an array of non-cardiac diagnoses can be eliminated, and the student can activate the newly stored knowledge of potential cardiac problems and interventions. Thus the student is helped to strengthen the cognitive connections among linked cue groups and to increase the accessibility of the information by establishing a related knowledge system.

Guided by the situation prime, the student begins to gather cues (pieces of information) that will help identify the specific patient problem. These may be laboratory or diagnostic test results, clinical signs and symptoms, physical assessment data and/or information from reports of other health care team members. Again, the situation prime has focused the student's investigation on a limited number of diagnoses. Cue gathering is the first step towards identification of the presenting problem from that limited list of possible diagnoses.

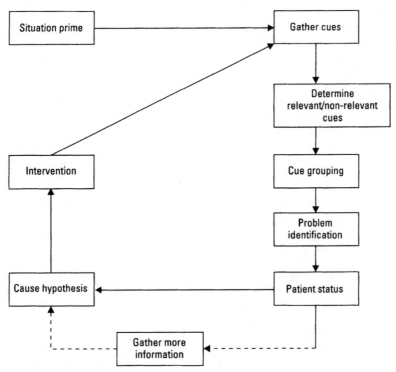

Figure 18.1 Clinical reasoning model

A critical feature of the cue gathering stage is the grouping and prioritizing of cues. Available patient information is examined and the discrimination between relevant and non-relevant cues is made. For example, shortness of breath is a relevant cue for a cardiac patient, whereas a slight rise in body temperature is usually an irrelevant cue for this type of patient. The outcome of this reasoning stage is a number of cues that the student has concluded are related to the situation prime or presenting problem.

Once these relevant cues are gathered, the student then begins to create relationships among cues and to group related cues together. These groupings may be made on the basis of subjective features, physical signs and symptoms, organ systems and/or potential clinical disease patterns. All the groups combine to build an accurate picture of the patient situation.

The process of cue grouping is guided by two factors: the situation prime and existing patterns of knowledge, or *schemata*, in memory. The situation prime has already introduced our hypothetical cardiac patient situation. This contextual clue has limited the list of possible presenting problems but still leaves a large number of potential causes for the current situation. It is now that the student begins to compare these relevant groups of cues to schemata of similar situations stored in memory. If those schemata are not present, the case study process encourages their creation by forcing the student to work with the information as a related whole, rather than isolated facts or unassociated data.

After cue grouping, the student considers possible hypotheses that might explain these groups. At this point, there may be more than one plausible hypothesis that may explain the patient's condition. A hypothesis is now retained or rejected depending on its alignment with the grouping of relevant cues. The goal is the identification of the problem. For example, the cues 'pallor' and 'diaphoresis' could indicate chest pain, a cardiac arrhythmia and/or hypotension. The instructor's input is critical at this point, to guide novices through the possible hypotheses, articulating the expert's thinking processes as he/she considers, discards or retains a potential clinical cause.

The instructor asks, 'Why is the patient experiencing this problem?' Obviously, determining the cause of the presenting problem is necessary to identify and select the appropriate interventions. The student continues to gather and group cues for ongoing evaluation of the correctness of the identified hypothesis and treatment. Once an intervention has been enacted, the reasoning process reiterates, and the student can gather and group additional cues, develop supplemental hypotheses, check on the status of the patient, and intervene as required by the patient situation.

Of obvious importance is the way in which this theoretical model can be translated into practice in the nursing school classroom. Research has shown that clinical reasoning skills are best acquired in settings that most closely approximate the real patient situations that the nursing student will face in clinical practice (Brown *et al.*, 1989; Resnick, 1982a; Resnick, 1982b; Tanner *et al.*, 1987). However, it is neither possible nor particularly desirable to duplicate the reality of the clinical situation in the classroom, especially for beginning nursing students. Despite the limitations of simulation as an educational methodology in health care settings, the rudimentary concepts of the clinical reasoning model can be instantiated through the use of case studies. This educational tool provides the nursing student with the closest approximation to real patient situations within the classroom.

There are many significant reasons for using a case study as an educational method to teach the clinical reasoning process to nursing students. When utilized with the appropriate guidance, questioning and feedback from experienced clinical nurse educators, case studies offer numerous opportunities for the student to exercise clinical reasoning in a simulation of a real situation, model exemplary decision-making behaviour, demonstrate accurate thought processes in solving clinical problems, make and correct mistakes in a controlled and safe situation, identify assumptions, biases and values that impact in a given situation, integrate information from the entire nursing curriculum, apply knowledge, acquire new knowledge, measure and evaluate knowledge acquisition, and measure and evaluate the outcomes of the clinical reasoning process.

Case studies have been used successfully as an educational method in the professions of medicine, law and business, engineering and education (Baxter, 1988; Bernheimer, 1982; Boehrer and Linsky, 1990; Boyce, 1992; Carter and Unklesbay, 1989; Christensen, 1987; Epstein, 1981; Feinstein and Veenendall, 1992; Gale, 1993; Gist, 1992; Harrington, 1991; Hartman, 1992; Kreps and Lederman, 1985; McCarthy, 1987; McWilliam, 1992; Merseth, 1991; Nagel, 1991; Oldham and Forrester, 1981; Rasinski, 1989; Sansalone, 1990; Taylor, 1989; Zarr, 1984). They are particularly useful in nursing education because the case study approach is one of the few educational methods that promotes the integration of the psychological, social, emotional, physical and affective aspects of patient care in a controlled situation that prevents harm to the patient. In addition, varying the complexity of case studies allows the instructor to help students progress in their ability to deal with increasingly difficult and complex clinical problems.

Case study development

The process of writing a valid and reliable case study is labour intensive but not complicated. The first and most important question the author needs to ask is, 'What is the purpose of this case study?' There are four major reasons for using a case study: (a) to teach students assessment and evaluation of patient data, (b) to promote integration and application of knowledge, (c) to teach specific content, and (d) to teach and evaluate reasoning skills.

The second step is to articulate clearly the specific instructional goals that the case study is designed to achieve. Next, the case study author needs to describe in detail the learners who will use the case study. Previous knowledge, age, level in school and timing during the semester all factor into the type and level of the case study used.

The priorities and constraints of the educational situation require serious consideration. First, the size of the class must be taken into account. An educator may use a case study as a small group or individual student written task, or may discuss it with all the students participating during class. Student participation could be difficult in large classes, but would work quite well in small ones. In addition, the classroom size and configuration should be examined. A large classroom with fixed chairs and desks does not lend itself to small group work.

Next, the case study author should determine the amount of time allotted for the class. The case study format may be determined by the time available to work on the case study. A more complex case study requires more time for effective use.

The purpose of the case study should be determined early in the development process. Does the instructor plan to use the case study instead of the content lecture, as a basis for the class discussion? Or does the instructor plan to use the case study as an example to illustrate the points made in the class presentation? The complexity and dynamism of the case study will be determined significantly by its purpose.

The educational materials that are currently available to both instructors and students need to be catalogued. Some universities have a rich library of print, audiovisual and computer-assisted case studies that can be easily integrated into the classroom. If appropriate materials are not easily available, the instructor will need the time and resources to develop them.

The delivery logistic of the case study needs to be determined. Options include handing out the written case study in class, handing out the written case study before class, handing out the case study after class, using the case study as an audiovisual display and presenting the case study verbally. If class time is limited, it is better to distribute the case study before class rather than using time in class for reading it. If a collaborative analysis of the case study by the entire class is planned, then using the case study as an audiovisual display or presenting the case study verbally would be most useful. Each option depends on the purpose of the case study and the logistics of the individual class.

The author also needs to consider the specific content to be included in the case study. Categories of information can include general information about the simulated patient such as name, age, gender, height, weight, social habits, profession/job and education, past medical/surgical history, the patient's current status, the chief complaint, physical examination results, lab values, medications, and psychosocial information. Information about the patient's environment, or perhaps a specific patient situation, can also be provided. This is information that the student would be expected to collect from the patient, the patient's chart or the patient's situation before providing care.

For classroom instruction, three major types of case study seem to be most useful. The selection of case study format will depend upon the purpose of the case study and the other considerations discussed previously. The first type of case study is the *stable case study*. This case presents a body of static information and then asks the student about that information. Its purpose is to transmit information, identify assumptions and/or allow assessment of general or specific information contained in the case study. Stable case studies are relatively easy to write and are the most effective type for beginning students. The most significant disadvantage of the use of stable case studies is their lack of approximation to a real, dynamic patient situation. That is, students are not required to judge

Table 18.1 Static case study example

Mrs Smith is a 47-year-old woman admitted with a pain in her left side. She has a 3 day history of nausea and vomiting. She complains of severe pain unrelieved by aspirin or Tylenol.

Vital signs: heart rate 112, blood pressure 145/72, respiratory rate 28, temperature 101.2°F
Labs: Na 144, K 4.9, glucose 122

1. List three important assessment cues about Mrs Smith
2. What would your most immediate nursing priority be for Mrs Smith?

what information is needed or to extract the information themselves. Stable case studies can be helpful to demonstrate reasoning about a set of patient data, but cannot demonstrate the clinical reasoning process over time. Table 18.1 gives an example of a static case study.

The *dynamic case study* is a more sophisticated presentation in which the students are given a body of patient information, questioned about it, then given more information and more questions. Built into this case study are changes in the patient's status over time. Dynamic case studies can be used to assess or predict changes in the patient's physical, emotional or psychological status over time, and are excellent tools to demonstrate and evaluate application and synthesis of complex information. They are more realistic and more sophisticated than stable case studies. Care must be taken to manage dynamic case studies so that students do not become lost or overwhelmed by the complexity of information provided. This is especially true if the case study is being used in a small group, and each student takes a different amount of time to answer the questions posed about the case. The amount of information provided and the level of probing questions used with the dynamic case study can vary with the level of student and the time available for case study analysis. Table 18.2 illustrates an example of a dynamic case study.

The third major case study format is the *dynamic case study with expert feedback*. This approach combines the advantages of the dynamic case study with the educational benefit of immediate feedback to student responses. It is an effective method to illustrate one or more satisfactory reasoning pathways by comparing student responses or decisions with satisfactory or exemplary decisions made by identified experts. While all case study formats provide feedback upon completion of the case study analysis, the dynamic case study with expert feedback builds in written or verbal expert feedback after students answer each set of questions. The case study analysis involves several sets of questions, as each new block of information is added to the case. By receiving feedback on their evolving thoughts and decisions, students are able to adjust their reasoning during the case and come to a solution along with the expert rather than simply be 'corrected' in hindsight. There may be more than one feasible reasoning pathway, of which the expert response is only one. Students are encouraged to examine both their own and the expert's responses and rationalize or explain their choice of response. Although the expert's answers are not the only correct answer, the expert's response provides a framework for students to study the method and outcome of the clinical reasoning process. Table 18.3

Table 18.2 Dynamic case study example

Mrs Smith is a 47-year-old woman admitted with a pain in her left side. She has a 3 day history of nausea and vomiting. She complains of severe pain unrelieved by aspirin or Tylenol.

Vital signs: heart rate 112, blood pressure 145/72, respiratory rate 28, temperature 101.2°F
Labs: Na 144, K 4.9, glucose 122

1. List three important assessment cues about Mrs Smith
2. What would your most immediate nursing priority be for Mrs Smith?

Three hours after admission, she vomits 250 cm³ of bright red blood.

3. What other information do you need to assess Mrs Smiths clinical status?
4. What is the first thing that you would do for her?

Table 18.3 Dynamic case study with expert feedback

Mrs Smith is a 47-year-old woman admitted with a pain in her left side. She has a 3 day history of nausea and vomiting. She complains of severe pain unrelieved by aspirin or Tylenol.

Vital signs: heart rate 112, blood pressure 145/72, respiratory rate 28, temperature 101.2°F
Labs: Na 144, K 4.9, glucose 122

1. List four important assessment cues about Mrs Smith
2. What would your most immediate nursing priority be for Mrs Smith?

Expert response: You have a lot of info about this patient. She has severe pain in her abdomen, nausea and vomiting. × 3 days and her vital signs (VS) are all elevated. The VS could be up because of her pain or because she is having some other sort of stress, like a peptic ulcer bleed. After 3 days of nausea and vomiting, I'd really worry that she was dehydrated – in fact, her Na is 144, probably due to fluid loss. My first concern would be for pain relief, but I would also want some more information about her fluid status.

Three hours after admission, she vomits 250 cm^3 of bright red blood.

3. What other information do you need to assess Mrs Smiths clinical status?

Expert response: Well, now we have a better idea of what's going on, I would immediately want a set of VS and to subjectively assess how Mrs Smith is doing.

---

provides an example of a dynamic case study with expert feedback.

Case study question development

The final step in constructing an educational case study is to formulate a list of questions that will help promote the critical understanding that will fulfill the purpose of the case study. The educational motive for the case study, whether to review important information, provide a knowledge application/integration opportunity or test clinical reasoning ability, will be an invaluable guide for structuring questions. The level of the student in his/her program of study and timing of the case study use within the specific course (early or late) will affect the questioning strategy. Beginning nursing students have less clinical experience than more advanced students. Their facility with medical terminology is often primitive, and they are less knowledgeable than more experienced students about lab values and medications. For these reasons, the case study should be carefully written and reviewed by several educators to make sure that the overall structure of the example (wording, content, and assumptions about supporting knowledge) is consistent with the level of the student group. Many students have not worked with case studies in previous classes, and take some time to become familiar with the process. Case studies used early in the course should be more straightforward and shorter in length than those used towards the end of the course.

The sequencing of questions about the case study can follow one of several formats. A hierarchical approach, such as Bloom's taxonomy (Bloom *et al.*, 1956) or Belenky's structure (Belenky *et al.*, 1986), can be useful to move from primitive, low cognitive level questioning, to more generalizable, sophisticated queries. Low cognitive level questions ask the learner to recall a fact in a similar form to that in which it was presented (What was the patient's blood pressure? Is this higher or lower than a normal blood pressure?). Higher cognitive level questions require some analysis, synthesis or evaluation of the information presented and the decisions made based on that information (How do you know that your intervention was effective? What would you tell the patient's family at this time?). A time-oriented questioning strategy (What comes first? What would you do next?) can help clarify and consolidate a dynamic case study. A priority-oriented strategy (What is your first concern? Next priority?) is useful to promote application, synthesis and problem formulation.

The following questioning sequence flows directly from the conceptual model of clinical reasoning (see Figure 18.1). The questions are structured as follows:

(a) State the situation prime. What does your knowledge of the patient's history, chief complaint, diagnosis and/or current situation lead you to suspect about the patient?
(b) List all the available cues that are present in the case study.

(c) In writing, categorize these cues into relevant and irrelevant cue categories based on the situation prime.

(d) Organize the cues into meaningful groups based on your previous knowledge. Do these relevant cues suggest a disease or patient condition? Does this sound like anything you already know?

(e) List all plausible hypotheses that you can think of that would fit (explain) these cues.

(f) Under each hypothesis, list all other information you would need to gather to accept or reject each of the alternatives.

(g) Based upon available and accessible information, select and state a problem/diagnosis hypothesis.

(h) List the status of the diagnosis as emergency (immediate intervention), high risk or low risk, or potential risk.

(i) Regroup available cues to develop a hypothesis about the possible cause(s) of the patient's condition.

Regardless of the case study format selected, the sequencing and alignment of questions with the conceptual model of reasoning presented in Figure 18.1 promotes modelling of orderly and effective reasoning, and provides frequent opportunities for the instructor to correct demonstrated errors in the student's reasoning process.

Application

What follows is an example of this case study process in an actual classroom situation. This particular case study is used to encourage knowledge acquisition and teach effective clinical reasoning about congestive heart failure (CHF) to nursing students in an undergraduate pathophysiology course.

Purpose

The purpose of this case study is to provide a model of the clinical reasoning process concerning the patient with CHF and to reinforce content about CHF.

Learners

The students using this case study are all first or second year undergraduate nursing students who have as general prerequisites an anatomy and physiology class, basic normal physical assessment

and basic lab value assessment skills including normal values for sodium (Na), potassium (K), glucose (gluc), blood urea nitrogen (BUN), creatinine and creatinine phosphokinase-myocardial band (CPK-MB). Specific prerequisite knowledge for this case study includes: anatomy of the cardiovascular system; the normal route of blood flow through the body, traced from the left ventricle; definitions of pre-load and after-load; how to calculate cardiac output (CO), stroke volume (SV), ejection fraction (EF), left ventricular end diastolic pressure (LVEDP); normal pressures in the four chambers of the heart and the pulmonary circulation; neural regulation of heart rate (HR), contractility and vascular diameter. Before the class in which this case study is to be used, students have completed reading assignments in the assigned pathophysiology text about CHF.

Objectives

The objectives of this case study are to:

(a) Identify the relevant cues that indicate the clinical status of a given patient with CHF.

(b) Identify all potential complications for the patient with CHF.

(c) Describe nursing interventions to manage these complications.

(d) Describe the expected medical interventions to treat these complications.

(e) Explain the pathophysiological cause of each sign and symptom of CHF.

(f) Relate the clinical signs and symptoms and treatments of CHF to the pathophysiology changes.

Priorities and constraints of situation

The priorities of the situation are the class size (40 students) and the timing of the class (halfway through a 15 week semester). The class is scheduled for 80 minutes in the late afternoon in a classroom with movable desks. The case study was developed by the instructor and is given to the students at the end of a lecture/discussion about congestive heart failure. In class, the students form small groups of five to six students. The groups work on the case study for about 20 minutes, then share their answers with the entire class. Because the learners are beginning nursing students and the case study is used about halfway through the semester, the instructor has chosen to use a stable case study. The focus of this exercise for these beginning students is identification and

Table 18.4 Congestive heart failure case study

Mr Jones is a 64-year-old man with a history or two prior myocardial infarctions. He is admitted to your unit complaining of extreme shortness of breath, dispnoea on exertion, 2–3 pillow orthopnoea and ankle oedema, all increasing over the last 3 days. He was a postal worker forced to retire after his second heart attack 3 years ago.

Physical exam: Elderly-looking man in moderate resiratory distress, sitting upright at side of bed; lung sounds – bilateral crackles 1/2 way up, heart sounds – inaudible because of loud lung sounds; + 3 oedema of lower extremities to knees, feet cool and unable to palpate pedal pulses, present with Doppler; Foley catheter to gravity draining scant amounts of dark yellow urine.

Psych/social: He lives in a third storey apartment with his wife of 42 years.

Meds: Digoxin 0.25 mg orally every day, Lasix 80 mg orally 3 times a day and as needed, KCl 40 mEq orally every day

Vital signs: heart rate 126, blood pressure 104/78, respiratory rate 28, temperature 99.6°F

Labs: Na 145, K 3.7, gluc 148, BUN 18, creatinine 1.9, CPK–MB 5%

Intake and output: 24 h intake = 800 cm^3 24 h output = 240 cm^3

Urinalysis: Sp.G 1.022, dark yellow, pH 5

1. What do you expect to find?
2. List all the available cues.
3. Categorize the cue:

   Relevant
   Non-relevant

4. The most likely explanation/diagnosis is:
5. Other explanations/diagnoses could be:

   (a)
   (b)
   (c)

6. List the additional information you would need to confirm/reject these alternative explanations.
7. The correct diagnosis is:
8. The status of this diagnosis is:

   ☐ emergency
   ☐ high risk
   ☐ low risk
   ☐ potential

9. Describe the probable cause of this diagnosis, based on available information.

interpretation of clinical cues and recognition of patterns in the information. In other activities where inquiry, planning and evolution of thought processes are stressed, a dynamic case study format would be preferred. Table 18.4 shows the case study information and the questions asked as they would appear on a single piece of paper for the student groups. Each student receives his/her own copy of the case study.

This case study aims to exemplify the patient with congestive heart failure, a common clinical situation encountered by nursing students. Numerous cues are presented that allow the students to think about the physical, emotional and psychosocial implications of this disease for this patient. His physical status is that of a stereotypic congestive heart failure patient. In addition, his laboratory values and vital signs provide information which is common for patients with this disorder. The

psychosocial information gives the student some ideas for discharge planning for this patient.

The systematic progression of students and instructor through the case study questions at the end of the case study gives opportunities to assess students' knowledge of CHF and their ability to apply this cognitive information to a simulated patient situation. Students can identify relevant and irrelevant cues and receive immediate feedback about those choices from the instructor. In addition, students can make incorrect decisions without harm to the patient.

Conclusions

The case study approach has been used successfully as an instructional method for undergraduate nursing students at the University of San Francisco.

Obviously, much more research needs to be done to investigate the educational possibilities of the case study method as a way to teach clinical reasoning. Case studies have been found to be an effective method for building cognitive schemata as demonstrated by increased knowledge acquisition and prolonged information retention in a small, quasi-experimental study with beginning nursing students (Prion, 1995). Until much more is known about how and why case studies succeed instructionally, we can only suggest that a carefully developed and thoughtfully implemented case study seems to be the best way to model clinical reasoning in a classroom setting.

Acknowledgement

The author gratefully acknowledges the contributions of Dr Robert P. Graby to the first edition of this chapter.

References

Albanese, M. A. and Mitchell, S. (1993) Problem-based learning: A review of literature on its outcomes and implementation issues. *Academic Medicine*, **68**, 52–81.

Andrews, M. and Jones, P. R. (1996) Problem-based learning in an undergraduate nursing programme: A case study. *Journal of Advanced Nursing*, **23**, 357–365.

Baxter, V. (1988) A case-study method for teaching industrial sociology. *Teaching Sociology*, **16**, 21–24.

Belenky, M. F., Clinchy, B. M., Goldberger, N. R. and Tarule, J. M. (1986) *Women's Ways of Knowing: The Development of Self, Voice and Mind*. New York: Basic Books.

Bernheimer, E. (1982) Teaching community agency referrals to medical students: The case method approach. *Journal of Medical Education*, **57**, 718–719.

Bloom, B. S., Engelhart, M. D., Furst, E. J., Hill, W. H. and Krathwohl, D. R. (1956) *Taxonomy of Educational Objectives*. New York: McKay.

Boehrer, J. and Linsky, M. (1990) Teaching with cases: Learning to question. *New Directions for Teaching and Learning*, **42**, 41–57.

Boyce, B. A. (1992) Making the case for the case-based method approach in physical education pedagogy classes. *Journal of Physical Education, Recreation and Dance*, **63**, 17–20.

Brown, J. S., Collins, A. and Duguid, P. (1989) Situated cognition and the culture of learning. *Educational Researcher*, **33**, 32–42.

Carnevali, D. L., Mitchell, P. H., Woods, N. F. and Tanner, C. F. (1984) *Diagnostic Reasoning in Nursing*. Philadelphia, PA: Lippincott.

Carter, K. and Unklesbay, R. (1989) Cases in teaching and law. *Journal of Curriculum Studies*, **21**, 527–536.

Chi, M. T. H., Glaser, R. and Farr, M. (1988) *The Nature of Expertise*. Hillsdale, NJ: Lawrence Erlbaum.

Christensen, R. (1987) *Teaching and the Case Method*. Boston, MA: Harvard Business School.

Corcoran, S. A. (1986) Planning by expert and novice nurses in cases of varying complexity. *Research in Nursing and Health*, **9**, 115–162.

Craik, F. I. M. and Tulving, E. (1975) Depth of processing and the retention of words in episodic memory. *Journal of Experimental Psychology: General*, **104**, 268–295.

Epstein, W. (1981) The classical tradition of dialectics and American legal education. *Journal of Legal Education*, **31**, 424–451.

Feinstein, M. C. and Veenendall, T. L. (1992) Using the case study method to teach interpersonal communication. *Inquiry: Critical Thinking Across the Disciplines*, **9**, 11–14.

Fonteyn, M. E. (1991) A descriptive analysis of expert critical care nurses' clinical reasoning. *Doctoral dissertation*. University of Texas, Austin, TX.

Frost, M. (1996) An analysis of the scope and value of problem-based learning in the education of health care professionals. *Journal of Advanced Nursing*, **24**, 1047–1053.

Gale, F. G. (1993) Teaching professional writing rhetorically: The unified case method. *Journal of Business and Technical Communication*, **7**, 256–266.

Gist, G. L. (1992) Problem-based learning: A new tool for environmental health education. *Journal of Environmental Health*, **54**, 8–13.

Harrington, H. (1991) The case as method. *Action in Teacher Education*, **12**, 1–10.

Hartman, L. D. (1992) Business communication and the case method: Toward integration in accounting and MBA graduate programs. *Bulletin of the Association for Business Communication*, **5**, 41–45.

Heliker, D. (1994) Meeting the challenge of the curriculum revolution: Problem-based learning in nursing education. *Journal of Nursing Education*, **33**, 45–47.

Kreps, G. L. and Lederman, L. C. (1985) Using the case method in organizational communication education: Developing students' insight, knowledge and creativity through experience-based learning and systematic debriefing. *Communication Education*, **34**, 358–364.

Mayer, R. E. (1992) *Thinking, Problem Solving, Cognition*, 2nd edn. New York: Freeman.

McCarthy, M. (1987) A slice of life: Training teachers through case studies. *Harvard Graduate School of Education Bulletin*, **22**, 7–11.

McWilliam, P. J. (1992) The case method of instruction: Teaching application and problem-solving skills to early interventionists. *Journal of Early Intervention*, **16**, 360–373.

Merseth, K. K. (1991) The early history of case-based instruction: Insights for teacher education today. *Journal of Teacher Education*, **42**, 243–249.

Nagel, G. K. (1991) The case method: Its potential for training administrators. *NASSP Bulletin*, **75**, 37–43.

Norman, G. R. (1988) Problem-solving skills, solving problems and problem-based llearning. *Medical Education*, **22**, 279–286.

Norman, G. R. and Schmidt, H. G. (1992) The psychological basis of problem-based learning: A review of the literature. *Medical Education*, **67**, 557–565.

Oldham, M. and Forrester, J. (1981) The use of case studies in pre-experience business education. *Vocational Aspects of Education*, **33**, 27–29.

Prion, S. K. (1995) The case method used inductively as an instructional approach to create cognitive schema in undergraduate nursing students. *Doctoral dissertation*. University of San Francisco, San Francisco.

Radwin, L. E. (1990) Research on diagnostic reasoning in nursing. *Nursing Diagnosis*, **1**, 70–77.

Rasinski, T. V. (1989) The case method approach in reading education. *Reading Horizons*, **30**, 5–14.

Resnick, L. (1982a) *Education and Learning to Think*. Washington, DC: National Academic Press.

Resnick, L. (1982b) Learning in school and out. *Educational Researcher*, **16**(9), 13–20.

Rumelhart, D. E. and Norman, D. A. (1981) Analogical processes in learning. In *Cognitive Skills and Their Acquisition* (J. R. Anderson, ed.). Hillsdale, NJ: Lawrence Erlbaum.

Sansalone, M. (1990) Teaching structural concepts through case studies and competitions. *Engineering Education*, **80**, 474–475.

Tanner, C., Padwick, K., Putzier, D. and Westfall, U. (1987) Diagnostic reasoning strategies of nurses and nursing students. *Nursing Research*, **36**, 359–363.

Taylor, W. C. (1989) A first-year problem-based curriculum in health promotion and disease prevention. *Academic Medicine*, 673–677.

Tichenor, C. J., Davidson, J. and Jensen, G. M. (1995) Cases as shared inquiry: Model for clinical reasoning. *Journal of Physical Therapy Education*, **9**(2), 57–62.

Vernon, D. T. A. and Blake, R. L. (1993) Does problem-based learning work? A meta-analysis of evaluative research. *Academic Medicine*, **68**, 550–563.

Walton, H. J. and Matthews, M. B. (1989) Essentials of problem-based learning. *Medical Education*, **23**, 542–558.

Watson, D. E. and West, D. J. (1996) Using problem-based learning to improve educational outcomes. *Occupational Therapy International*, **3**(2), 81–93.

Zarr, M. (1984) Learning criminal law through the whole case method. *Journal of Legal Education*, **34**, 697–701.

19

Teaching clinical reasoning to medical students

Ann Sefton, Jill Gordon and Michael Field

Clinical reasoning represents the process by which medical practitioners make decisions on diagnosis and management of a patient who may present with what has been described as an ill-structured problem (Barrows and Feltovich, 1987). Substantial interdisciplinary research has focussed on clinical reasoning with the result that different descriptions and models have been proposed (see, e.g. Barrows and Feltovich, 1987; Boshuizen and Schmidt, 1995; Grant, 1989; Kassirer, 1989; Schmidt *et al.*, 1990, and earlier chapters of this book). One common finding is that clinical reasoning does not develop in isolation: it is associated with increasingly refined and elaborated medical knowledge (Schmidt *et al.*, 1990). Problem solving is domain-specific and not generic (Chi *et al.*, 1982), so the challenge for medical educators is not only to make explicit the processes of reasoning (Kassirer, 1995), but also to identify the necessary content.

To a beginning medical student, a patient presents with a bewildering array of complex information (clinical, personal, social, emotional) of uncertain relevance. How can teachers encourage the skills of ordering the information, identifying the more important elements, generating, testing and refining hypotheses, and formulating clear, specific, answerable diagnostic or therapeutic questions? What are the most appropriate strategies and how are they made explicit to students?

Clinical reasoning and its components

As noted, reasoning alone is inadequate for clinical decision making; knowledge and understanding of basic mechanisms of human functioning are essential. The linking of the basic biomedical sciences with clinical and epidemiological information is crucial, as is the capacity to organize these data into coherent representations of disease processes (Boshuizen and Schmidt, 1992; Schmidt *et al.*, 1990). Thus, recently, debate has centred around the effectiveness of different methods to ensure that the acquisition of knowledge is associated with the development of reasoning.

What are the components of the diagnostic and management skills of the expert? A diagnosis often represents an explanation of an illness (Elstein, 1995), emphasizing the need for mechanisms of health and disease to be understood. Associations of symptoms and signs generate patterns that experts recognize quickly; for students, the patterns are less apparent. Increasing medical knowledge must be integrated into logically organized and elaborated structures or 'illness scripts' (Schmidt *et al.*, 1990); which structures aid rapid, accurate and relevant retrieval. Effective clinical reasoning is based on iterative information gathering as hypotheses are framed, tested, modified or discarded (Kassirer, 1995). This process requires skills in communication and physical examination, as well as the selective ordering and interpretation of investigations, using the best evidence available (Sackett *et al.*, 1997).

One difficulty in generalizing from existing research is that only the initial patient encounter has been scrutinized; management and continuing care have been less often studied (Barrows and Feltovich, 1987). Management requires more than understanding processes of disease, mechanisms for repair and means of alleviating symptoms; it demands a deep and empathic understanding of the patient's perspectives and needs. Such understanding derives from face-to-face encounters and so the effectiveness of bilateral communication becomes an issue. Another problem lies in the fact that in general, information is available from practitioners who – generally by introspection – describe the experience of reasoning in various clinical contexts. Such descriptions are largely phenomenological and characteristically highly individual.

Yet another difficulty is the number of perspectives which researchers employ. Each viewpoint offers insights which can be helpful when designing appropriate teaching, but significant differences in initial starting conditions and ongoing interpretation make it difficult to synthesize the various data into a single coherent model or strategy. Some elements, however, are common: the need to collect observations and information which is often disordered and not expressed in medical terms; the ordering of that information into more or less formal hypotheses based on existing medical knowledge and experience; further inquiry for clarification; expression of diagnostic possibilities that can be eliminated; a plan for further investigation and/or immediate management. An experienced clinician often undertakes some of the processes in parallel, rather than sequentially.

What can teachers do?

Medical teachers are faced with various descriptions of clinical reasoning, which they are assured can be taught (Kassirer, 1995), and no shortage of advice on educational strategies. They must determine overall curricular goals, identify essential content and design the processes for learning which will best support the development of an effective medical professional. Not all teachers acknowledge the need to make educational strategies explicit to students. However, we argue that it is *essential* to focus explicitly both on the processes of clinical

reasoning itself and on the educational methods that support its development. Students need to be engaged actively as informed partners.

Since experts process information and seek further inputs to clarify, reinforce or discard possibilities, communication becomes a focus for learning. For the novice with limited knowledge, the parallel processing of information is restricted and so some structure to information gathering is essential. Templates are useful initially to ensure that information is not missed, but rigid adherence to them is inefficient in the long term. Their uncritical use may obscure the recognition of priority issues and impede the development of appropriately structured knowledge (Schmidt *et al.*, 1990).

Given that experts are highly individual, are there useful general strategies for teaching clinical reasoning? Grant (1989) has encouraged students to share experiences and articulate the processes they use to work through diagnostic problems. In a supportive and safe atmosphere, her students express themselves honestly and receive specific, sensitive feedback; they also observe and model the strategies of others. Perhaps the most important benefit is the development of metacognitive skills which ensure that self-aware learners identify their thinking processes and monitor their own progress. The strategy may well appeal to those who are convinced of the individuality of mental processes or who question the notion of imposing a single best reasoning process.

Traditional curricula

Most medical schools this century have featured defined preclinical years, focussing on basic sciences, which are separated from clinical years when illness is emphasized and clinical reasoning introduced. Students learn science by reasoning from first principles (Niaz, 1993). These hypothetico-deductive processes are appropriate to the biomedical or physical sciences (Patel and Kaufman, 1995). Similar strategies are used by skilled medical practitioners only when problems are particularly difficult or obscure (Norman *et al.*, 1994). It is not surprising, therefore, that students find it difficult to reason backwards when confronted with patients with ambiguous symptoms and signs (Barrows and Feltovich, 1987; Patel *et al.*, 1991).

In traditional curricula, individual subjects are often taught in isolation so that little information is transferred between them. Thus conceptual linkages necessary for effective clinical problem solving (Schmidt *et al.*, 1990) are not readily established. Indeed, many teachers report anecdotes of students unable to relate fundamental concepts: e.g. in physiology to anatomy; or in pathology to microbiology. The recent information explosion within existing disciplines and the inclusion of new areas (e.g. molecular biology, new imaging techniques) have increased the overload of the curriculum (Bordage, 1987), militating against the thoughtful reflection required for deep understanding. Pushed to master an increasing volume, students resort to surface learning, at the expense of critical analysis and thinking. When assessments value recall, students are discouraged from reasoning at all (Ramsden, 1992). The resulting deficiencies hamper the later development of effective clinical reasoning when basic and clinical subjects must be interrelated.

Some medical sciences are well explained from the perspective of the abnormal (e.g. endocrine excess and deficiency help in understanding normal balances and controls; the function of neuroanatomical structures is illustrated by lesions). Such examples can introduce students to aspects of clinical reasoning. Since fewer medically qualified staff now teach in early years, examples of conceptual links between basic and clinical sciences are less accessible to the teachers. Specific approaches to integrating clinical experiences and basic sciences include those of Coles (1990), in which basic science examinations were delayed until after the first clinical attachments, and Patel and Dauphinee (1984), in which students learned some basic science during clinical years. In both examples, students had elaborated their knowledge and demonstrated an enhanced ability to retrieve and use basic information in clinical settings.

Hospital and community settings can be used to provide clinical examples for students in early years of traditional programs. At their best, such stimulating experiences provide not only a sense of relevance to the basic studies but also opportunities for students to see and model aspects of clinical reasoning. In order to be effective rather than tokenistic, however, the exposure must be well planned, explicit in its aims and directly related to other concurrent learning.

Problem-based learning

Those who introduced problem-based learning at McMaster University included clinical thinking as a high priority (Neufeld and Barrows, 1974). This educational method also removes the separation between basic sciences and clinical applications; students use the vocabulary of both and integrate their understanding across discipline boundaries. Problem-based learning encourages relevant reasoning, since students' learning is triggered by clinical problems (Engel, 1992) and supported by a facilitator (Barrows, 1983). Models of clinical reasoning are frequently used as a framework for group discussion (Barrows, 1985; McPherson and Murphy, 1997; Neame, 1989), making the process more explicit. The tutorial provides a safe environment in which issues brought into discussion are subjected to scrutiny. Knowledge brought to the tutorial by students is valued, a characteristic of adult learning (Boud and Griffin, 1987). Evidence suggests that the clinical-reasoning skills of such students are enhanced (de Vries *et al.*, 1989; Patel *et al.*, 1991), although not without some costs.

Content and coverage is important. If students are to develop a strong base of clinically elaborated knowledge (Patel *et al.*, 1991) or 'illness scripts' (Schmidt *et al.*, 1990), they need to be exposed to a variety of common and important clinical presentations and problems. Specialized teaching hospitals for clinical education can restrict the students' experience to the rare, complex and serious. In problem-based curricula, a careful choice of cases ensures that common and preventable conditions are emphasized appropriately.

Some strengths of integrated curricula, whether traditional (discipline based) or problem based, include the breaking down of artificial barriers between disciplines. Students may, however, have less opportunity to build a secure, sequential understanding of key concepts. Boundaries still exist in problem-based curricula so that students may be inhibited from truly free-ranging explorations of issues because problems are usually collated into blocks of related material. Such criticism clearly relates more to the early years of learning; a less structured clinical environment encourages broader thinking.

Since knowledge is an essential substrate of clinical reasoning, the problems chosen for study must reflect an adequate range, cover important content and encourage students to understand mechanisms. Computers now offer excellent opportunities for tracking content and ensuring that staff consult adequately in order to provide feedback to colleagues. Up-to-date information allows teachers to demonstrate how their topic contributes to an integrated understanding of medicine (Field and Sefton, 1998).

Teaching methods have been criticized in both traditional programs (e.g. Neame, 1989) or problem-based curricula (e.g. Patel *et al*., 1991). Faced with an array of potential models of clinical reasoning, and demands from content experts, how do planners embark on a problem-based approach? We suggest that it is useful to select one model of clinical reasoning (e.g. Kassirer, 1989) and base the tutorial discussion on it. The precise model is less important than its generic use as a framework to structure the flow of discussion and encourage the development of metacognitive skills. It later serves as a fall-back strategy in complicated clinical situations.

Could some advantages of problem-based learning be grafted on to a traditional curriculum? Many programs are 'hybrid' in the sense of providing structured sessions which support the learning actively generated by the problems (Armstrong, 1991; Sefton, 1997). Not only self-direction, but the processes of identifying cues and searching for associations and explanations would be muted if the problems were encountered only after formal study of the elements. Introducing disciplines followed by problem-based learning to illustrate applications fails to recognize the importance of active inquiry learning. Discipline-based teaching which follows problem-based learning may, however, be more effective. Some problem orientation has been introduced into more traditional programs in either subject-specific or integrated contexts but they have not yet been extensively reviewed and evaluated. The danger lies in overwhelming the time available for independent learning.

Computers, evidence-based medicine and clinical reasoning

Current imperatives exert pressure on doctors to practise medicine efficiently and cost-effectively (Towle, 1998). Access to ever-increasing investigations and treatments poses problems of choice and equity (Wolf *et al*., 1985). Guidelines are advocated, encouraging optimal use of resources. Patients now have unprecedented access to information through the Internet (Carlile and Sefton, 1998). It is imperative that students learn to respond to these changing expectations and pressures and use technology to assist their reasoning. Thus, they must frame appropriate questions, access relevant information, appraise it critically and apply the data to clinical decisions (Sackett *et al*., 1997).

Essential information is now available to guide clinical judgement and monitor practice. Computers open access to large databases, library resources and other information for students as well as for practising doctors, with significant implications for medical education (Coiera, 1997). Such ready access to on-line information is revolutionizing medical practice and decision making (Carlile and Sefton, 1998), although some of the obstacles highlighted by Balla *et al*. (1989) remain.

Computer programs are now being specifically designed to encourage students' diagnostic-reasoning skills (Bryce *et al*., 1998). Standardized and 'realistic' clinical situations can offer students and teachers rare insights into the processes of clinical thinking. A student's reasoning path through each problem is tracked and recorded, without risking harm or embarrassment to a patient. The sequential steps are accessible to student and teacher who review and discuss the process in detail. Areas of strength are recognized and concerns identified, enhancing the student's metacognitive skills. Remedial assistance is then designed as needed.

Learning clinical reasoning in practice settings

Regardless of experiences in the early years of a medical curriculum, all students quickly recognize certain fundamental differences in cognitive approach once they enter practice settings more or less full-time. Experienced clinicians, as teachers and *de facto* role models, may appear to 'short circuit' the reasoning process in routine encounters with patients. They may seem to students to be neither building on basic sciences to deduce the underlying pathophysiology of a patient's complaint, nor constructing an orderly series of hypotheses that are systematically considered and tested. Rather, they are observed to move quickly to an early working hypothesis on the basis of a few fragments of clinical information, taking in the context of the patient's age, sex, race and overall appearance (how 'ill' he or she looks). The subsequent refinement of this hypothesis by focussed clinical questioning, examination and investigations may give all the appearances of inspired guesswork to the novice clinical student.

That skilled clinicians use such abridged strategies in the efficient pursuit of a final diagnosis has been well documented (Glass, 1996; Kassirer,

1989; Kassirer and Kopelman, 1991; Newble and Cannon, 1994; Ridderikhoff, 1991; Rimoldi, 1988). They typically establish an early 'context' for continuing investigation and management by invoking one or more initial working diagnoses, often arrived at by the recognition of a familiar 'set' of data from a background of extensive knowledge of clinical features and prevalence of disease. In contrast to the formal process of problem-based learning, many rules of thumb, short-cuts or 'heuristics' (Kassirer and Kopelman, 1991) are used in recognizing clinical patterns which are not taught as such formally. Moreover, clinicians will be observed frequently to discard, replace and revive hypotheses as data accrue, seemingly making 'intuitive' judgements on the utility of specific tests or interventions.

In this setting, it is not surprising that many students rethink their approach to clinical problems in acquiring this practice style. They may feel caught between the admonition to be thorough and systematic in gathering and presenting clinical data, on the one hand, and the pressure to reach efficient but appropriate diagnostic endpoints, on the other. While they are exhorted to avoid 'premature closure' in the diagnostic process, they may feel that senior practitioners do this regularly.

This dilemma in the transition to clinical settings is resolved by implementing an educational model in which the underlying basis of real-world clinical reasoning is made explicit. Teaching formats used for decades in ward environments are not successful in achieving this aim. The traditional case presentation, in which all the data concerning a patient's admission is assembled and delivered without interruption is unlikely to lead to significant insights by any students present into how diagnostic and management decisions were made. Even less useful are fact-based 'topic tutorials' in which textbook summaries of specific diseases are presented.

Two approaches have emerged over recent years which promote better acquisition of clinical reasoning. First, the structure of clinical case presentations should change so that 'iterative hypothesis testing' is modelled (Kassirer, 1983). Here the student in possession of the details of the case releases only small packets of information to a group of peers, who form appropriate hypotheses and justify the need for further specific data on this basis. The clinician acts as a supportive facilitator of the interactions among the students, injecting where necessary the

knowledge base or 'experience' needed to reject some directions of inquiry and reinforce others. There are analogies here to models of problem-based learning.

The second approach calls for more explicit use of Bayesian analysis[1] in justifying the use of clinical and investigative data (Kassirer and Kopelman, 1991; Glass, 1996). While the formalities of this approach are not known to many practising clinicians, they make implicit use of these principles (to a greater or lesser extent) in interpreting individual items of clinical information and in ordering diagnostic tests, based upon long familiarity with their utility and performance. Since students cannot have instant access to this experience-based behaviour pattern, they should be encouraged to seek the underlying data justifying the use of specific pieces of information for confirming or rejecting a diagnosis. To this end, basic textbooks of clinical epidemiology (Sackett *et al.*, 1991) and targeted journal articles (e.g. Sackett and Rennie, 1992) are invaluable adjuncts to appropriate training in the principles of evidence-based medicine as they apply to clinical practice.

Concluding statement

Regardless of the model of curriculum, if clinical reasoning is incorporated as an explicit goal, appropriately staged teaching strategies and effective feedback to students are required. Students must be encouraged and rewarded by assessments which measure their development in reasoning skills as well as knowledge in the progression from novice to expert. These conclusions imply substantial commitments to communication with students and adequate staff development, so that all are aware of the values assigned to the process of clinical reasoning.

References

Armstrong, E. G. (1991) The Harvard Medical School curriculum: A hybrid model of problem-based learning. In *The Challenge of Problem-based Learning* (D. Boud and G. Felletti, eds), pp. 137–149. London: Kogan Page.

[1] An epidemiological approach based on a theorem in probability theory named after Thomas Bayes (1702–1761). In clinical decision analysis, it is used for estimating the probability of a particular diagnosis given the appearance of some symptom, sign or test result in a specific patient (Last, 1995).

Balla, J. I., Elstein, A. S. and Christensen, A. (1989) Obstacles to acceptance of decision analysis in clinical settings. *British Medical Journal*, **298**, 579–582.

Barrows, H. S. (1983) Problem-based, self-directed learning. *Journal of the American Medical Association*, **250**, 3077–3080.

Barrows, H. S. (1985) How to design a problem-based curriculum for the preclinical years. New York: Springer.

Barrows, H. S. and Feltovich, P. J. (1987) The clinical reasoning process. *Medical Education*, **21**, 86–90.

Bordage, G. (1987) The curriculum: Overloaded and too general? *Medical Education*, **21**, 183–188.

Boshuizen, H. P. A. and Schmidt, H. G. (1992) On the role of biomedical knowledge in clinical reasoning by experts, intermediates and novices. *Cognitive Science*, **16**, 153–184.

Boshuizen, H. P. A. and Schmidt, H. G. (1995) The development of clinical reasoning expertise. In *Clinical Reasoning in the Health Professions* (J. Higgs and M. Jones, eds), pp. 24–32. Oxford: Butterworth-Heinemann.

Boud, D. and Griffin, V. (1987) *Appreciating Adults Learning: From the Learners' Perspective*. London: Kogan Page.

Bryce, D. A., King, N. J., Graebner, C. F. and Myers, H. J. (1998) Evaluation of a diagnostic reasoning program (DxR): Exploring student perceptions and addressing faculty concerns. *Journal of Interactive Media in Education*, **1**, http://www-jime.open.ac.uk/98/1/

Carlile, S. C. and Sefton, A. J. (1998) Medical education for the information age. *Medical Journal of Australia*, **168**, 340–343.

Chi, M. T. H., Glaser, R. and Rees, E. (1982) Expertise in problem solving. In *Advances in the Psychology of Human Intelligence* (R. J. Sternberg, ed.), pp. 7–75. Hillsdale, NJ: Lawrence Erlbaum.

Coiera, E. (1997) *Guide to Medical Informatics, the Internet and Telemedicine*. London: Chapman & Hall.

Coles, C. R. (1990) Elaborated learning in undergraduate medical education. *Medical Education*, **24**, 14–22.

de Vries, M. W., Schmidt, H. G. and de Graaff, E. (1989) Dutch comparisons: Cognitive and motivational effects of problem-based learning on medical students. In *New Directions for Medical Education* (H. G. Schmidt, M. Lipkin Jr, M. W. de Vries and J. M. Greep, eds), pp. 230–238. New York: Springer.

Elstein, A. S. (1995) Clinical reasoning in medicine. In *Clinical Reasoning in the Health Professions* (J. Higgs and M. Jones, eds), pp. 49–59. Oxford: Butterworth-Heinemann.

Engel, C. E. (1992) Not just a method but a way of learning. In *The Challenge of Problem-based Learning* (D. Boud and G. Felletti, eds), pp. 23–33. London: Kogan Page.

Field, M. J. and Sefton, A. J. (1998) Computer-based management of content in planning a problem-based medical curriculum. *Medical Education*, **32**, 163–171.

Glass, R. D. (1996) *Diagnosis: A Brief Introduction*. Melbourne: Oxford University Press.

Grant, J. (1989) Clinical decision making: Rational principles, clinical intuition or clinical thinking? In *Learning in Medical School: A Model for the Clinical Professions* (J. I. Balla, M. Gibson and M. Chang, eds), pp. 81–100. Hong Kong: Hong Kong University Press.

Kassirer, J. P. (1983) Teaching clinical medicine by iterative hypothesis testing: Let's preach what we practice. *New England Journal of Medicine*, **309**, 921–923.

Kassirer, J. P. (1989) Diagnostic reasoning. *Annals of Internal Medicine*, **110**, 893–900.

Kassirer, J. P. (1995) Teaching problem-solving – how are we doing? *New England Journal of Medicine*, **332**, 1507–1509.

Kassirer, J. P. and Kopelman, R. I. (1991) *Learning Clinical Reasoning*. Baltimore, MD: Williams & Wilkins.

Last, J. M. (1995) *A Dictionary of Epidemiology*, 3rd edn. Oxford: Oxford University Press.

McPherson, J. and Murphy, B. (1997) Preparing problems for an integrated, problem-based curriculum. In *Imperatives in Medical Education* (R. Henry, C. Engel and K. Byrne, eds), pp. 180–191. University of Newcastle: Faculty of Medicine and Health Sciences.

Neame, R. L. B. (1989) Problem-based medical education: The Newcastle approach. In *New Directions for Medical Education* (H. G. Schmidt, M. Lipkin Jr, M. W. de Vries and J. M. Greep, eds), pp. 112–146. New York: Springer.

Neufeld, V. and Barrows, H. (1974) The McMaster philosophy: An approach to medical education. *Journal of Medical Education*, **49**, 1040–1050.

Newble, D. and Cannon, R. (1994) *A Handbook for Medical Teachers*, 3rd edn. Dordrecht: Kluwer.

Niaz, M. (1993) Problem solving in science. *Journal of College Science Teaching*, **23**, 18–23.

Norman, G. R., Trott, A. L., Brooks, A. R. and Smith, E. K. M. (1994) Cognitive differences in reasoning related to postgraduate training. *Training and Learning in Medicine*, **6**, 114–120.

Patel, V. L. and Dauphinee, W. D. (1984) Return to basic sciences after clinical experience in undergraduate medical training. *Medical Education*, **18**, 244–248.

Patel, V. L., Groen, G. J. and Norman, G. R. (1991) Effects of conventional and problem-based medical curricula on problem-solving. *Academic Medicine*, **66**, 380–389.

Patel, V. L. and Kaufman, D. R. (1995) Clinical reasoning and biomedical knowledge: Implications for teaching. In *Clinical Reasoning in the Health Professions* (J. Higgs and M. Jones, eds), pp. 117–128. Oxford: Butterworth-Heinemann.

Ramsden, P. (1992) *Learning to Teach in Higher Education*. London: Routledge.

Ridderikhoff, J. (1991) Medical problem-solving: An exploration of strategies. *Medical Education*, **25**, 196–207.

Rimoldi, H. J. (1988) Diagnosing the diagnostic process. *Medical Education*, **22**, 270–278.

Sackett, D. L. and Rennie, D. (1992) The science of the art of the clinical examination. *Journal of the American Medical Association*, **267**, 2638–2644.

Sackett, D. L., Richardson, W. S., Rosenberg, W. and Haynes, R. B. (1997) *Evidence-based Medicine: How to Practice and Teach EBM*. New York: Churchill Livingstone.

Sackett, D. L., Rosenberg, W. M., Gray, J. A., Haynes, R. B. and Richardson, W. S. (1996) Evidence based medicine: What it is and what it isn't. *British Medical Journal*, **312**, 71–2.

Schmidt, H. G., Norman, G. R. and Boshuizen, H. P. A. (1990) A cognitive perspective on medical expertise: Theory and implications. *Academic Medicine*, **65**, 611–621.

Sefton, A. J. (1997) From a traditional to a problem-based curriculum: Estimating staff time and resources. *Education for Health*, **10**, 165–178.

Towle, A. (1998) Changes in health care and continuing medical education for the 21st century. *British Medical Journal*, **316**, 301–304.

Wolf, F. M., Gruppen, L. D. and Billi, J. E. (1985) Differential diagnosis and the competing hypothesis heuristic: A practical approach to judgement under uncertainty and Bayesian probability. *Journal of the American Medical Association*, **253**, 2858–2862.

20

Teaching clinical reasoning to occupational therapists

Judy Ranka and Chris Chapparo

Occupational therapists are viewed as successful clinical reasoners if they can identify the problem, understand the client's view of the problem, decide on which is the best, most just and non-harmful course of action, and predict the outcome of therapy for the client. These skills involve multiple processes that result in ongoing decision making that is characterized by dimensions of knowledge, reflection and intuition. As Rogers (1983, p. 615) has stated, these dimensions 'are inextricably entwined' in a clinician who is simultaneously a scientist, ethicist and artist: a clinical reasoner.

If clinical reasoning is the core of occupational therapy practice, the occupational therapy curriculum is responsible for guiding students to become effective clinical reasoners. To do this, opportunities for participants to develop the knowledge, skills and attitudes associated with being a clinical reasoner are essential. We believe there are five core dimensions to the process.

(a) Participants need to develop and learn to use knowledge stores that contain information about occupational therapy theory, health and disability, and the tools of occupational therapy practice, as well as experiential knowledge of outcomes.
(b) Participants need to develop the specific interpersonal skills required to glean information about another person's perspective of illness and the skill to effect change.
(c) Participants need to develop insight and the use of intuition to create images of future potential for clients with disability.

(d) Participants need to become cognisant of their own moral positions and ways of dealing with ethical dilemmas that arise during the course of therapy.
(e) Participants need to be able to reason a best course of action within the context of restrictions imposed by current health care systems.

The purpose of this chapter is to describe examples of learning units that facilitate the development of clinical reasoning in undergraduate and graduate occupational therapy participants. The units focus on procedural reasoning, reasoning that enables an understanding of the client's perspective, ethical reasoning and the use of multiple reasoning modes. An outline of the aims, structure and content is presented for each unit.

Facilitating procedural reasoning: learning to use knowledge to develop a picture of the problem

Various conceptualizations of what Fleming (1991, 1994a) refers to as procedural reasoning have been described in occupational therapy literature (Bridge and Twible, 1997; Dutton, 1996; Pelland, 1987; Rogers and Holm, 1997; Rogers and Masagatani, 1982). The units described in this section have been constructed largely through a synthesis of this and other occupational therapy literature presented by Ranka and Chapparo (1995; Chapter 13), literature from the field of education specifically concerned with adult, self-directed and lifelong learning, and our own ideas.

Aim and structure of learning experiences

The aim of these units is to provide participants with a model for procedural reasoning. This model includes a problem solving structure and a strategy for using the directions provided by theory and personal views of practice. Evaluating the effectiveness of these units involves assessing how well participants can construct a comprehensive occupational therapy program to manage problems, a program that is framed by theory and reflects a critical appraisal of the literature. Three sequential phases involved in teaching procedural reasoning are described.

Using knowledge to construct a picture of the problem

This learning unit is organized around incomplete and 'ill-structured' case studies in the form of referrals to occupational therapy. Some clients are individuals while others are groups, organizations or communities; some cases focus on the major occupational areas affected while others focus on the causes of dysfunction in occupational performance (e.g. psychosocial, biomechanical, environmental). The teachers and learners in each group form small collaborative groups that constitute 'the occupational therapist'.

In this initial problem sensing stage, each 'therapist' begins to formulate hypotheses about the problems in occupational performance, the nature of dysfunction and/or disease, tentative theoretical frameworks for practice, and ideas about suitable occupational therapy programs, by answering the questions, '*What do I know?*' (What knowledge do I have? What cues have I noted?), '*What do I need to know?*' (What knowledge is lacking?) and '*How can I find out?*' (Who may provide information? How do I consult them? What tangible material and electronic resources may expand my knowledge or confirm my impressions? How do I access them?). These questions form the substrate of each successive stage in procedural reasoning from initial assessment through to the conclusion of therapy.

As the unit progresses through the stages of procedural reasoning, decisions made by each group influence the type of supplemental information provided. In this way, each case becomes unpredictable and several courses of action may be

appropriate. For example, one group may decide to assess the home environment of their client, while another may focus on upper limb function. Based on these decisions each group receives different information and pursues different lines of reasoning. Additional cues are introduced through combinations of written case notes, videotaped excerpts of client performance and/or experiential role plays involving the use of actors or former occupational therapy clients employed as tutor assistants for this purpose.

Using theory to complete the picture

This phase requires that participants apply conceptual models of occupational therapy practice to the process of procedural reasoning. Participants examine the philosophical bases of a variety of conceptual models of practice, identify and define the dominant concepts and constructs of each model, and outline major principles and describe underlying assumptions of selected models. Cases are used to explore the process of procedural reasoning under each model. Participants have an opportunity to select and apply an appropriate occupational therapy conceptual model to an ill-structured case study similar to those described in the previous phase. Comparing and contrasting various models and their applications provides participants with an opportunity to examine the ways in which various theories can shape the process of procedural reasoning.

Using experience to construct a personal theory

Phase three of developing procedural reasoning is necessarily the most mature phase. Again, a case-based approach is used. In this unit collaborative groups of participants examine complex cases that contain many conflicting cues. Participants then attempt to link their acquired knowledge of health and disease, knowledge of occupational therapy conceptual models for practice, and knowledge gained from experience, to construct individual 'pictures' of the problem and a proposed course of action. We refer to these individual pictures as 'personal theories'. Participants are helped to develop a supporting rationale for their personal views and to present it to the other learners in the group. Through this process participants learn to present incomplete ideas and discuss conflicting viewpoints, articulating their own views and respecting the views of others.

Facilitating understanding of the client's perspective through clinical reasoning

As detailed by Ranka and Chapparo (1995; Chapter 13), creating an image of the meaning of disability and illness from the client's perspective is a primary goal of clinical reasoning in occupational therapy. Critical self-reflection is central to this outcome. Communication and dialogue become salient factors in the process of critical reflection, because this type of reasoning involves testing the justification or validity of presuppositions or assumptions about the client. It is through the interactive system of skilled communication that occupational therapists attempt to understand what is valid in the assertions made by others and attempt to achieve consensual validation for their own assertions about clients' problems and potential. Fleming (1991, 1994b) referred to this process as 'interactive reasoning'.

Research about the process of reflective judgement from the field of adult education indicates that participants at different ages and educational levels enter courses with markedly different assumptions about what and how something can be known or understood (Mezirow, 1991). Our experience in teaching undergraduates suggests that many first year participants in occupational therapy enter the course believing that they can 'know' through concrete observation and knowledge about what is the 'right' thing to do in therapy. Some participants at this level view clinical reasoning as discovering 'the truth'. Others rely on occupational therapy educators to explicate it. However, many of the problems faced by occupational therapists involve uncertainty, are incomplete, or cannot be articulated by clients (Chapparo, 1997; Rogers, 1983). If participants are to develop clinical reasoning strategies that are based on understanding the client's perspective of the problem, they must learn to construct a therapeutic solution to the existing problem that is justifiable after consideration of all perspectives of the problem and all interpretations of the problem. This can occur only if participants begin to accept that for some problems there are no uniquely 'true' answers.

Aim and structure of learning experiences

The aim of these learning experiences is for participants not only to understand the perspectives of others but also to be challenged to examine their own perspectives about illness, therapy and disability. These challenges, along with appropriate environmental support, promote an interactive clinical reasoning style that is based on reflective thinking. The effectiveness of these learning experiences can be judged by assessing how well participants are able to communicate effectively with a variety of people. Specific to clinical reasoning, critical communication skills include identifying and interpreting another person's beliefs and values about disability, phrasing interpretations of another person's views of disability in non-judgemental terms, and comparing and contrasting client problems from the perspectives of the medical diagnosis, the occupational diagnosis and the client who is ill.

Three increasingly complex stages of interactive reasoning as described by Chapparo (1997) are addressed. First, participants work on developing the antecedent skills required for client-focused communication. These antecedent skills are largely interpersonal and include observation, listening, questioning and feeling at ease with entering purposive social interactions within the context of an interview. Second, participants work on developing the ability to accurately record and interpret information they obtain from others during discourse. This phase could be conceptualized as testing out the interpretations of other people's stories and metaphors of illness and disability. Third, participants engage in the process of exploring what is meaningful for other people, for themselves and differentiating between the two. This involves participants engaging in purposive discourse in which the structure, duration, context and conditions are set by the client's situation. The primary function of this aspect of interactive reasoning is to let the participant explore issues of maintaining and relinquishing control and authority, thereby enabling clients and others to become participants in the reasoning process.

Antecedent phase

Developing communication skills within the context of interactive reasoning consists of intensive practice in interacting with others, with the goal being to understand other people's perspectives about disability. Participants are required to encourage others to voice their views about disability and illness. These practice interview sessions are videotaped and then discussed by the whole tutorial group. Ultimately, participants obtain a range of different perspectives of disability that are held by different individuals. In such situations the risks and pressures of voicing personal opinions are minimized by the educator who models the kind of listening, observing and interviewing that is essential to the participant's role as an interactive reasoner, encouraging the participant to examine information gathered and to identify gaps that pose problems in creating a picture of another person's perspective.

Interpretation phase

During this interactive phase of learning, facilitators question participants about the dimensions of the information obtained through interviews and observations of clients and others. Prompting is used when information has been missed or when assumptions have been made in the absence of direct information from the client. Participants are encouraged to interpret the narratives of others and rephrase them in a form that they understand. They are encouraged to identify aspects of client narratives that are puzzling, and to create an explanation that could account for the puzzling phenomena.

Meaning and differentiation phase

In this aspect of developing interactive reasoning skills, participants engage in exploration of the perspectives of others in situations that are characterized by risk taking, pressure and accountability. Participants participate in a series of 'hypotheticals' that require them to role-play various dichotomous scenarios (Donelly, 1992). The technique of dichotomous scenarios employs a forced-choice format, where the participant is assigned one of a number of alternative perspectives concerning some aspect of a situation. An example involves a case history of an occupational therapist who is engaged in helping parents place their child with developmental disability into a mainstream school. Participants are required to take the part of the child, the parents, the classroom teacher, the school principal and the occupational therapist. They develop arguments for and against such a placement from the perspective of a particular person in the scenario. Underpinning the development of these positions is information regarding ideology, educational policy, hegemony, general views of people about children with developmental disability, the participants' views about developmental disability and their interpretations of videotapes of interviews with parents of children with developmental disability. The purpose of these exercises is to help participants learn to develop a client-centred reasoning process. Facilitation includes (a) helping participants identify and confront the issue of their degree of commitment to the clients' perspectives, goals and needs versus other participants' perspectives, goals and needs, (b) helping each other confront and understand hostile judgements and reactions, and (c) helping each other expand the extent to which they are conscious of client-centred issues in their reasoning processes.

Facilitating ethical reasoning in occupational therapy

Although occupational therapy interventions are not often directly concerned with ethical issues of life and death, they are concerned with issues of quality of life and the consequences of many modern life saving techniques. The commonest ethical question to be answered by occupational therapy practitioners today is concerned with 'who will be treated when not all can be treated' (Neuhaus, 1988, p. 288). Having the knowledge, the clinical judgement and the clinical skill but not the funding, the time or resources to enhance a client's quality of life is a constant dilemma for today's practising therapist.

The reality of these ethical dilemmas is often far removed from the idealism that is a feature of many curricula. Participants often report back from fieldwork sites about difficulties they had with clinical reasoning that led to decisions about the amount, type and intensity of actual treatment versus the treatment that should have been given. Participants in these situations speak of feelings of helplessness, ineffectiveness and in many cases anger towards therapists, clients, educators and the health system or other systems and organizations in general. They have difficulty using their reasoning processes to imagine how they, as future therapists, will work in environments where such decisions must be made. Participants often lack three ingredients that offer a sense of direction to experienced therapists: facts, experience (Neuhaus, 1988), and wisdom.

It is clear that participants need useful and timely learning experiences that bring ethical questions closer to reality. These learning experiences can illustrate how decision making must always be tempered with open acknowledgement that it may not always be possible to decide the 'right' thing to do in a situation. In many instances, it is a matter of accepting that one decision is better than other less desirable options.

Aim and structure of learning experiences

The general aim of these learning experiences is to help participants consider in a systematic way alternative solutions to problems involving ethical dilemmas, and to increase participants' understanding of the psychological dimensions of ethical decision making. We evaluate these learning experiences by identifying how well participants are able to (a) identify ethical issues in therapy situations, (b) articulate ethical reasons for treatment choices they make, (c) appropriately tolerate and/or resist ethical disagreement and ambiguity in therapy situations, and ultimately (d) articulate a personal ethical framework that can guide decision making.

There are two primary processes involved in ethical reasoning. One involves a cognitive process whereby participants identify and understand ethical principles and issues that relate to health care and disability. The other involves interpersonal and intrapersonal processes that incorporate individual values, perceptions, opinions and feelings. As with the development of interactive reasoning, learning experiences that facilitate ethical reasoning are structured in consideration of participants' levels of maturity and their increasing ability for self-reflection. Harnessing the interpersonal communication skills acquired in other parts of the curriculum, together with knowledge about disability, participants can begin to engage in the process of ethical reasoning.

Ethical imagination is stimulated

This occurs by increasing participants' knowledge of key ethical principles (autonomy, beneficence, truthfulness and justice) and by exposing them to many ethical issues in occupational therapy practice. One of the most effective teaching tools to stimulate ethical imagination is the use of case studies. Through case studies, participants can be guided to identify ethical issues, apply ethical principles to real-life therapy situations and determine their own ethical position. Supervision in these learning experiences requires an educator who can create a 'safe' learning environment where participants are free to express their own opinions and feelings rather than asserting the 'correct' ethical position.

Decision making that involves ethical reasoning

Structures for facilitating this level of reasoning again involve case studies. One example is an exercise where participants are asked to determine who will be treated in an occupational therapy program that is limited by staff shortages. Out of five clients of varying age, sex and disability, participants are to choose which two will receive immediate therapy. Each participant is required to outline the line of reasoning that led to this choice and articulate how the choice reflects his or her personal, ethical and moral values. Using case studies, another exercise also contributes to helping the participant become aware of the ethical issues implicit in reasoning a course of action. After presentation of a case, participants are required to analyse the implied contract between the occupational therapist and client(s) in the case. This analysis incorporates such aspects of ethical action as rights, obligations of the therapist and client, the nature of the relationship, determining who makes the decisions about the course of action and the handling of conflicting ethics (Haddad, 1988). Participants are then required to articulate how the implicit ethics of the situation impact on the clinical-reasoning process that culminates in treatment.

Appreciation of emotional and affective reactions that accompany ethical dilemmas and channelling these responses into a feeling, but logically reasoned response

As with interactive reasoning, role-playing dichotomous scenarios allows participants to simulate therapy experiences initially within a safe environment. As Haddad (1988) reports, role-playing demonstrates the difference between doing and thinking. It permits participants to practise developing the reasoned affective responses that are often required for maintaining good interpersonal relationships among health care workers who have disparate ethical positions. It illustrates how a therapist's behaviour is a function not only of personality but also of role expectation. Participants become aware of the feelings of others and learn that it is usual for others to hold different points of view. In using this method, participants are encouraged to display genuine responses and to ask questions as the scenario unfolds. Volunteers for each scenario are sought while others act as participant observers of the decision making process. The primary focus of the technique at this level is that it is focused on process rather than solution (Donelly, 1992).

Putting it all together using multiple reasoning modes

Ultimately participants require opportunities to orchestrate multiple reasoning modes and learn about the 'art' of clinical reasoning. Functional performance requires motivation, physical action and understanding of social meaning within social and cultural contexts. It is necessary, therefore, that participants engage in learning experiences that challenge them to consider all aspects of the client and the presenting problem.

Aim and structure of learning experiences

Of the clinical reasoning modes described, this is perhaps the most difficult for undergraduate participants, as it requires professional and life experience to construct images of client potential. We expect that participants will be able to change from one reasoning mode to another in describing a course of action in therapy.

The stimulus used to promote the development of multiple reasoning modes is a detailed case history that incorporates complex and conflicting information about diagnosis, client perceptions, social, physical and cultural environments and organizational variables. Participants are encouraged to use multiple reasoning modes by answering questions such as:

- '*What is the problem?*' Answers to this question are identified from several perspectives: the client, caregiver, doctor, and therapist, thereby challenging the participant to use both procedural and interactive modes of reasoning.
- '*What should be done?*' and '*What can be done?*' Answers to these contrasting questions challenge participants to shift from procedural modes of reasoning to making ethical decisions about what can be done within the social and economic constraints imposed by the variables in the case.
- '*What will I do?*' and '*Why?*' Answers to these questions challenge participants to make decisions about their own actions based on the information at hand and to give reasons for their choice based on personal theoretical and ethical notions of the case.

- '*What will be the outcome?*' The ability to answer this question develops later in the curriculum when participants have had considerable fieldwork experience. At earlier stages of learning it is important that educators provide this part of the story of cases presented. Through experiential narratives from educators and from clinicians, participants develop images of therapy outcomes. Story-telling within the context of case scenarios becomes a useful technique in developing skill at this stage of developing clinical reasoning.

Conclusion

Facilitation of clinical reasoning incorporates scientific and artistic elements that are directed to a specific conclusion: the most appropriate action for a particular client. Since this process calls for judgement and decision making as well as science, the ethical and intuitive elements of the reasoning process must be equally recognized as significant facets of the educational process. We have described in this chapter learning units that facilitate both specific modes and integrative modes of clinical reasoning.

References

Bridge, C. and Twible, R. (1997) Clinical reasoning: Informed decision making for practice. In *Occupational Therapy: Enabling Function and Well-being* (C. Christiansen and C. Baum, eds), pp. 158–180, Thorofare, NJ: Slack.

Chapparo, C. (1997) Influences on clinical reasoning in the occupational therapy practice area of neurology. *Doctoral dissertation*. Macquarie University, Sydney.

Donelly, M. (1992) *Integration Issues in Occupational Therapy: OTIV Hypotheticals*. Sydney: School of Occupation and Leisure Sciences, The University of Sydney.

Dutton, R. (1996) *Clinical Reasoning in Physical Disabilities*. Baltimore, MD: Williams & Wilkins.

Fleming, M. H. (1991) Clinical reasoning in medicine compared with clinical reasoning in occupational therapy. *American Journal of Occupational Therapy*, **45**, 988–996.

Fleming, M. H. (1994a) Procedural reasoning: Addressing functional limitations. In *Clinical Reasoning: Forms of Inquiry in a Therapeutic Practice* (C. Mattingly and M. Fleming, eds), pp. 137–177. Philadelphia, PA: F. A. Davis.

Fleming, M. H. (1994b) The therapist with the three-track mind. In *Clinical Reasoning: Forms of Inquiry in a Therapeutic Practice* (C. Mattingly and M. Fleming, eds), pp. 119–136. Philadelphia, PA: F. A. Davis.

Haddad, A. M. (1988) Teaching ethical analysis in occupational therapy. *American Journal of Occupational Therapy*, **42**, 300–304.

Mezirow, J. (1991) How critical reflection triggers transformative learning. In *Fostering Critical Reflection in Adulthood* (J. Mezirow, ed.), pp. 122–137. San Francisco: Jossey-Bass.

Neuhaus, B. (1988) Ethical considerations in clinical reasoning: The impact of technology and cost containment. *American Journal of Occupational Therapy*, **42**, 288–292.

Pelland, M. J. (1987) A conceptual model for the instruction and supervision of treatment planning. *American Journal of Occupational Therapy*, **41**, 351–359.

Ranka, J. and Chappero, C. (1995) Teaching clinical reasoning to occupational therapy students. In *Clinical Reasoning in the Health Professions* (J. Higgs and M. Jones, eds), pp. 212–223. Oxford: Butterworth-Heinemann.

Rogers, J. C. (1983) Eleanor Clarke Slagle lectureship 1983: Clinical reasoning: The ethics, science and art. *American Journal of Occupational Therapy*, **37**, 601–616.

Rogers, J. C. and Holm, M. (1991) Occupational therapy diagnostic reasoning: A component of clinical reasoning. *American Journal of Occupational Therapy*, **45**, 1045–1053.

Rogers, J. C. and Masagatani, G. (1982) Clinical reasoning of occupational therapists during the initial assessment of physically disabled patients. *Occupational Therapy Journal of Research*, **2**, 195–219.

21

Learning reasoning in physiotherapy programs

Judi Carr, Mark Jones and Joy Higgs

Human activity is essentially instructive activity
(Mageean, 1991).

The physiotherapist's activities of clinical assessment and intervention form a cycle of problem formulation and re-formulation.[1] This cycle fits closely with models of experiential learning such as the one developed by Kolb (1984). These learning models emphasize that it is not the experience in itself that results in learning, but the processing of new information encountered and the cognitive effort of trying to make sense of it on the basis of past experience. Clinical reasoning may be compared to the 'processing' part of this learning activity, clinical data about the client to the 'new information encountered' and the physiotherapist's existing knowledge to the 'past experience' with which this new information is to be integrated.

The learning that results from clinical experience means that each physiotherapist constructs an *own reality*, not just by adding extra bits of information to an existing knowledge bank, but also by assimilating and integrating new information into existing organized knowledge structures (referred to as 'schemas'), and by creating new schemas which take account of the newly acquired information (Anderson, 1990). Hence, knowledge base and cognitive processing skills are interdependent, not independent, factors in further developing the clinician's knowledge; reasoning cannot take place in isolation from content.

[1] Refer to Chapter 1.

If it is agreed that the possession of and ability to use an extensive, context- and domain-specific knowledge base is what characterizes the expert (Boshuizen and Schmidt, 1992; Patel *et al.*, 1986), then major aims of professional preparation programs should be to foster effective learning strategies in students and to help them to learn about how they learn. The authors of this chapter are involved in physiotherapy education programs at undergraduate, postgraduate and continuing professional education levels. These programs emphasize that a clinical reasoning process is required for effective clinical learning. They aim to produce graduates who can be self-reliant in their learning, with the ability to evaluate their knowledge, reasoning and other clinical skills as a basis for further learning. The sections below outline the content and processes that our students use in learning to reason in clinical practice, and examples of how such content and process are incorporated in our educational programs.

Educational content and process – What do we want our students to learn?

Five major aspects of learning are addressed in our programs (Carr *et al.*, 1995). These are:

- The *cognitive skills* which allow the intellectual processing to occur, such as cue perception, data evaluation, hypothesis generation, deductive and inductive reasoning, pattern recognition.

Problem formulation or problem setting (Schön, 1983) is a particularly important skill here, as the initial conceptualization of the person and the problem confronting the physiotherapist will determine the line of inquiry to be followed in further assessment, and hence will affect the type of information that is fed into the clinical reasoning process during both assessment and treatment phases (Jones *et al.*, 1995).

- The *knowledge base* which supports reasoning. This knowledge base includes the physical and biomedical sciences (anatomy, physiology, pathology, kinesiology) and professional knowledge (clinical facts, principles, concepts and procedures of importance to the physiotherapist) (Higgs and Titchen, 1995). New knowledge encountered during clinical reasoning is likely to remain more accessible to memory because of the relevance of the context in which it is gained (Cervero, 1988), in contrast to the limited clinical relevance of the classroom in which these subjects are normally taught.

- *Metacognition and self-evaluation.* Because most physiotherapists practise independently, they must be able to monitor and judge their own performance. There is no external assessor to assist with this process in real-life clinical practice as there is in the normal classroom. A major skill required by physiotherapists, then, is the ability to engage in reflective practice (Schön, 1983). In the simplest sense, this means acting as the 'fly on the wall' during clinical practice, observing their own actions and reviewing their knowledge and thinking processes in a clear and dispassionate way. The awareness and monitoring of one's thinking is called metacognition, and it requires the clinician to be able to process two types of information simultaneously. On one level clinicians are gathering, analysing and synthesizing data related to the client being assessed, but on another level they are evaluating the quality of their information processing.

- *Interpersonal and verbal communication skills.* Much of the information used in clinical problem solving is obtained through interviewing the client, and collaborative decision making, teaching and counselling are essential aspects of clinical practice. The physiotherapist must establish a climate in which clients feel comfortable to speak freely and must communicate clearly with them, in order to attain satisfactory treatment outcomes.

- *Other skills* which support clinical reasoning effectiveness. These include, for example, manual or other technical skills used in assessment or treatment, and the ability to critically read and extract relevant information from laboratory reports and X-rays.

Educational programs – How do our students learn these things?

Our students learn 'reasoning' not in isolation, but during a variety of activities which encourage them to practise and recognize elements of clinical reasoning which we believe can lead to expert performance. These activities include real-time clinical practice and clinical simulations, with case studies having a high profile. Three sections of our programs are described by way of illustration.

First-year undergraduate preclinical learning

Physiotherapy Studies 100/101 is a subject taught in the first year of the Bachelor of Applied Science (Physiotherapy) course at the University of South Australia. This subject exists within a fairly traditional course, where the majority of the first-year curriculum is dedicated to the teaching of basic physical, social and biomedical sciences, through lectures and practical classes. The aims of this subject are multiple, but fall within four broad goals: to introduce students to the complex role of the physiotherapist, to give students a clinical focus for their other first-year learning, to help students develop a positive attitude to independent learning and acquire skills which facilitate independent learning, and to introduce students to a basic clinical problem-solving model so that they start to develop clinical reasoning skills which will be further developed in later years of the course.

The central feature of the subject design is the small group problem-based tutorial, modelled on the format used in a growing number of medical schools (e.g. Henry *et al.*, 1997). A variety of physiotherapy cases is used in this subject to introduce students to orthopaedic, cardio-respiratory, neurological, paediatric and psychosocial topics. Each case is addressed over two tutorial sessions, separated by several days.

At the beginning of each case, the student group is given a trigger containing some information about the client and the presenting problem, and a task to work on. Students list any cues that they can identify in the trigger, make reasonable inferences based on the cues (e.g. 'looks fit', 'looks like it's just her shoulder'), and then develop an initial summary of the client and the problem which attempts to encapsulate and categorize all the important information so far (e.g. 'an elderly woman with a problem of general stiffness and discomfort'). The group then generates a set of hypotheses which they think may explain the client's problem, and sets about trying to clarify which of the possibilities is correct through interviewing and examining the client (role played by the tutor). In discussing how the information gained seems to support or negate these hypotheses, the list of possibilities may be added to, refined or reduced and cues that initially were not perceived as relevant may be recognized as such. At the end of the first session, students identify the information the group needs in order to further clarify the problem, and learning goals are allocated to individual group members. The research required usually includes aspects of anatomy, physiology, kinesiology and pathology, together with aspects of physiotherapy assessment and treatment.

In the second tutorial session, students summarize for the group any new information they found, commenting on how they think it contributes to clarifying the problem and suggesting any further questions that need to be asked of the client or additional aspects of the physical examination that should be performed. Again, cues that were originally missed may be identified as relevant in the light of new information, or discussion from the previous session may be revisited in more detail, sometimes resulting in quite different conclusions. The examination of the client is continued (albeit in an abbreviated and superficial way because of the students' inexperience) and this additional information is incorporated into the group's evolving concept of the problem. At the end of this second tutorial session, the group constructs a final client/problem summary and records the argument which led to that conclusion.

The emphasis during these tutorials is on the students identifying what is known (individually or collectively), what they need to know to be able to progress towards the problem solution, the use of evidence and sound reasoning to support or negate hypotheses, and student responsibility for their learning. The tutor acts as a resource person, giving client information through role play, keeping students reasonably 'on track', modelling how to present, for example, an argument or a clinical

summary, suggesting alternative learning resources, providing feedback on group performance and, especially early in the year, helping the group to establish a productive working pattern.

The group tutorial program is complemented by written assignments designed to lead students through other clinical cases. These mirror the group format as closely as possible while allowing students to complete the tasks alone and obtain feedback about their individual achievement and progress.

At the beginning of the year tasks are diagnostic in nature and straightforward, e.g. 'work out what is wrong with this boy'. Other types of task related to management are then introduced, e.g. 'what issues would you/other professionals need to consider in planning to have Simon go home from the rehabilitation unit independent of other people's assistance?' The cases used early in the year assume some student knowledge at a lay level only, such as common sports injuries and arthritis. These topics are treated fairly simply with the aims of familiarizing students with the problem solving format to be used, and starting the move away from the use of lay knowledge to more scientific knowledge such as the structure of muscles, the mediation of pain, the biochemical nature of the inflammatory process and how physical assessment (e.g. movement and palpation) can be used to analyse the cause of the presenting problem. All the early problems use visual triggers in the form of brief video clips. They are deliberately rich in cues and a relatively large proportion of time is spent on the perception-evaluation-analysis of these cues. As the year progresses, the problems themselves become more complex and there is a shift in emphasis from consideration of initial cues and derivation of reasonable inferences to the planning and carrying out of interviews and physical examinations, progressive reasoning through those assessments, and planning approaches to intervention based on decisions made.

Throughout the year, students are asked to reflect on questions such as 'What did I learn from working on this problem?', 'What learning resources that I used were most helpful?', 'How have I done this assignment differently/better compared to the previous one?', 'What is it that contributes to this learning group working well or working poorly?', 'How has our learning been helped or hindered by the tutor?' In addition to promoting self-appraisal in a non-threatening manner, aspects of these reports form part of the evaluation of the subject. Subject evaluation has been multi-faceted, incorporating not only regular reviews of this student feedback, but also methods such as anonymous student questionnaires and observation by other members of the university staff and by outside observers. Resulting data have been used both formatively to develop and improve the subject, and also summatively to judge the subject's worth as an ongoing component of the undergraduate curriculum. It is considered that Physiotherapy Studies 100/101 has been successful in achieving its aims and similar curriculum designs are being introduced progressively in later years of the course.

Postgraduate clinical reasoning program in manipulative physiotherapy

Two subjects, Clinical Reasoning I and II, have been taught for several years within the Graduate Diploma and Master of Applied Science (Manipulative Physiotherapy) courses at the University of Sydney. These courses are designed for qualified physiotherapists, and the curricula therefore build on the students' considerable base of professional knowledge and skill. Other subjects include applied sciences, physiotherapy theory and practice. All subjects are closely integrated with clinical education, to enhance the transfer of knowledge and skills from the classroom into clinical practice. The specific aims of the clinical reasoning subjects are to enable students to become aware of how they reason in relation to clinical problems, to understand the theoretical processes of clinical reasoning, and to develop skills in the areas of clinical reasoning, self-evaluation of reasoning abilities and communication of reasoning to others.

These aims highlight the need for students to become aware of their thinking, and to practise, describe, examine and receive feedback on their reasoning. If clinical decisions are to be explored in depth and students are to be free to attempt and evaluate different reasoning strategies and decision alternatives, the real-life clinical setting with time pressures and possible negative consequences for clients is not ideal. A classroom setting permits 'time-out' to discuss students' thinking and consider the potential consequences of their decisions. It also allows students to hear the different reasoning and decisions of others so they can consider the relative merits of alternative positions. In the classroom, students can discuss their reasoning in groups and receive feedback from their peers and teachers. Classroom activity, followed by subsequent integration of reasoning skills into clinical education, is therefore used as the format for Clinical Reasoning I.

Early in the course, several classes examine theories and research associated with clinical reasoning. Students are encouraged to compare their reasoning strategies to models identified in the literature. They are also involved in drawing cognitive maps which represent their knowledge of a particular topic in diagrammatic form. This activity helps students assess and revise their knowledge base in terms of accuracy, comprehensiveness and organization. The process of map drawing can also help students learn how to organize their knowledge so it can be accessed more readily.

Later, another experiential learning strategy is used. The class is set up with a 'fish bowl' or discussion group facing the audience. The discussion group comprises (a) two groups of students, (b) an expert panel, and (c) a chairperson who manages time use, directs the questions and promotes discussion on the nature of clinical reasoning as well as the case under consideration. One group of three students (the 'student panel') is rostered each session to act as the physiotherapist whose task it is to work through and discuss a hypothetical client case. The second group of two to three students represents the client in the activity. These students have previously prepared a case study in consultation with an experienced physiotherapist.

The expert panel consists of experienced physiotherapists and, at times, other clinicians such as rheumatologists. Their particular role is to help students to evaluate the validity of their knowledge and their use of knowledge, and to critically review their own clinical strategies. They engage students in exploration of the relative advantages of different inquiry methods, investigation techniques and intervention strategies. They challenge students' reasoning and investigations via questions such as 'What information would you like to obtain next and why?' and 'What use can you make of the data you have just received in relation to your working hypotheses?' Questions such as these require students to become more conscious of what and how they are thinking, and to express and critique their thoughts. The questioning itself and the subsequent feedback to the students encourage them to use and develop their ability in reflective self-awareness/metacognition and self-evaluation.

The teacher/expert clinicians assess the student panel participants during the class on their reasoning, knowledge and ability to communicate their reasoning. The student panel also receives feedback from their peers in the audience during a general discussion at the end of the session. The teacher/clinician then meets with individual students after the class to give feedback on their performance.

The subject Clinical Reasoning II involves a higher level of student responsibility for the design and implementation of learning activities. Students conduct classes incorporating, e.g. role plays, debates and panel discussions. As well as continued exploration and articulation of students' clinical reasoning this subject gives greater attention to interpersonal interaction in the clinical role, the patient's role in clinical decision making, legal/ethical issues and communication. Classes during this subject examine errors in clinical reasoning and strategies for avoiding or dealing with them, and strategies for enhancing clinical reasoning expertise.

Evaluation of the subject has included student evaluation questionnaires, an open discussion session at the end of the course and review of student results by the teachers involved. Results indicate that participants have learned a great deal about the nature of clinical reasoning, about how they reason and about the soundness, relevance and breadth of their knowledge. They have developed skills in metacognition and in communicating their reasoning, a necessary part of being a collaborative and credible member of the health care team. Further, they have had opportunities to explore their attitudes and values regarding clinical practice and clinical decision making, to experience the client's role, and to examine how the client participates in reasoning and decision making.

Postgraduate supervised clinical practice in manipulative physiotherapy

The clear intent of the preceding examples of experiential learning activities is to help students recognize and develop skills in the process of clinical reasoning. Clinical simulations have distinct advantages over real-life clinical practice as a medium for teaching, such as better control over problem type and complexity, and avoidance of the safety risks associated with incorrect clinical decisions. However, students will eventually be required to function in the clinical setting, and no degree of simulation can replicate the unpredictability and variability which exists in real-life client presentations. This third example describes learning during supervised clinical education in the

Master of Applied Science (Manipulative Physiotherapy) course at the University of South Australia.

Clinical placements are an integral component of physiotherapy curricula at both undergraduate and postgraduate levels. They always involve teaching students safe and effective client care based on accepted modes of practice, but they do not necessarily identify the development of clinical reasoning as an educational objective. However, it is a stated major aim of the supervised clinical practice component of the postgraduate programs at the University of South Australia. Incoming students have varying levels of skill in problem solving or critical thinking which they can apply to the physiotherapy domain, and so are introduced to the concept and a process of clinical reasoning in physiotherapy during preclinical learning activities.

Students are then encouraged to work within a coherent clinical-reasoning framework in their clinical work on course.[2] This framework integrates hypothetico-deductive reasoning and pattern recognition with interviewing, manual assessment and treatment procedures.

In order to facilitate the development of better clinical reasoning, supervisors must have means of accessing students' thoughts. One way of doing this is via a clinical reasoning worksheet. Students are required to pause at key points, such as after taking a history, and complete relevant sections of the worksheet. These enforced periods of time-out encourage the student to review information that has just been found and to plan the next section of assessment or management. Such planning can be critical, not only for the student's reasoning but also for the client's well-being, as excessive examination or treatment can result in worsening of some symptoms. However, too many interruptions can be time consuming and disturbing to the student's flow of thought.

Ideally, the supervisor will review all worksheets immediately on completion and provide students with feedback. Even when time does not allow this, experience has shown that the process of reflecting on the client examination or management in order to answer the worksheet questions is in itself an excellent independent learning activity. Students may recognize, through their difficulty in answering certain questions, that they have insufficient information or understanding about the case.

[2] For discussion of this physiotherapy reasoning process the reader is referred to Chapter 12 and Jones (1992).

While the clinical reasoning form is designed for postgraduate manual therapy students, the concept of such a worksheet which encourages retrospective reflection together with planning for future action is applicable to all areas of physiotherapy practice and all levels of professional education.

Another way of accessing student thinking is by discussion during the actual clinical encounter. Clearly it is neither practical nor desirable to interrupt the student after every inquiry to question interpretation of information, but strategically placed pauses at key stages of the examination and treatment can be effective: students can be encouraged to make interpretations of their observations, formulate hypotheses, identify interview or physical examination measures that could be used to test those hypotheses, consider the examination and management implications associated with different hypotheses, or specify supporting or negating evidence to substantiate their judgements. In addition to these planned time-outs, students are interrupted if it appears they are following incorrect or unexplained lines of inquiry. Clients usually co-operate with the interruptions if they are aware of their purpose, and informal contracts negotiated beforehand between individual students and supervisors are used to delineate the extent and method of such discussions. When the discussions are an agreed part of the learning process and when they are conducted in a non-threatening manner, students enjoy the opportunity for ongoing reflection during the clinical encounter.

The extent and nature of the interaction, guidance and feedback provided during clinical sessions varies considerably. For example, working interpretations or hypotheses are based on the student's conceptualization of the client data. Students' ability to perceive and evaluate relevant cues is influenced by their existing knowledge schemas. Schemas are developed partly by common classroom activities conducted during the course, but they also depend on each individual's unique base of knowledge and experience gained from previous academic education, clinical experience and life in general. Therefore, supervisors must deal with each student according to level of knowledge and reasoning ability. To further their learning, students also need to be able to test for themselves the implications of their own decisions. This process can be difficult in the clinical setting where there is always some degree of ethical constraint for the correct solution to the client's problem to be obtained as quickly as possible. Thus, supervisors must balance their involvement in the clinical decision making process to ensure that safe and reasonable judgements are reached and acted upon while at the same time enabling students to experience the results of their reasoning.

Because reasoning proficiency and knowledge base are viewed as interdependent factors, another major aim of clinical practice in the postgraduate manual therapy programs at the University of South Australia is to promote students' acquisition of declarative knowledge such as clinical patterns of presentation (e.g. syndromes) and of procedural knowledge such as 'if/then' guides to action.

Students are required to maintain a 'Diary of Clinical Patterns'. They are provided with forms on which to record the typical features of the most common clinical patterns presenting in manual therapy practice. Students keep the diary for the duration of the course, adding information to it as the year progresses. These patterns are not taught directly to students, rather students are expected to extract the relevant information from their involvement in classroom activities, private reading, and their clinical practice with real clients. The diaries serve several purposes. Firstly, they provide a form of advanced organizer for learning, priming students to look for information to add to their evolving diary during clinical practice and other learning activities. The exploration of clinical patterns through a hypothetico-deductive reasoning process encourages students to test the consistency of the patterns and their response to alternative treatment approaches. The diaries also provide a stimulus for independent study, with students seeking additional information from other sources (textbooks, journals, peers, experienced therapists) to support their clinical observations. Lastly, the inevitable overlap in clinical patterns that emerges assists students to learn not only the classical features of a pattern, but also the range of features which may be shared by several patterns, the variation of features within one pattern that are encountered in real clients, and treatment principles and techniques associated with effective management of the different patterns.

Evaluation of the supervised clinical practice component of the course is undertaken as a round table student-staff discussion at the end of the course. This clinical practice is almost always cited as the most valuable component of the course because of the way it encourages students to think logically and because of the attention it provides to individual needs. Course review sessions are also conducted among staff members, usually with an independent facilitator. Developments in the program, such as modifications to the clinical reasoning worksheet, have been outcomes of these review sessions.

Conclusion

Clinical reasoning proficiency is central to the physiotherapist's ability to manage clients efficiently and effectively because this thinking process guides the entire clinical encounter. Each treatment session and each case are powerful sources of learning for the physiotherapist if a clinical-reasoning process is followed and the therapist engages in reflection and self-evaluation during and after the process. Such experiential learning facilitates the building of an extensive body of clinically relevant declarative and procedural knowledge, and develops the ability to readily access this knowledge during clinical practice. If these are hallmarks of expertise, then the educational programs described above are devised to move students closer to that position by encouraging learning within simulated and actual clinical contexts and by promoting reflective and independent learning skills, which will ensure that students' knowledge acquisition does not stop on completion of their university courses.

References

Anderson, J. R. (1990) *Cognitive Psychology and its Implications*, 3rd edn. New York: Freeman

Boshuizen, H. P. A. and Schmidt, H. G. (1992) On the role of biomedical knowledge in clinical reasoning by experts, intermediates and novices. *Cognitive Science*, **16**, 153–184.

Carr, J., Jones, M. and Higgs, J. (1995) Teaching clinical reasoning expertise in physiotherapy practice. In *Clinical Reasoning in the Health Professions* (J. Higgs and M. Jones, eds), pp. 235–245. Oxford: Butterworth-Heinemann.

Cervero, R. M. (1988) *Effective Continuing Education for Professionals*. San Francisco: Jossey-Bass.

Henry, R., Byrne, K. and Engel, C. (eds) (1997) *Imperatives in Medical Education. The Newcastle Approach*. Callaghan, NSW: Faculty of Medicine and Health Sciences, University of Newcastle.

Higgs, J. and Titchen, A. (1995) Propositional, professional, and personal knowledge in clinical reasoning. In *Clinical Reasoning in the Health Professions* (J. Higgs and M. Jones, eds), pp. 129–146. Oxford: Butterworth-Heinemann.

Jones, M. A. (1992). Clinical reasoning in manual therapy. *Physical Therapy*, **72**, 875–884.

Jones, M., Jensen, G. and Rothstein, J. (1995) Clinical reasoning in physiotherapy. In *Clinical Reasoning in the Health Professions* (J. Higgs and M. Jones, eds), pp. 72–87. Oxford: Butterworth-Heinemann.

Kolb, D. A. (1984) *Experiential Learning – Experience as the Source of Learning and Development*. Englewood Cliffs, NJ: Prentice-Hall.

Mageean, B. (1991) Self-rapport: A note on psychology and instruction. *Australian Journal of Education*, **35**, 41–49.

Patel, V. L., Groen, G. J. and Frederiksen, C. H. (1986) Differences between medical students and doctors in memory for clinical cases. *Medical Education*, **20**, 3–9.

Schön, D. (1983) *The Reflective Practitioner: How Professionals Think in Action*. New York: Basic Books.

22

Speech-language pathology students: Learning clinical reasoning

Lindy McAllister and Miranda Rose

Writing this chapter posed something of a dilemma because, in general, speech-language pathologists do not talk about clinical reasoning. As we searched the literature to identify this concept and practice in our profession we discovered interesting findings which are the subject of this chapter. Firstly, speech-language pathologists (educators and clinicians) may well discuss or write about differential diagnosis, problem solving, decision making, critical thinking, professional judgement and diagnostic reasoning; they rarely discuss clinical reasoning.[1] Secondly, the processes involved in clinical reasoning in our profession have been poorly researched and are little understood within the profession. Thirdly, the scene is changing, and exciting challenges are being posed to clinicians, educators and researchers alike, with a demand for more research and understanding of clinical reasoning in speech-language pathology.

Seeking clinical reasoning in speech-language pathology

In this chapter we make a distinction between clinical decision making and clinical reasoning. We see clinical decision making as an end-product of

clinical reasoning; the generation of tangible decisions about clinical management. In contrast we see clinical reasoning as the often intangible, rarely explicated thought processes that lead to the clinical decisions we make. We suggest that clinical reasoning utilizes *metaprocesses*, including an awareness or a becoming conscious of what we are thinking and what thought processes we are using. Reflection in and on action (Schön, 1987) has a major role to play in clinical reasoning. In speech-language pathology, we have found that clinical decision making is discussed and described more often than clinical reasoning. The following section highlights the confusion in terminology found in the speech-language pathology literature.

Based on our critical reading of the literature, we could describe the process of clinical reasoning in speech-language pathology as the 'black box' of information processing occurring between the input phase of data gathering and the output phase of producing decisions (concerning diagnosis and treatment) and taking action (see Figure 22.1). The reasons for this black box state of affairs lie in the history and operation of our profession wherein clinical reasoning, being (broadly) the thinking associated with clinical practice, was assumed to be a skill that could be absorbed without explication. Kamhi (1998, p.102), for instance, argues that 'as clinicians become more experienced, they gradually internalize the framework of an assessment protocol and become proficient at analysing and interpreting test information and observational data'. The speech-language pathology profession seems to have adopted what Bridge and Twible

[1] There are, of course, exceptions in the specially commissioned chapters on teaching clinical reasoning to speech-language pathology students in the earlier and current editions of this book, by Doyle (1995) and Edwards *et al.* (1995), as well as the chapter by Higgs (1997).

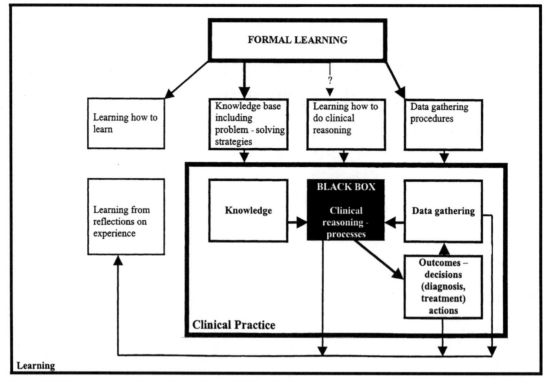

Figure 22.1 Clinical reasoning in speech pathology – the 'black box'

(1997) refer to as a content-oriented approach to clinical reasoning. This approach assumes that knowledge and reasoning are interdependent. There is an expectation that with increasing knowledge and clinical experience, students and clinicians will be better able to reason and make clinical decisions. Undergraduate curricula have concentrated more on knowledge acquisition and skills development. Records *et al.* (1994, p. 74) note that 'issues related to gathering information have been the central focus in the speech-language pathology literature, whereas issues specific to the decision making process are relegated to the periphery of discussion'.

Another focus of our profession has been on solving problems in clinical practice (i.e. on the outcome, not the process of clinical thinking). Consider the recent sources in speech-language pathology literature:

● Dodd's 1995 text *Differential Diagnosis and Treatment of Children with Speech Disorder* contains a chapter on a problem-solving approach to clinical management. This problem solving model begins at the stage of description

of the current communication status (after diagnosis). While an excellent model for problem solving in client management, it offers no clues to the clinical reasoning which lies behind the clinical problem solving.

● The *Pocket Reference of Diagnosis and Management for the Speech-Language Pathologist* (White, 1997) contains a wealth of useful information to assist in clinical problem solving or decision making. It does not consider the clinical reasoning thinking processes underpinning diagnosis and management.

Another factor leading to the neglect of understanding of the processes involved in speech-language pathology clinical reasoning is that decision making in speech-language pathology has been seen as a linear or logical process, which obscures the 'messiness' of clinical reasoning in action. Duffy (1998, p. 96) suggests that the processes of decision making 'became obscured with training that views diagnosis as a linear, test-oriented, and mechanistic process, and that often "teaches" diagnosis by starting with the target disorder (the diagnosis) and then proceeding back to its defining symptoms and signs'. Yoder and Kent (1988) published a series of decision-making trees for the diagnosis and management of communication disorders. They stated that the trees are not to be seen as recipes, but rather as a series of guidelines and prompts for the clinician engaged in decision making. 'Cookbooks cannot deal with the unknown or the uncertain, but clinical decision making frequently encounters them' (Yoder and Kent, 1988, preface). This approach has the advantage of providing guidance without rigidity and recognizing the need for professional judgement as part of decision making. However, the focus is again on the decision steps to be taken rather than on the nature of thinking in which clinicians engage and how they might respond to the prompts provided. The approach reinforces the view that clinical reasoning and decision making are basically linear and logical, which they are not. Further, the responsibility for learning how to think lies with the clinician. It is not made explicit.

Emerging directions and challenges in speech-language pathology clinical reasoning

In their edited text *Differential Diagnosis in Speech-Language Pathology*, Philips and Ruscello (1998) provide a broader picture of the process of diagnosis. Whilst they refer readers to decision-making trees, such as those of Yoder and Kent (1988), they move beyond a formulaic data collection approach to an acknowledgement that 'the speech-language pathologist's curiosity and inquisitiveness drive the process of differential diagnosis. The clinician who accepts diagnostic challenges, is curious about missing information and inconsistencies, constantly questions, and searches for possible answers is most likely to solve puzzles presented by difficult problems' (Philips and Ruscello, 1998, p. 3). It is argued here that the clinician needs to be aware of missing information and inconsistencies and to be thinking about them, questioning self, the process and the data. In other words, the clinician needs to be engaged in metacognition, or thinking about thinking, a key component in the Higgs and Jones (1995) definition of clinical reasoning.

Deputy and Weston (1998, p. 143) 'invite readers to foster their own critical thinking and consider how their own current clinical procedures could contribute to the description and decisions for each case'. Here again is evidence of an acknowledgement of thinking about our clinical thinking, without exploration of that thinking.

Kamhi (1988) and Deputy and Weston (1998) remind readers of the importance of asking causal questions but caution them about assuming linear causality. Asking questions about factors that may or may not cause communication disorders and that contribute to the data obtained in evaluation is an important component of what we would call clinical reasoning.

Records *et al.* (1994) discuss clinical judgement and provide an illustrative case study. They emphasize not only the objective aspects of data collection, but also the subjective aspects of the decision-making process; the gut feelings, expertise and insights which are aspects of clinical reasoning. They consider clinical judgement to be a process poorly understood by speech-language pathologists.

Current circumstances also frame our attitudes to and practice of clinical reasoning. Funding pressures create 'clinical practices whose explicit demands are heavily weighted toward management and productivity rather than diagnosis and understanding' (Duffy, 1998, p. 96). Such practices are not conducive to thinking about our understanding. In such a climate, the call for research into clinical reasoning (or clinical decision making, as advocated by McCauley and Baker, 1994) may be difficult to advance. However, we remain undaunted.

How do speech-language pathologists reason?

There is a paucity of literature directly dealing with clinical decision making and clinical reasoning in speech-language pathology. Three recent sources were located. The entire first issue of Volume 19 of *Seminars in Speech and Language* (1998) is devoted to case studies of diagnostic decision making by eminent clinicians, who discuss puzzling cases and their thinking and reflections on these cases. The articles in that issue and those of Records *et al.* (1994) and McCauley and Baker (1994) cited above are rare in the speech-language pathology literature in that they seek to make explicit their thinking about the nature and process of clinical decision making.

In the relative absence of research to address this topic directly, writers in our discipline have resorted to supposition or analogy, drawing on research in other professions. The guest editor Campbell (1998), in his introduction to the journal *Seminars in Speech and Language,* outlines four approaches to what he refers to as diagnostic decision making found in clinical medicine: pattern recognition, decision-making trees, diagnosis by exhaustion (collecting all possible data) and hypothetical-deductive reasoning. Such approaches are referred to as clinical reasoning models in medicine. Campbell makes the assumption that those approaches also apply to speech-language pathology. Duffy (1998, p. 97), in reflecting on his diagnostic decision making, states that 'most good diagnosticians reach conclusions through a hypothetical-deductive strategy, with frequent reliance on pattern recognition'. The paucity of research into decision making and clinical reasoning in the speech-language pathology profession does not provide the data to test Campbell's or Duffy's assumptions. However, in reflecting on comparisons with reasoning approaches in other disciplines, Campbell and Duffy begin to question possible reasoning strategies in speech-language pathology.

A useful starting point for investigation of clinical reasoning in speech-language pathology is a model from occupational therapy (Fleming, 1991). The model describes 'therapists with three track minds' who use a number of clinical reasoning approaches, depending on the client, presenting problems and contexts. Given the similarities in values and beliefs about clients and therapy between occupational therapy and speech-language pathology, it could serve as a useful starting point for research in speech-language pathology.

Teaching clinical reasoning in professional entry curricula

Considering the historical frame of reference above it is not surprising that there is little evidence or recognition of the need for teaching clinical reasoning in professional entry curricula. Doyle (1995) in fact argues against having units within a speech-language pathology program titled 'clinical reasoning', arguing that there is little evidence that a theoretical coverage of the area will generalize to clinical practice. In one of the most influential texts in the area of education of speech-language pathologists, Rassi and McElroy (1992) make no more than passing mention of clinical reasoning and do not advocate its inclusion in speech-language pathology curricula. Most programs (with a few exceptions[2]) designed to prepare speech-language pathology students do not include in the curriculum subjects which seek to make the process of clinical reasoning explicit for students.

Some curricula do teach decision analysis. Syder (1996), for instance, discussed how by engaging with simulated patients, students' differential diagnosis and complex problem-solving skills can be developed.[3]

In the absence of research and debate to guide us, it may well be that as a profession, speech-language pathology adopts a content-oriented approach to clinical reasoning and that we mainly use hypothetico-deductive and pattern recognition approaches, with little attention to the metacognitive aspects of our reasoning. The clinical reasoning in which we undoubtedly engage is not discussed or made explicit. Most speech-language pathology students develop clinical reasoning abilities without having the process made explicit. However, in any program there will be marginal students who have difficulty with the development of clinical competence (Maloney *et al.*, 1997). Nemeth and McAllister (1995) have shown that for at least some of these students the difficulty lies in how they think about their clinical work. Certainly, as experienced managers of large speech-pathology clinical education programs, we can attest to the challenges presented by those students who 'don't know how to think' about their clinical work. We believe that these students in particular, as well as other students who appear to learn well through knowledge building and experience, benefit from having the processes of clinical reasoning made explicit as a routine part of clinical education. To this end, Rose and colleagues have developed a stream within their clinical education program which builds clinical-reasoning skills from first to final year of their 4 year undergraduate degree. This approach is described below.

An approach to teaching clinical reasoning in speech-language pathology

The Bachelor of Speech Pathology course at La Trobe University is a 4 year undergraduate degree, the entry level qualification for practice in Australia. The course has four major divisions: basic biological sciences and psychological sciences (e.g. anatomy, developmental processes); specific subjects in communication development and disorders (e.g. voice and laryngectomy, phonology); clinical practicum which is spread throughout the 4 years; and a professional practice and clinical

---

[2] See, e.g. Edwards *et al.* (1995) and McCabe *et al.* (1998).

[3] See also Chapter 30.

problem solving stream. It is the latter stream we proceed to discuss in this chapter, but first a brief note about nomenclature.

Clinical problem solving or clinical reasoning?

The term 'clinical problem solving' has been the term of choice to date in this program. Students' clinical problem-solving skills are formally assessed during clinical placements and students must reach competence in these skills before graduation. Why has the term clinical problem solving been used and not 'clinical reasoning'? It is not just a matter of semantics; rather, until very recently it has been indicative of the curriculum focus and a specific conceptualization of the diagnostic process. Prior to recent curriculum changes (see below), the focus has been on 'a clinical problem to be solved' and its possible solutions, rather than the processes that are being used to solve the problem, that is, clinical-reasoning processes. A consequence of the recent move toward teaching and facilitating clinical reasoning rather than clinical problem solving is a greater emphasis on reflective practice and a heightened consciousness about the cognitive processes being used by practitioners and students in client management. Such awareness may assist both practitioners who are generalizing their existing knowledge base into complex and novel situations and teachers who are assisting students to develop adequate clinical-reasoning skills. In this program the shift to clinical reasoning nomenclature is likely to occur in the near future, as the processes employed in the clinical problem solving stream have become clinical-reasoning processes.

Development of the stream

During a recent curriculum review, staff identified the need to include a series of subjects that allowed for explicit clinical reasoning activity. In previous curricula, clinical reasoning instruction was presumed to occur in clinical practicum subjects and in case discussions during lectures and tutorials. While many students were able to take their theoretical knowledge about communication disorders and integrate it into a holistic view of clients and client management, others found such integration *in situ* difficult. For many students the clinical practicum is the place where they make the cognitive shifts from purely theoretical knowledge bases to practical and client-centred clinical knowledge bases (Edwards, 1996).

Anxiety about harming a client can make clinical reasoning a difficult activity for students while they are interacting with the client (Carter *et al.*, 1994). During a clinical practicum students' clinical-reasoning skills are assessed, and for many students this domain has been the source of failure of a clinical subject. In addition, following funding cutbacks and major restructures in health services, speech pathologists in the field advised that they had less time available for non-client contact and therefore less time to devote to facilitating and teaching students skills (Rose *et al.*, 1996).

With these points in mind a clinical reasoning stream was developed across the 4 years of the course with the following principles guiding the design:

- Make clinical reasoning a more conscious process for students in the belief that this consciousness would enable better clinical reasoning in novel or complex situations
- Utilize adult learning principles that recognize prior learning and one's personal constructs of the world (Knowles, 1990)
- Utilize clinical-reasoning processes that stress hypothetico-deductive reasoning (Elstein *et al.*, 1978), pattern recognition (Barrows and Feltovich, 1987), reflective practice (Schön, 1987) and client-centred practice (Egan, 1990)
- Demonstrate the similarities in the clinical-reasoning process regardless of client disorder type and age group
- Provide explicit opportunities to develop links across student knowledge bases in order to facilitate a more integrated overall knowledge base
- Provide opportunities for metacognitive processing (see Higgs and Jones, 1995) about the clinical-reasoning process.

Structure of the clinical reasoning stream

Year 1

The stream begins in the first year of the course with introductory exercises in basic clinical decision making, utilizing simple case examples. The basic philosophy and principles of speech-language pathology assessment and treatment are presented and a flow chart is discussed which details the usual activities involved in these activities. During such presentations the lecturer carefully and liberally illustrates each phase in the assessment or therapy procedure with examples from client practice. As each phase is presented, the lecturer poses questions about the clinical decision making that is occurring. The case exemplars are simple, straightforward examples of communication impairment involving a single parameter or modality (e.g. developmental articulation delay). In addition, principles of adult learning, learning style and reflective practice are introduced briefly, with the major emphasis being on client observation, description of client presentation, and awareness of self in the therapeutic role. Students attend speech pathology clinics in the field to observe clients and the roles and practices of the clinical educator. They write reflective journals about these experiences and present their reflections to the class.

Year 2

In the second year, students develop a deeper understanding of adult learning principles, reflective practice, learning styles and the need for self-evaluation skills. These concepts are presented through didactic lecture material, experiential learning activities such as role play, and critique of videotaped student/clinical educator interactions. At this stage in the stream the emphasis in the clinical reasoning activity is on a slightly narrower aim of integration into practice of theory about the communication disorder and its management. Thus integration of the psychosocial and environmental issues of client management and dealing with complex symptom clusters are left to the third and fourth year. Relatively straightforward cases involving both developmental and acquired disorders are contrasted, and the reasoning applied to each is highlighted to demonstrate the similarities and differences in the clinical reasoning used. Clients' communication skills are compared and contrasted, while expert clinicians verbalize their reasoning skills and the rationales for their chosen approaches to the clinical problem solving tasks.

Students are encouraged to extend their knowledge bases beyond the disorder-specific context in which they acquired the knowledge to a more integrated and client-centred conceptualization. For example, students acquire disorder-specific knowledge in theory subjects that are developed along specific communication parameters, such as voice and laryngectomy, fluency, language and phonology. In the first 3 years of the course, students develop deep veins of knowledge along a particular communication parameter but do not necessarily transfer learning from one theory subject to another or apply the theory learnt in one

subject to a client with impairments in multiple parameters. Hence, we select case examples where several parameters are involved, and students are required to integrate chunks of knowledge that previously may have been encapsulated in isolated streams. The following are specific examples.

Two cases are used with the aim of integration and knowledge base extension. Case One is a child born with a cleft palate who has both phonetically-based speech production errors arising principally from structural changes to the articulators, and phonologically-based speech production errors arising from failure to learn appropriate phonologic rules for speech production. Case Two is a 21 year old who sustained a mild closed head injury in a motor vehicle accident and has speech production errors resulting from a mild dysarthria. The following clinical reasoning activities are undertaken:

- The students are provided with case history information for both cases and, working in small groups, are asked to generate a speech pathology assessment plan for both clients.
- The plans are then compared and contrasted through discussion facilitated by expert clinicians. This discussion draws out the similarities and differences between the developmental and the acquired case.
- The group reflects on the processes being used to generate the assessment plans, and rationales for a particular approach are developed.
- A summary of the relevant assessment data is then provided for the students and they are asked to review the data and develop a differential diagnosis for each client.
- The diagnoses are then discussed and debated. Students are asked to be explicit about why certain presenting signs are seen to be indicative of a certain level of breakdown in the speech production system and to consider alternative explanations and conclusions.
- Treatment options are discussed and contrasted. The therapeutic strategies involved are highlighted, e.g. reconstitutive versus compensatory therapies.
- Having worked through this exercise, expert clinicians facilitate discussion about the clinical reasoning utilized and reiterate the processes used.

Year 3

During the third year of the program students are introduced to increasing case complexity and are expected to take into consideration the psychosocial and environmental issues that impact on client management. Students work in small groups and select from a list of options a complex case which interests them. The cases are complex in the degree of disorder present, the number of co-occurring disorders, the social and cultural background of the client, and the ease of access to speech pathology services. The students interview a practising clinician about the case, gather relevant information about the case, research the disorder type, and the social, emotional, and environmental impacts of the communication disorder. The students present a synopsis of their work to their peers in a verbal class presentation and prepare a detailed written case study for formal assessment.

Further, students work with simulated clients who demonstrate communication disorders of acquired neurological origin and have impairments in multiple communication parameters. They have social and emotional issues that significantly impact on assessment and treatment strategies. The use of a simulated patient allows for considerable metacognitive processing to take place. At any time the client (simulated) interaction can be stopped through the 'time-out' facility and the group can discuss the situation, reflect on current feelings and actions, brainstorm possible solutions, evaluate courses of action and trial them. In discussions about clinical reasoning facilitated by the lecturer, students are encouraged to be conscious of the approach and the process they are using to formulate a diagnosis or devise a treatment plan.

Issues considered include:

- Selecting testing materials and procedures: students are asked to critically evaluate the test batteries they have chosen, identifying the type of information they are likely to collect and considering its applicability to this case.
- Deciding where to begin to analyse the assessment data: students are asked questions such as 'where do we begin and why?', in order to promote their clinical reasoning strategy from the start, being conscious of the logic behind a particular strategy. We believe this facilitates a deeper understanding of the strategy and assists better retrieval of the clinical reasoning strategy for subsequent consideration.
- Developing an appropriate treatment plan for the client: students are asked to consider the client's communication strengths and weaknesses and identify any hierarchy in behaviours that require treatment in advance of others.

- Tailoring basic therapeutic processes to the individual client: students develop task descriptions, reinforcements, strategies for timing and sequencing of procedures, and response monitoring systems appropriate to the particular client. Discussion includes the importance of client preferences, and the role of the speech-language pathologist in adult versus paediatric therapeutic interactions.
- Identifying the psychosocial needs of the client: Students need to consider their intervention strategies carefully and tailor them to meet individual needs.
- Considering students' views of client management in conflict with clients' views: students are encouraged to reflect on and discuss their views of impairment, disability, handicap, and illness, and contrast them with the views of the client. The impacts of potential mismatches for client management are discussed.

During this process students have been encouraged to attach personal meaning to the clinical reasoning strategies used and to make committed choices. This method contrasts with teaching which emphasizes the expert's practice, e.g. 'do as I do', 'current convention dictates'. The latter leads to the recipe-like approach about which we were critical in an earlier section. The former student commitment approach encourages students to creatively generate potential courses of action and to evaluate them critically. Students are given the freedom to choose the way they would like to proceed and then to be explicit about why they have chosen that course of action. They are expected to articulate the likely benefits and disadvantages of their choice. During feedback from the simulated patient, students can check their reality against that of the client, and become more conscious of the factors at play in the particular context.

Year 4

In year 4 the emphasis shifts from clinical reasoning applied to particular clients to clinical reasoning about professional issues such as the workplace environment, professional ethics, staff management issues, legal and safety requirements and quality management practices, and the impact these have on clinical reasoning. Students attend a series of lectures which provide basic information on these topics and then select a particular topic to research with a small group. The group makes a class presentation toward the end of the academic year in which the practical implementation of the knowledge they have researched is stressed. Specific cases are used to illustrate the importance of these various professional issues and the impact they have on clinical reasoning, e.g. the choice of service delivery model for a client being constrained by staffing levels rather than client need.

Clinical reasoning beyond the formalized curriculum stream

In addition to this graded 4 year stream in clinical reasoning, individual lecturers continue to develop case discussion and client problem-solving activities within their theoretical subjects. The clinical practicum continues to offer the opportunity for rich clinical-reasoning experiences. In particular, students in years 2 and 4 are paired and attend a university based clinic. This peer-learning model encourages the participants to reason together, verbalize their decision making, reflect on their interactions and question their actions. The year 2 students are expected to keep a reflective journal throughout the placement and to bring their reflections to their peer and clinical educator interactions. Clinical educators in the field are encouraged to assist students to be reflective practitioners, e.g. through using reflection-after-action, reflective diary writing and video analysis of performance, and to help students self-evaluate.

Recent research has highlighted the lack of theory-based discussion that clinical educators undertake with their students during clinical placements (Kenny, 1996; Rose *et al.*, 1996). This state of affairs is unfortunate, as the clinical learning environment offers rich opportunity for clinical reasoning activity and learning. The vast majority of speech pathology clinical educators would not have had undergraduate experiences or subjects which emphasized clinical reasoning and the metacognitive processes associated with it, as opposed to clinical problem solving. It is therefore not surprising that these clinical educators do not naturally emphasize this activity with their students.

Conclusions

This chapter had several aims. The first was to highlight the confusion in terminology used in discussion of clinical decision making and clinical reasoning in speech-language pathology. The second aim was to highlight the lack of discussion about clinical reasoning in speech-language

pathology education and practice. The current assumptions in speech-language pathology seem to be those of 'knowledge banking', which assumes that clinical decisions are made more easily with more knowledge, and that the making of decisions is a linear and logical process. There is little attention paid to the processes which lead to clinical decisions, that is, clinical-reasoning processes. The third aim was to present an argument for making the clinical-reasoning process more explicit. Research into the clinical-reasoning process in speech-language pathology is required. The fourth aim was to present a curriculum for speech-language pathology students which systematically seeks to develop clinical-reasoning skills. Different approaches to clinical reasoning (discussed in other chapters in this book) are used, building on the traditional methods of clinical decision making typically found in the speech-language pathology profession. We hope that this chapter will serve both as a catalyst for discussion of clinical reasoning in our profession and as a model for developing clinical-reasoning skills in students.

Acknowledgements

The clinical reasoning stream described in this chapter was jointly developed by Beverly Joffe, Georgia Dacakis, Miranda Rose (Lecturers) and Louise Brown (Senior Lecturer and Chief Speech Pathologist, Mount Eliza Centre, Melbourne), School of Human Communication Sciences, La Trobe University, Melbourne.

References

Barrows, H. S. and Feltovich, P. J. (1987) The clinical reasoning process. *Medical Education*, **21**, 86–91.

Bridge, C. and Twible, R. (1997) Clinical reasoning: Informed decision making in practice. In *Occupational Therapy: Enabling Function and Well Being* (C. Christiansen and C. Baum, eds), pp. 158–179. Thorofare, NJ: Slack.

Campbell, T. (1998) Themes in diagnostic decision making. *Seminars in Speech and Language*, **19**, 3–6.

Carter, S., Chan, J. and McAllister, L. (1994) Contributors to anxiety in clinical education in undergraduate speech-language pathology students. *Australian Journal of Human Communication Disorders*, **22**, 57–73.

Deputy, P. and Weston, A. (1998) A framework for differential diagnosis of developmental phonological disorders. In *Differential Diagnosis in Speech-Language Pathology* (B. J. Philips and D. Ruscello, eds), pp. 113–158. Boston, MA: Butterworth-Heinemann.

Dodd, B. (1995) A problem solving approach to clinical management. In *Differential Diagnosis and Treatment of Children With Speech Disorder* (B. Dodd, ed.), pp. 149–165. London: Whurr.

Doyle, J. (1995) Issues in teaching clinical reasoning to students of speech and hearing science. In *Clinical Reasoning in the Health Professions* (J. Higgs and M. Jones, eds), pp. 224–234. Oxford: Butterworth-Heinemann.

Duffy, J. (1998) Stroke with dysarthria: Evaluate and treat; garden variety or down the garden path. *Seminars in Speech and Language*, **19**, 93–98.

Edwards, H. (1997) Clinical teaching: An exploration in three health professions. *PhD thesis*. University of Melbourne.

Edwards, H., Franke, M. and McGuiness, B. (1995) Using simulated patients to teach clinical reasoning. In *Clinical Reasoning in the Health Professions* (J. Higgs and M. Jones, eds), pp. 269–278. Oxford: Butterworth-Heinemann.

Egan, G. (1990) *The Skilled Helper: A Systematic Approach to Effective Helping*, 4th edn. Pacific Grove, CA: Brooks/Cole.

Elstein, A. S., Shulman, L. S. and Sprafka, S. S. (1978) *Medical Problem Solving: An Analysis of Clinical Reasoning*. Cambridge, MA: Harvard University Press.

Fleming, M. (1991) The therapist with the three track mind. *American Journal of Occupational Therapy*, **45**, 1007–1014.

Higgs, J. (1997) Learning to make clinical decisions. In *Facilitating Learning in Clinical Settings* (L. McAllister, M. Lincoln, S. McLeod and D. Maloney, eds), pp. 130–153. Cheltenham: Stanley Thornes.

Higgs, J. and Jones, M. (1995) Clinical reasoning. In *Clinical Reasoning in the Health Professions* (J. Higgs and M. Jones, eds), pp. 3–23. Oxford: Butterworth-Heinemann.

Kamhi, A. (1998) Differential diagnosis of language learning disabilities. In *Differential Diagnosis in Speech-Language Pathology* (B. J. Philips and D. Ruscello, eds), pp. 87–112. Boston, MA: Butterworth-Heinemann.

Kenny, B. (1996) An investigation of self-evaluation by speech pathology students during supervisory conferences. *Masters thesis*. University of Sydney.

Knowles, M. (1990) *The Adult Learner: A Neglected Species*, 4th edn. Houston, TX: Gulf Publishing.

Maloney, D., Carmody, D. and Nemeth, E. (1997) Students experiencing problems learning in clinical settings. In *Facilitating Learning in Clinical Settings* (L. McAllister, M. Lincoln, S. McLeod and D. Maloney, eds), pp. 185–213. Cheltenham: Stanley Thornes.

McCabe, P., McAllister, L., Winkworth, A. and Maloney, D. (1998) Assessment clinic: a powerful learning experience. Paper presented at the *Annual Conference of Speech Pathology Australia*, Fremantle.

McCauley, R. and Baker, N. (1994) Clinical decision making in specific language impairment. *National Student Speech Language Hearing Association Journal*, **21**, 50–58.

Nemeth, E. and McAllister, L. (1995) Students experiencing difficulties in clinical education: their perspectives. Paper presented at the *Annual Conference of the Australian Association of Speech and Hearing*, Brisbane.

Philips, B. J. and Ruscello, D. (1998) *Differential Diagnosis in Speech-Language Pathology*. Boston, MA: Butterworth-Heinemann.

Rassi, J. and McElroy, M. (1992) *The Education of Audiologists and Speech-Language Pathologists*. Timonium, MD: York Press.

Records, N., Jordan, L. and Tomblin, J. B. (1994) Clinical judgement: A familiar concept, but a poorly understood process. *National Student Speech Language Hearing Association Journal*, **21**, 74–81.

Rose, M., McGartland, M. and Joffe, B. (1996) Current supervisory practice. In *Proceedings of the 2nd Biennial Conference of the Foundation for Quality Supervision*, pp. 78–94. Melbourne.

Schön, D. A. (1987) *Educating the Beginning Practitioner*. San Francisco: Jossey-Bass.

Syder, D. (1996) The use of simulated clients to develop the clinical skills of speech and language therapy students. *European Journal of Disorders of Communication*, **31**, 181–192.

White, P. (1997) *Pocket Reference of Diagnosis and Management for the Speech-Language Pathologist*. Boston, MA: Butterworth-Heinemann.

Yoder, D. and Kent, R. (1988) *Decision Making in Speech-Language Pathology*. Toronto: BC Decker.

23

Using mind mapping to improve students' metacognition

Mary Cahill and Marsha Fonteyn

Have you ever thought about creative ways to enhance your students' learning, or help them have more fun and enjoy their learning, even if the subject matter seems difficult or dry? Are there better ways to learn than just memorizing facts and theories? Is it possible to stimulate students' minds to think and learn in more global, associative ways? This chapter introduces a teaching strategy known as mind mapping, and examines its relationship to critical thinking and a closely aligned concept called metacognition. We demonstrate how this strategy can improve the way your students think and learn, and present a pilot study examining the use of mind mapping as a tool to improve the metacognitive skills of nursing students.

A mind map or concept map is a graphic representation of information or the thought processes of an individual (Buzan and Buzan, 1996; Novak and Gowin, 1984). There are several approaches to teaching students how to build mind maps. In some instances, especially in natural science education, a group of related words or concepts is presented to the student accompanied by a lecture and the students are then asked to create a mind map. The concepts or words are connected with arrows and sometimes there are words along the arrows such as 'leads to', 'causes', 'is related to', 'becomes', 'is needed for' (Jegede *et al.*, 1990; Novak, 1990; Okebukola and Jegede, 1989). In other instances, an idea or a concept is placed centrally on a piece of paper and students participate in an activity similar to brainstorming, making multiple outward connections from that central point to elucidate how ideas or concepts are related (Dorough and Rye, 1997; Novak and Gowin, 1984; Regis *et al.*, 1996).

The authors of this chapter were particularly interested in whether mind mapping could improve the critical thinking and metacognitive abilities of nursing students. The importance of teaching nursing students sound critical-thinking skills and the applicability of critical thinking to the generation of clinical decisions resulting in favourable patient outcomes have been documented in the nursing literature (Alexander and Giguere, 1996; Baker, 1996; Conger and Mezza, 1996; Degazon and Lunney, 1995; Fonteyn, 1995; Oermann, 1997; Whiteside, 1997). Degazon and Lunney (1995, p. 271) refer to critical thinking as a 'multidimensional cognitive and perceptual process, including intuition, that involves reflective thought for decision making'. They assert that critical thinking is correlated with nursing competence, and that in order to advance to higher levels of clinical competence, ever increasing and sharpened critical thinking skills are needed. Alexander and Giguere (1996, p.16) maintain that the development of critical thinking skills in nursing education fosters 'therapeutic nursing interventions that promote the health of the whole individual'. They define critical thinking as an 'analytic process addressing not only problem solving but also the ability to raise pertinent questions and critique solutions' (Alexander and Giguere, 1996, p. 16).

To teach a purely linear, reductionist type of reasoning style provides nursing students with only some of the skills they will need to arrive at prudent clinical decisions. Critical thinking allows decisions to be made through a more reflective and multidimensional thinking process. The student is thus provided with the skills necessary to weigh the importance and relevance of large amounts of data, consider alternatives and options, and ultimately to arrive at sound and logical decisions (Baker, 1996; Degazon and Lunney, 1995; Oermann, 1997). Fonteyn (1995, p. 60) views critical thinking and clinical reasoning as the essence of nursing practice, stating that 'it is intrinsic to all aspects of care provision, and its importance pervades nursing education, research and practice'. She stresses the need for the teaching of critical thinking in nursing curricula, in order to produce graduate nurses with the skills necessary to function effectively and competently in the ever changing, demanding and increasingly complex health care setting.

A concept closely aligned with, and often equated with critical thinking, is that of metacognition. Metacognition 'refers to an awareness of our own cognitive processes (thinking and learning abilities) or knowing about what we know' (Gordon and Braun, 1985, p. 2). Yussen (1985, p. 253) adds the following remarks:

> Metacognition, broadly speaking, is identified as that body of knowledge and understanding that reflects on cognition itself. Put another way, metacognition is that mental activity for which other states or processes become the object of reflection. Thus, metacognition is sometimes referred to as thoughts about cognition, or thinking about thinking.

The educational psychologists Gavelek and Raphael (1985), in their investigation of metacognitive processes, describe two critical areas of learning where metacognition plays a key role. The first area relates to the active role of the learner in guiding his or her own learning process. It is metacognitive self-knowledge which enables the student to function as an independent learner.

The second area in which metacognition plays a key role is in the concept of transfer. Gavelek and Raphael (1985, p. 103) pose the question: 'To what extent are individuals able to apply what and how they have learned across different settings?' and respond that metacognition is the central way in which a learner is able to apply, consider, modify and reflect upon cognitive activity across varying tasks. Indeed, it is this process which allows the learner a deeper understanding and awareness of the interactive nature of the learning process.

Degazon and Lunney (1995, p. 271) define metacognition as 'the ability to recognize, analyze and discuss thinking processes' and suggest that as learners increasingly focus on their thinking processes, their metacognitive abilities likewise improve. They state further that due to the nature of metacognition as a tool for self modification, development of this skill 'provides a basis for growth as a thinking professional' (Degazon and Lunney, 1995, p. 272).

Many of the tenets of mind mapping find their roots in Ausubelian (Ausubel, 1963) learning theory. This theory states that human thinking and understanding is based not only on understanding concepts, but also on understanding the relationships between concepts. In other words, concepts do not exist in isolation, but rather depend on others for meaning.

Ausubel (1963) distinguished between rote learning and meaningful learning. Meaningful learning occurs when learners are able to take new concepts and incorporate or relate them to concepts or knowledge structures already possessed. Thus learners are able to widen and enhance their existing knowledge domains. Rote learning, on the other hand, involves an arbitrary assignment of new concepts or knowledge into the present cognitive structure, without consideration of how this new knowledge may relate to, enhance or advance the existing cognitive structure held by the learner. Okebukola and Jegede (1988, p. 490) state that concept mapping is an effective way to attain meaningful learning because 'each concept depends upon its relationships to many others for meaning'. Heinze-Fry and Novak (1990) compare students who learn meaningfully to those who employ rote learning. They state, 'in contrast to students who learn by rote, students who employ meaningful learning are expected to retain knowledge over an extensive time span and find new, related learning progressively easier' (Heinze-Fry and Novak, 1990, p.463).

Proponents of the mind map as an educational aid point to the similarities between the radiant, associative nature of the brain and the graphic representation of knowledge through a mind map. Buzan and Buzan (1996) describe the highly complex biochemical pathways and architecture of the brain. They assert that these internal brain pathways function associatively and radiantly, and that any outward expression of this internal structure, such as mind mapping, serves to enhance creativity, learning and higher orders of thinking. Buzan and Buzan (1996, p.100) suggest that association is one of the major ways to improve memory and creativity, and that 'it is the integrating device our brains use to make sense of our physical experience, the key to human memory and understanding'. They discuss the inadequacies of traditional note taking as a means to learn, organize and create, stating 'by its very nature, the linear presentation of standard notes prevents the brain from making associations, thus counteracting creativity and memory' (Buzan and Buzan, 1996, p. 50).

Learning theorists Novak and Gowin (1984), in their classic text *Learning How to Learn*, encourage the use of mind mapping as a way to represent relationships between concepts. These authors maintain that the best way to help students to learn meaningfully is to allow them to see explicitly the nature of the relationship between concepts as they exist within and outside their minds. They point to the mind map as a means to externalize relationships and connections between concepts and ideas. They describe the mind map as a 'visual road map showing some of the pathways we may take to connect meanings of concepts' (Novak and Gowin, 1984, p.15). Additionally, Novak and Gowin assert that in the process of drawing mind maps, new relationships and new meanings between concepts may arise or become evident in ways that were not readily apparent prior to construction of the mind map.

A large body of research has emerged from the science education field, examining the efficacy of mind mapping as an educational tool. Findings indicate that mind mapping increases achievement, decreases perceived anxiety and promotes meaningful learning. Albertazzi *et al.* (1996, p. 1088) reported positive outcomes from using the mind map as a 'metacognitive tool to help chemistry teachers and learners to improve teaching and learning'. Barenholz and Tamir (1992) compared learning and achievement outcomes for 'mappers' versus 'non-mappers' in a high school microbiology program. They found that post-test scores compared with pre-test scores were higher for those in the 'mapping' group. Jegede *et al.* (1990) investigated the usefulness of mind mapping as a means of decreasing student anxiety and increasing achievement in biology. Based on the pre- and post-test scores on both achievement and anxiety scales, mind mapping, as compared to traditional instruction, was found to enhance learning and decrease anxiety within the context of biology study.

Heinze-Fry and Novak (1990) found that meaningful learning was enhanced using mind mapping.

The students in their study described mind mapping as 'an integrated educational experience', and said it helped them 'make sense out of the material' (Heinze-Fry and Novak, 1990, p. 471). Additionally, students in this study reported that mind mapping gave them insight into how they learned and helped to clarify connections.

Okebukola and Jegede (1989) investigated the usefulness of mind mapping as a way to decrease perceived anxiety in the study of ecology and Mendelian genetics. They found a significant decrease in anxiety and perception of subject difficulty among the students employing mind mapping compared with the control group. The authors contend that one of the mechanisms accounting for these results is the acquisition of meaningful learning. If students are unable to understand a subject, especially one traditionally perceived as difficult, they are likely to exhibit higher levels of anxiety and perceive greater subject difficulty. On the other hand, if students can identify the intricate relationships and connectedness between concepts and ideas, a greater depth of understanding is attained. Okebukola and Jegede remark, 'by making the student feel comfortable when working within intricate and interconnected systems of thought, concept mapping could be said to depress anxiety levels toward such intricate and originally perceived as difficult concepts' (Okebukola and Jegede, 1989, p. 90).

Study of the nursing literature reveals scant information about using mind mapping as an educational tool. Irvine (1995) asks whether concept mapping could be used to promote meaningful learning in nurse education. This nurse educator describes how the focus of nursing education has shifted from rote learning to methods which help students learn how to learn. Rather than merely transmitting facts, nursing education has become more concerned with facilitating learning. Irvine maintains that the information nurses will need to contend with continues to increase in both size and complexity, and thus promoting meaningful and effective learning is an issue of importance. She suggests that mind maps be used as a metacognitive strategy to promote meaningful learning in nursing education.

All and Havens (1997) encourage the use of mind maps to help nursing students approach and make sense out of large amounts of highly technical and complex text book material. They advocate mind mapping as a means to enhance understanding of classroom activities and to help organize data obtained before and after the clinical day. They discuss the obsolescence of rote learning in nursing education, and advocate the use of alternative methods of learning which promote the development of the sound critical-thinking skills that nurses will need to deal effectively with the complex clinical situations they will encounter in their practice.

A mind mapping pilot study

The use of mind maps was introduced to a group of nine nursing students during a 15-week clinical practicum at a large western American teaching hospital. These students were in their third year of a 4-year baccalaureate nursing program. For this clinical practicum, the students did not 'pre-lab' [i.e. they did not come into the hospital the day before clinical to receive a patient assignment and review that patients' charts; and they did not develop nursing processes (written care plans) on each patient to guide their care on the following day]. Fonteyn and Flaig (1994) have challenged nursing educators to question their continued use of this 'sacred cow' that may not be as effective for developing students' metacognitive skills as other teaching strategies, such as clinical logs and mind maps.

For this practicum, each student arrived in time for the morning report and was assigned to work with one of the registered nurses (RNs) on duty, who then gave the student a patient assignment. After report, the student quickly looked up the essential information needed to care safely for the patient(s) and then proceeded to do a complete assessment on each patient. From this assessment, the student identified priority problems to be addressed that day, determined a plan of care, and then articulated these findings to both the RN and to the clinical staff. Thus, instead of using a deductive approach to patient care, the students utilized a more inductive methodology, combining new pieces of data with those previously acquired, thus furthering their understanding of the patient case as the shift progressed.

For the first 10 weeks of the clinical practicum, students recorded their thoughts about each patient case in a clinical log which they completed at the end of each clinical week, and handed to their clinical instructor for review and feedback. Fonteyn and Cahill (1998) have recommended reflective writing in clinical logs as a means of improving students' metacognition. During the last 5 weeks of the semester, instead of writing in clinical logs, students drew a graphic representation of their thinking about a patient case, a mind map, after having been provided with some explanatory information about mind maps from their clinical instructor. The mind maps were intended to illustrate the mental organization of the students' thoughts about their plan of care for a particular patient.

Examples of student mind maps

Figures 23.1 and 23.2 provide examples of the students' mind maps; a general discussion of each follows.

The central focus of the student's mind map illustrated in Figure 23.1 is the patient (56-year-old female) and her diagnosis (perforated diverticulitis; sigmoid colectomy). The primary problem identified (stated as a nursing diagnosis) is anxiety relating to knowledge deficit secondary to emergency surgery (a causal relationship). Pain relating to surgery, although stated in nursing diagnostic terms and associated with nursing actions (assessment and reassessment of level of pain, and encouraging the use of Patient Controlled Analgesia morphine), is not specifically labelled as a problem and is not ranked in terms of priority. Other patient problems are implied by the data displayed in the map, but are not stated, e.g. ineffective gas exchange (see upper right of mind map), impaired skin integrity (lower right) and potential alteration of cardiac output (left side of mind map).

The data in the student's mind map depicted in Figure 23.2 is organized quite differently from the previous one. Although the central focus of this mind map is also the patient's medical diagnosis, other major concepts are represented as equally important. These include: assessment, report, nursing interventions and goals. Data related to each of these primary concepts radiate to form a cluster of associated details.

Examination of the mind maps

Students' completed mind maps were examined with their clinical instructors so that students could improve their thinking about future patient cases. During this activity, the instructor posed a series of questions to elucidate how patient data were structured and inter-related in the student's

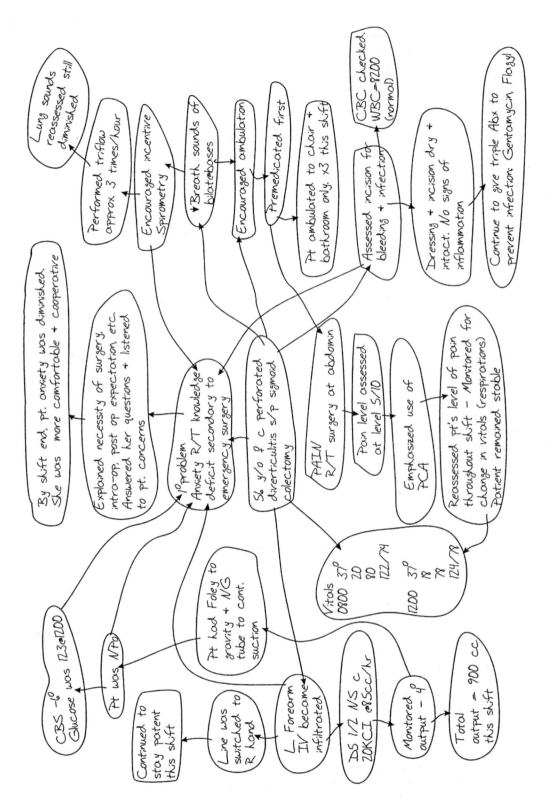

Figure 23.1 Mind map 1

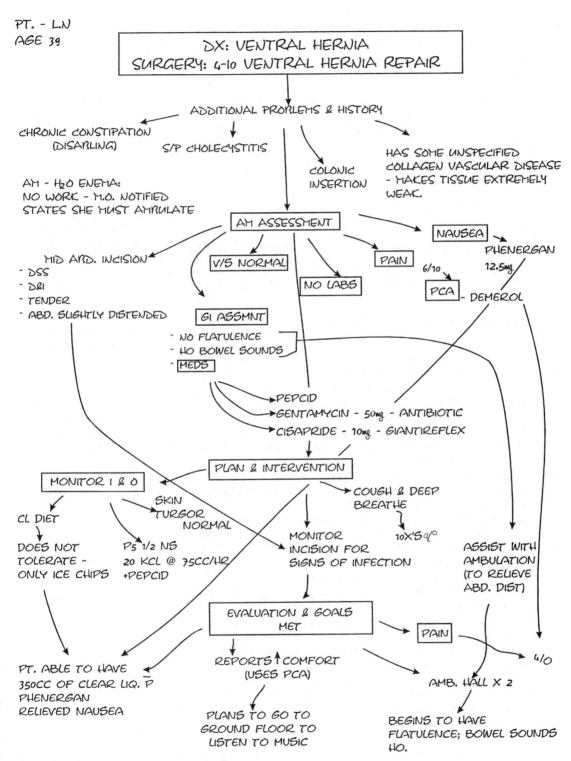

PT. - L.N
AGE 39

DX: VENTRAL HERNIA
SURGERY: 6-10 VENTRAL HERNIA REPAIR

ADDITIONAL PROBLEMS & HISTORY

CHRONIC CONSTIPATION
(DISABLING)

S/P CHOLECYSTITIS

COLONIC
INSERTION

HAS SOME UNSPECIFIED
COLLAGEN VASCULAR DISEASE
- MAKES TISSUE EXTREMELY
WEAK.

AM - H2O ENEMA:
NO WORK - M.O. NOTIFIED
STATES SHE MUST AMBULATE

AM ASSESSMENT

NAUSEA

PHENERGAN
12.5mg

MID ABD. INCISION
- DSS
- D&I
- TENDER
- ABD. SLIGHTLY DISTENDED

V/S NORMAL

NO LABS

PAIN

6/10

PCA - DEMEROL

GI ASSMNT

- NO FLATULENCE
- HO BOWEL SOUNDS
- MEDS

PEPCID
GENTAMYCIN - 50mg - ANTIBIOTIC
CISAPRIDE - 10mg - GIANTIREFLEX

PLAN & INTERVENTION

MONITOR I & O

SKIN
TURGOR
NORMAL

COUGH & DEEP
BREATHE

CL DIET

DOES NOT
TOLERATE -
ONLY ICE CHIPS

P5 1/2 NS
20 KCL @ 75CC/HR
+PEPCID

MONITOR
INCISION FOR
SIGNS OF INFECTION

10X'S q°

ASSIST WITH
AMBULATION
(TO RELIEVE
ABD. DIST)

EVALUATION & GOALS
MET

PAIN

PT. ABLE TO HAVE
350CC OF CLEAR LIQ. P̄
PHENERGAN
RELIEVED NAUSEA

REPORTS↑COMFORT
(USES PCA)

4/0

AMB. HALL X 2

PLANS TO GO TO
GROUND FLOOR TO
LISTEN TO MUSIC

BEGINS TO HAVE
FLATULENCE; BOWEL SOUNDS
HO.

Figure 23.2 Mind map 2

thoughts that were graphically represented in the mind map. The questions included:

- What is the quality and quantity of data included in your mind map? What does this tell you about your thinking?
- What is the quality and quantity of data omitted from your map? What does this tell you about your thinking? What data are missing that might be important to the case? Why do you think these data are missing?
- What data are linked and what is the significance of these connections?
- What data are not linked and what is the significance of this?
- What other questions arise from examining your map?
- Overall, what have you learned from examining your mind map that could help improve your thinking about future patient cases?

Student evaluation of improvement in their thinking

Students' perceptions of how their thinking had improved during this clinical practicum were evaluated using a 'Thinking Assessment' instrument. This tool comprised 10 Likert scale questions assessing the extent to which students perceived that various activities improved their thinking. Data collected from nine student evaluations were analyzed and represented by an average ranked score (out of a possible 5.0) and a percentage of agreement (out of 100%) with each response.

Results indicated that students' thinking about patient data and care had improved a great deal. [The average response score was 4.9 (out of five) or 98% and 4.2 or 84% respectively, for the first two questions.] Students' comments supported these findings, e.g. 'I'm finally able to make sense of all the pieces of the puzzle, to form relationships (among pieces of data)'.

Students perceived that their thinking had improved by not 'pre-labbing', an approach that was new for the students in this clinical practicum. Analysis of students' responses to questions 3–6 revealed that their thinking had improved considerably. (The average response score was 4.2 or 84%.) Comments included, 'Not pre-labbing is helpful because it prepares students for real life as a nurse' and 'If something was not clear, the nurse (RN) made sure to explain it clearly'.

Students considered that their confidence in their thinking had improved considerably since the

beginning of the semester. (The average score for this question was 4.2 or 84%.) In comparing three different cognitive tools (written nursing care plans, clinical logs and mind maps) with regard to how well each improved their thinking, students' response scores indicated they considered that mind maps improved their thinking more than care plans (average score of 4.4 or 88%) and more than clinical logs (average score of 4.2 or 84%).

Summary

Learning is an interactive, dynamic process. Providing students with learning techniques which will reflect the way in which their minds perceive and connect information helps them to become more creative and efficient in their learning. Mind mapping assists students to understand how they link related data for meaning and understanding, and encourages creative and divergent thinking.

Mind mapping shows promise for enhancing the reasoning and metacognitive skills of students, and for decreasing anxiety and fear towards subjects often perceived as difficult. The description of the use of mind maps in a clinical practicum confirms the value of this unique and creative tool. We encourage the use of this metacognitive teaching strategy and suggest its use in nursing education as a means to enhance the learning and critical thinking abilities of nursing students.

References

Alexander, M. K. and Giguere, B. (1996) Critical thinking in clinical learning: A holistic perspective. *Holistic Nursing Practice*, **10**(3), 15–22.

All, A. C. and Havens, R. L. (1997) Cognitive/concept mapping: A teaching strategy for nursing. *Journal of Advanced Nursing*, **25**, 1210–1219.

Ausubel, D. P. (1963) *The Psychology of Meaningful Verbal Learning*. New York: Grune & Stratton.

Baker, C. R. (1996) Reflective learning: A teaching strategy for critical thinking. *Journal of Nursing Education*, **35**, 19–22.

Barenholz, H. and Tamir, P. (1992) A comprehensive use of concept mapping in design instruction and assessment. *Research in Science and Technology Education*, **10**, 37–52.

Buzan, T. and Buzan, B. (1996) *The Mind Map Book*. New York: Plume/Penguin.

Conger, M. M. and Mezza, I. (1996) Fostering critical thinking in nursing in the clinical setting. *Nurse Educator*, **21**(3), 11–15.

Degazon, C. E. and Lunney, M. (1995) Clinical journal: A tool to foster critical thinking for advanced levels of competence. *Clinical Nurse Specialist*, **9**, 270–274.

Dorough, D. K. and Rye, J. A. (1997) Mapping for understanding. *The Science Teacher*, **64**, 37–41.

Fonteyn, M. E. (1995) Clinical reasoning in nursing. In *Clinical Reasoning in the Health Professions* (J. Higgs, J. and M. Jones, eds), pp. 60–71. Oxford: Butterworth-Heinemann.

Fonteyn, M. E. and Cahill, M. E. (1998) The use of clinical logs to improve nursing students' metacognition: A pilot study. *Journal of Advanced Nursing*, **28**, 149–154.

Fonteyn, M. and Flaig, L. (1994) The written nursing process: Is it still useful to nursing education? Journal *of Advanced Nursing*, **19**, 315–319.

Gavelek, J. R. and Raphael, T. E. (1985) Metacognition, instruction, and the role of questioning activities. In *Metacognition, Cognition, and Human Performance, Vol. 2: Instructional Practices* (D. L. Forrest-Pressley, G. E. MacKinnon and T. G. Waller, eds), pp. 103–136. Orlando, FL: Academic Press.

Gordon, C. J. and Braun, C. 1985. Metacognitive processes: reading and writing narrative discourse. In *Metacognition, Cognition, and Human Performance, Vol. 2: Instructional Practices* (D. L. Forrest-Pressley, G. E. MacKinnon, and T. G. Waller, eds), pp. 1–75. Orlando, FL: Academic Press.

Heinze-Fry, J. A. and Novak, J. D. (1990) Concept mapping brings long term movement toward meaningful learning. *Science Education*, **74**, 461–472.

Irvine, L. M. C. (1995) Can concept mapping be used to promote meaningful learning in nurse education? *Journal of Advanced Nursing*, **21**, 1175–1179.

Jegede, O. J., Alaiyemola, F. F. and Okebukola, P. A. O. (1990) The effect of concept mapping on students' anxiety and achievement in biology. *Journal of Research in Science Teaching*, **27**, 951–960.

Novak, J. D. (1990) Concept mapping: A useful tool for science education. *Journal of Research in Science Teaching*, **27**, 937–949.

Novak, J. D. and Gowin, D. B. (1984) *Learning How to Learn*. New York: Cambridge University Press.

Oermann, M. H. (1997) Evaluating critical thinking in clinical practice. *Nurse Educator*, **22**(5), 25–28.

Okebukola, P. A. and Jegede, O. J. (1988) Cognitive preference and learning mode as determinants of meaningful learning through concept mapping. *Science Education*, **72**, 489–500.

Okebukola, P. A. and Jegede, O. J. (1989) Students' anxiety towards and perception of difficulty of some biological concepts under the concept mapping heuristic. *Research in Science and Technological Education*, **7**, 85–92.

Regis, A., Albertazzi, P. G. and Roletto, E. (1996) Concept maps in chemistry education. *Journal of Chemical Education*, **73**, 1084–1088.

Whiteside, C. (1997) A model for teaching critical thinking in the clinical setting. *Dimensions of Critical Care Nursing*, **16**, 152–165.

Yussen, S. R. (1985) The role of metacognition in contemporary theories of cognitive development. In *Metacognition, Cognition, and Human Performance, Vol. 1: Theoretical Perspectives* (D. L. Forrest-Pressley, G. E. MacKinnon and T. G. Waller, eds), pp. 253–283. Orlando, FL: Academic Press.

24

Facilitating the acquisition of knowledge for reasoning

Angie Titchen and Joy Higgs

In Chapter 3, we made explicit our valuing of a view of knowledge in which both personal and public validation are sought, where propositional, professional and personal knowledge are granted validity, and where knowledge is seen as a dynamic phenomenon undergoing constant change and testing. The focus of this chapter is on ways of helping students generate their knowledge bases through knowledge construction and an increased awareness of the different forms of knowledge, and how these forms of knowledge need to be used in harmony in clinical reasoning. It is also concerned with helping students to gain understanding of the way they generate knowledge in practice through testing and retesting their knowledge base to justify knowledge claims. We explore critical companionship as an approach for facilitating the acquisition and harmonious use of the three types of knowledge, and for promoting critical reflection on past experience, the development of cognitive and metacognitive skills, and the ability to be a skilled companion to patients and families.

A theoretical framework for facilitating acquisition of knowledge

Studying conceptions of knowledge

Studying conceptions of knowledge (or acquiring *knowledge about knowledge*) can contribute to effective learning and clinical reasoning. Research demonstrates that the relevance and depth of knowledge content, the structure of individuals' knowledge bases and the learner's ability to organize knowledge in a meaningful way are of major importance to clinical reasoning ability (Grant and Marsden, 1987; Norman, 1988). This information can be applied to teaching and learning strategies by:

- Making the relevance of knowledge explicit in the classroom or clinical setting, so that knowledge can be described, reflected upon and analysed in relation to a specific experience or case.
- Explicitly valuing different types of knowledge through analysis of experience, feeling and thinking.
- Helping students articulate the structure of their knowledge bases to develop an understanding of their own knowledge and knowledge of their field. The domains of professional craft knowledge in nursing and patient-centred nursing outlined by Benner (1984) and Titchen (1998a) respectively offer frameworks for such analysis. Johns (1995) and Boykin and Schoenhofer (1991) applied Carper's (1978) empirical, personal, aesthetic and ethical ways of knowing for this purpose also. This kind of analysis differs from the way in which traditional case studies focus on medical, psychological, sociological and epidemiological features, hindering articulation of the structure and essence of the pertinent discipline knowledge.
- Integrating the different types of knowledge used in clinical cases, leading to meaningful organization of knowledge.

- Demonstrating the depth and complexity of knowledge to learners.
- Facilitating understanding of the content and structure of knowledge so that learners can more easily judge its validity.

Constructing knowledge from experience

The assertion that learners construct knowledge from experience has significant implications for curriculum planners. Opportunities need to be made available for learners to experience and construct their own realities through critical reflection upon, and theorization about, their practice. There is a variety of suitable approaches to achieve this goal, including experiential learning, inquiry learning and problem solving, co-operative group learning, and negotiating curricula with students (see Boud and Feletti, 1997; Graves, 1993; Mulligan and Griffin, 1992). A deep approach to learning is desirable and can be promoted by helping students to search actively for meaning, for an understanding of what they are learning and for links within their knowledge bases. Discussion of ideas with others and individual reflection upon experiences assists students to own the knowledge acquired and to use it in their clinical reasoning in a way that is compatible with autonomous behaviour.

Reflection (or conscious review) upon experience is a key element in helping learners to make sense of learning experiences and construct their own realities, and according to Engel (1991) in promoting a deep approach to learning. Learning experiences in themselves do not guarantee learning. Instead it is reflection, or the processing of experiences and the search for meaning within them, which promotes learning (Boud and Walker, 1991; Schön, 1987). Similarly, metacognition (or reflective self-awareness and *thinking about thinking*) is an important element of effective learning, knowledge generation and practice. Research in this area identifies the value of metacognition in helping learners to develop learning and problem solving skills (Biggs and Telfer, 1987). Fostering the use of both cognitive and metacognitive skills will help learners to learn to conceptualize, test and construct their knowledge.

Learning from the experiences of professional practice is a means of generating knowledge (Carr and Kemmis, 1986; Elliott, 1991; Eraut, 1985; Schön, 1983), particularly personal and professional craft knowledge. When students or practitioners encounter a puzzle or find that what

normally works is not working in a particular case, they can stop and reflect in order to develop an idea of what might work. The idea is then tested and if it works, new knowledge is generated. Schön (1983) calls this process *on-the-spot experimentation* and describes it as a form of *reflection-in-action*. Titchen's (1998a) research in nursing supports this assertion and has demonstrated that the knowledge creation skills of less experienced nurses are enhanced by having an expert nurse (who is prepared for the role) working alongside and engaging in critical reflection and debate with them.[1] This finding suggests that students' learning should be facilitated by practitioners as well as by academics, so that knowledge creation skills and knowledge use in clinical reasoning can be demonstrated and developed. This learning is facilitated by clinicians who adopt a relationship which is parallel to skilled companionship (Binnie and Titchen, 1998; Titchen, 1998a), i.e. critical companionship.[2]

Locating learning experiences in the context of practice

We argue that educational strategies designed to promote the construction and generation of all types of knowledge, and thinking should offer experiences located within practice contexts and should engage with the whole person (in order to strengthen links between knowledge and the contextual factors influencing its interpretation and use). Such strategies would counter the traditional educational strategies which tend to decontextualize knowledge and divide the patient into component parts to be learned and treated. By tending to focus on linear, rational models of clinical reasoning, traditional health sciences education has neglected holistic thinking and intuition (Benner and Tanner, 1987; Rew and Barrow, 1987).

We consider that attention to contexts and the person will enhance the construction and generation of the different types of knowledge and thinking. Furthermore, while propositional knowledge and rational thinking can be acquired through reading, literature review, case studies, essays, discussion, lectures and seminars, the construction of professional and personal knowledge, and the development of holistic and intuitive thinking

---

[1] For further discussion of learning partnerships in clinical settings, see Titchen and Binnie (1995).
[2] For further exposition of the relationship domain of critical companionship, see Titchen (1998a,b).

cannot be easily be acquired in these ways, either because they remain embedded in practitioners' accumulated experience or because they cannot be easily expressed in words. Instead, these goals can be facilitated by learning strategies (such as observing, listening and questioning, and story-telling) which are derived from interpretive research methodologies used by such phenomenological researchers as Benner (1984), MacLeod (1990), Mattingly (1991), Titchen and Binnie (1993), Brown and McIntyre (1993) and Titchen (1996). To develop an understanding of the lived experience of practice, these researchers used approaches which involved seeing the situation through the eyes of the actors in the situation, and retaining contextual and experiential integrity and wholeness. Titchen (1998a, b) has built on these methodologies in her creation of critical companionship strategies (presented below).

Creating a climate of challenge, open-mindedness and critical debate

To be successful, educational strategies need to be located in learning climates in which the different types of knowledge used and the distinct ways of generating knowledge are genuinely valued. Such learning climates are characterized by curiosity, challenge, open-mindedness and critical debate. Different strategies, including reflection, high challenge/high support, conceptualisation, theorization from practice, experimentation and critical dialogue need to be used to foster these goals. Learning experiences are facilitated within relationships which build on the humanness and wholeness of relationships. In other words, these are relationships in which the critical companion (whether educator or practitioner) uses the self-facilitatively to model the parallel process of therapeutic use of self with patients. Learners are helped to examine how their own beliefs, values, perceptions and interpretations influence their clinical reasoning. In this way self-evaluation and an understanding of the need to test and retest knowledge and to justify knowledge claims are promoted.

Educational strategies for developing knowledge

Within the theoretical framework presented above, a number of educational strategies can be adopted to help learners develop their knowledge bases and increase their awareness of the ways they use their knowledge in clinical reasoning. The strategies presented here are role modelling and articulation of knowledge, observing, listening and questioning, feedback on performance, critical dialogue, story telling, conceptual mapping, acquiring and expressing knowledge through arts, and use of different milieux. These strategies are based on empirical work [such as Titchen's (1998a) work on critical companionship] and are designed to realize the concepts of consciousness-raising, problematization, self-reflection and critique. Other strategies for fostering knowledge acquisition include small group, experiential, problem-based, and self-directed/learner managed learning discussions.

Role modelling and articulation of knowledge

Role modelling has long been recognized as an effective, if unconscious, way of facilitating others' learning (e.g. Estabrooks and Morse, 1992; Pembrey, 1980; Runciman, 1983). However, Titchen (1998a) found that even if used consciously and intentionally by experienced practitioners, without an articulation of the craft knowledge being used, role modelling did not realize its full potential. She describes four ways in which practitioners can make their craft knowledge more accessible:

- Story-telling (in which they analyse and interpret their own experiences).
- Suggestions (based on their craft knowledge) offered after analysis and interpretation of the less experienced practitioner's current experience.
- Analysis, interpretation and evaluation of shared experiences (informed by craft knowledge)
- Non-specific maxims.

Role modelling, combined with articulation of both propositional and non-propositional knowledge, can be used consciously by experienced practitioners. For instance, they can ensure that students have the opportunity to observe them as they go about their everyday work and *intentionally* create opportunities in which they can articulate their knowledge. This particularly applies to the more embedded, tacit and usually unexplicated aspects of practice, in addition to routine events such as handover reports, informal conversations over breaks and formal case presentations.

Observing, Listening and Questioning

The observing, listening and questioning strategy is closely linked to the previous strategy and can be used by students to access the knowledge of the experienced practitioner (or critical companion, as per Titchen 1998a,b) and make it available for critical reflection and discussion. (The guidelines in Table 24.1 can be helpful here.) In an experiential learning or clinical education setting, observing, listening and questioning can be used to facilitate articulation and discussion of the educator's, practitioner's or student's embedded knowledge and the deepening, refinement and generation of professional and personal knowledge.

Feedback on performance

On the basis of Titchen's (1998a) findings, we encourage critical companions to stimulate recall of observed events or stories and give feedback in detail. This enables learners to evaluate themselves, and serves as a device for identifying and naming professional and personal knowledge. Learners are helped to cope with constructive criticism by being given the opportunity to evaluate their own performance and self-diagnose learning needs before the teacher's feedback and diagnosis of learning needs are offered. Where appropriate, self-evaluation and diagnosis are validated, making any further critique more tolerable. It may also be necessary for the critical companion (or educator) to draw salient information together for the learner in a non-critical way, to facilitate self-evaluation, as illustrated in the following reflections of a clinical educator:

> When Harriet told me the situation . . . I asked in a non-critical voice, 'How long has Daisy been in?' So I was planting or bringing to the surface information and putting it together in Harriet's

mind, in a way, so the information was then in front of her. So I was making her think: Daisy has been in for a week – has she got a district nurse (yes she has) – two bits of information there. Then she's almost there herself, thinking, 'Well, I haven't actually spoken to her myself'. So I didn't need to say, 'You should have phoned the district nurse', because by the time I had drawn up the relevant bits of information in a cluster, she was able to make the judgement. (Titchen, 1998a)

Critical dialogue

Material revealed through the above strategies and through stories can be used by critical companions and learners to engage in a dialogue in which critical companions encourage learners to question, criticize and doubt their own perceptions, look for personal meaning, interpret the data and examine their beliefs and values (Titchen, 1998a,b). Critical companions promote collaborative critical analysis of and debate about the data, and also promote collaborative evaluations, interpretations and validations. They also facilitate the generation of emerging professional craft knowledge and theory, and the use of existing formal theory to inform further action, and assist in creating a vision for change and action. To effectively implement this strategy with students, it is likely that the (educator) critical companion will need to stimulate the student's self-awareness, reflective, critical and creative thinking, and particularization of research-based knowledge. In the following extract the educator helped the inexperienced nurse to particularize her general knowledge and to see how using research-based knowledge required the development of craft knowledge.

> You've probably heard of Dave Thompson's work . . . When he measured anxiety levels in patients after coronaries, the spouse had significantly

Table 24.1 Guidelines for helping experienced practitioners to articulate their professional and personal knowledge

After observing the experienced practitioner in the clinical setting, an opportunity is sought to talk with the practitioner, as soon as possible after the observation, using the following guidelines:

- Focus questions to the practitioner on the events just observed.
- Avoid framing questions in a generalized form.
- Concentrate on what has gone well during the observation period and avoid adverse criticism of the practitioner.
- Aim to probe and find out what the practitioner has done in achieving success.
- Enquire about how the practitioner made various judgements.
- Phrase questions in open rather than closed ways.
- Be supportive and willing to accept the practitioner's responses.
- Allow plenty of time for the practitioner to respond to questions.

Adapted from McAlpine *et al.* (1988).

higher anxiety than the patient themselves which is always worth bearing in mind . . . I often think it's worth offering the spouse some time on their own because they may be worried about things that they don't want to say in front of their husband because they think they may worry him more. But you've got to do that in such a way that you've got permission from the patient. What's quite a good idea is . . . (Titchen, 1998a)

Story-telling

Narrative approaches or story-telling in qualitative research (see Benner, 1984; Binnie and Titchen, 1998; Sandelowski, 1991; Uden *et al.*, 1992) have re-opened consideration of perhaps the oldest way in which human beings make sense of themselves and their worlds. Stories concern action and are dynamic accounts of things changing as a result of people's actions. Although stories do not to capture the whole of the lived experience of the situation, the story-teller conveys the essence of the experience, leaving out unnecessary detail (Boykin and Schoenhofer, 1991). The focal point of concern is the motives and intentions of the actors (Mattingly, 1991). Boykin and Schoenhofer found that stories are valuable for the insights and deepened understanding they bring practitioners concerning the meaning of their practices. Mattingly reports that reflective stories of occupational therapists provided an avenue for identifying multiple interpretations of events which facilitated reflective thinking and captured a level of complexity of clinical work that biomedically oriented accounts of practice could not depict. Dolan (1984) found that stories enabled nurses to abandon the often sterile language of case presentation as they began to use a more expressive style that incorporated the context and a holistic grasp of the situation, enriching both their practice and their sense of self as a nurse.

We propose that story-telling facilitates the construction and creation of knowledge and study of the conceptions of knowledge. It also offers opportunities for exploration and critical debate about the knowledge and reasoning of experienced practitioners. Story-telling can be facilitated both informally in the staff room and formally in the classroom. Spontaneous story-telling will become more reflective if colleagues and students ask *why?* and seek and offer interpretations. Formally, it can be used in seminars, group work and clinical supervision, using the processes of representing, interpreting and envisioning (Smith, 1992).

Conceptual mapping

Conceptual mapping provides another way of processing practice experiences and prior knowledge, and subjecting them to conscious appraisal. It allows for the exploration of students' knowledge underpinning hypothetical cases. A concept map is an external representation of internal ideas, and commonly refers to a visual representation of one or more areas of an individual's unique knowledge base. Cognitive maps can be formulated in many ways, such as flow charts, annotated diagrams, images or maps illustrating interconnected ideas (Novak and Gowin, 1984). They represent the way individuals conceptualize and organize their knowledge about their environment, their discipline and their experiences, and they offer an opportunity for learners to think about their thinking (metacognition) and to analyse their clinical knowledge and reasoning (Higgs, 1992).

Involvement of learners in conceptual mapping enables them to analyse, explore and discuss their concepts, and the way those concepts are linked and their knowledge is organized (Gowin, 1981). Conceptual mapping promotes critical self-reflection by students and re-construction of their knowledge bases (Deshler, 1990). Learners can assess and revise their knowledge bases in terms of accuracy, comprehensiveness and organization, and can learn how to organize and access their knowledge more effectively. They can be encouraged to think about the knowledge they have which is beyond propositional knowledge. Cognitive maps enable others to appreciate and evaluate what the learner knows and how the learner has organized his/her knowledge; and they provide feedback to the learner.

Acquiring and expressing knowledge through the arts

Literary texts, visual art, music, dance and drama can be used to help learners to explore, experience, express and create aesthetic, personal and ethical knowledge, and to understand the place of this knowledge in practice. It is likely that each health profession has rich sources of insights hidden away in reflective accounts in the form of stories, poems, diaries and anecdotes. For example, there are increasing numbers of published narratives (e.g. Benner, 1984; Dyck, 1989; Emanuel, 1994; Hedges, 1993; Miller, 1992) which focus attention on the characteristically human aspects of health care and which offer opportunities to explore our practice, selves and relationships with others (Holmes, 1992) and to explore our practice in relation to the person receiving our care.

Thow and Murray (1991), Robb and Murray (1992) and Darbyshire (1994) explore the use of literary texts, films, plays, novels, short stories, newspaper articles, drawings, paintings and photography to help learners engage with a variety of experiences, analyse attitudes, values and ethics, encourage reflection and promote self-awareness and alternative experiences of thinking and learning. As well as using the work of others to learn, we encourage students' expression and generation of knowledge through writing poetry (see, e.g. Bowe, 1994), dancing, painting, etc. As an example of this approach, Pearson (1992) used professional actors as lay teachers in his action research, and gave them patient profiles, constructed from real patients, from which to develop their characters. The aim was to help the nurses relate to their patients through empathizing with them. Visual art forms particularly can be useful to explore knowledge which cannot be described in words. Promoting understanding, creativity and expression through the arts may require educators to be courageous, to take risks and to be creative themselves. We have found that taking the plunge brings a new dimension to the educational experience; a dimension of soulfulness, spirituality and graceful care (in both physical and metaphysical senses). Graceful care is one of the concepts of skilled and critical companionship (Titchen, 1998a,b).

Milieux

The strategies presented above could be used in a number of milieux including clinical education and the classroom. This section presents some principles which could be used in learning programs to help educators (and critical companions) develop their skills in promoting students' knowledge generation, acquisition, critique and articulation.

To foster their skills in promoting learning, educators need to:

- Recognize their skills and expertise and have confidence that they can share them with others, including the next generation of health professionals. Benner (1984) proposes that clinicians at proficient and expert levels will benefit from clinical case studies and participation in research programs investigating clinical

problems, to develop their capacity to communicate knowledge and to gain positive reinforcement.

- Note the positive aspects of their teaching. This has been found to have a motivating effect on educators (Brown and McIntyre, 1993; Titchen, 1998a; Titchen and Binnie, 1993).
- Focus on understanding the learning event (e.g. observation, story or reflective diary) from the perspective of the actor (e.g. patient or student).
- Learn from each other. In particular, academic and clinical educators (i.e. critical companions or clinical educators) need a new collaborative learning relationship which recognizes each other's strengths. Not only educators but also students would benefit from this approach. Students on clinical placements would have the fruitful experience of watching experienced practitioners and educators learning from practice and analysing their knowledge generation and knowledge use in practice.
- Develop critical companionships with other educators to help each other benefit from planned and opportunistic learning and feedback activities.

Conclusion

In this chapter we have examined a theoretical framework and strategies for fostering knowledge development for clinical reasoning. It is important that knowledge be articulated, to enable educators and learners to gain insights into their knowledge and the knowledge of others. Another key part of gaining knowledge is critical feedback (from self and others) about knowledge development. The notions of critical companions and communities of practitioners and academics/educators have been suggested as a means of meeting both these needs. Students who develop a sense of other practitioners' knowledge and ways of thinking in relation to specific cases, and who are helped to explore their knowledge, will be assisted in developing and organizing their own knowledge bases. Educators and clinicians working within such a community would be able to deepen, refine and generate knowledge by making it available for self-reflection and evaluation and for debate and critique by colleagues, and would thereby enhance their effectiveness as practitioners and educators.

Putting these ideas and their underpinning values into practice may involve a number of actions. The climate in academic and clinical settings may need to be examined, and people's beliefs and values about the different types, use and generation of knowledge may need to be made explicit. Any dissonance between individual and institutional beliefs and values will need to be addressed. Practitioners will probably need help from colleagues and educators to become critical companions or clinical educators who can make their professional and personal knowledge accessible to learners, and who can facilitate learners' knowledge use and generation through reflection and metacognition. Practitioners and educators could be helped to develop their expertise and knowledge through collaborative in-service education programmes and through clinical supervision or critical companionship.

References

Benner, P. (1984) *From Novice to Expert: Excellence and Power in Clinical Nursing Practice*. London: Addison-Wesley.

Benner, P. and Tanner, C. (1987) Clinical judgment: How expert nurses use intuition. *American Journal of Nursing*, January, 23–31.

Biggs, J. B. and Telfer, R. (1987) *The Process of Learning*, 2nd edn. Sydney: Prentice-Hall.

Binnie, A. and Titchen, A. (1998) *Patient-Centred Nursing: An Action Research Study of Practice Development in an Acute Medical Unit*. Report. Oxford: Royal College of Nursing Institute.

Boud, D. and Feletti, G. (eds) (1997) *The Challenge of Problem Based Learning*, 2nd edn. London: Kogan Page.

Boud, D. and Walker, D. (1991) In the midst of experience: Developing a model to aid learners and facilitators. *A Quarterly Experience*, **27**, 5–9.

Bowe, G. (1994) Viewpoint: Nursing arts. *Nursing Standard*, **8**(23), 48–49.

Boykin, A. and Schoenhofer, S. O. (1991) Story as link between nursing practice, ontology, epistemology. *IMAGE: Journal of Nursing Scholarship*, **23**, 245–248.

Brown, S. and McIntyre, D. (1993) *Making Sense of Teaching*. Milton Keynes: Open University Press.

Carper, B. A. (1978) Fundamental patterns of knowing. *Advances in Nursing Science*, **1**, 13–23.

Carr, W. and Kemmis, S. (1986) *Becoming Critical: Education, Knowledge and Action Research*. London: Falmer Press.

Darbyshire, P. (1994) Understanding caring through arts and humanities: A medical/nursing humanities approach to promoting alternative experiences of thinking and learning. *Journal of Advanced Nursing*, **19**, 856–863.

Deshler, D. (1990), Conceptual mapping: Drawing charts of the mind. In *Fostering Critical Reflection in Adulthood* (J. Mezirow and Associates, eds), pp. 296–313. San Francisco: Jossey-Bass.

Dolan, K. (1984) Building bridges between education and practice. In *From Novice to Expert: Excellence and Power in Clinical Nursing Practice* (P. Benner, ed.), pp. 275–284. London: Addison-Wesley.

Dyck, B. (1989) The paper crane. *American Journal of Nursing*, June, 824–825.

Elliott, J. (1991) *Action Research for Educational Change*. Buckingham: Open University Press.

Emanuel, P. M. (1994) A gesture of humility. *Journal of Clinical Nursing*, **3**, 3–4.

Engel, C. E. (1991) Not just a method but a way of learning. In *The Challenge of Problem-Based Learning* (D. Boud and G. Feletti, eds), pp. 23–33. London: Kogan Page.

Eraut, M. (1985) Knowledge creation and knowledge use in professional contexts. *Studies in Higher Education*, **10**, 117–133.

Estabrooks, C. A. and Morse, J. M. (1992) Toward a theory of touch: The touching process and acquiring a touching style. *Journal of Advanced Nursing*, **17**, 448–456.

Gowin, D. B. (1981) *Educating*. New York: Cornell University Press.

Grant, J. and Marsden, P. (1987) The structure of memorized knowledge in students and clinicians: An explanation for diagnostic expertise. *Medical Education*, **21**, 92–88.

Graves, N. J. (1993) *Learner Managed Learning*. Leeds: World Education Fellowship.

Hedges, J. (1993) Into new life: A reflective account. *Journal of Clinical Nursing*, **2**, 194–195.

Higgs, J. (1992) Developing knowledge: A process of construction, mapping and review. *New Zealand Journal of Physiotherapy*, **20**, 23–30.

Holmes, C. A. (1992) The drama of nursing. *Journal of Advanced Nursing*, **17**, 941–950.

Johns, C. (1995) Framing learning through reflection within Carper's fundamental ways of knowing in nursing. *Journal of Advanced Nursing*, **22**, 226–234.

MacLeod, M. (1990) Experience in everyday nursing practice: A study of 'experienced' ward sisters. *PhD thesis*. University of Edinburgh.

Mattingly, C. (1991) Narrative reflections on practical actions: Two learning experiments in reflective storytelling. In *The Reflective Turn: Case Studies in and on Educational Practice* (D. Schön, ed.), pp. 235–257. London: Teachers College Press.

McAlpine, A., Brown, S., McIntyre, D. and Haggar, H. (1988) *Student–Teachers Learning from Experienced Teachers*. Edinburgh: The Scottish Council for Research in Education.

Miller, A. (1992) From theory to practice. *Journal of Clinical Nursing*, **1**, 295–296.

Mulligan, J. and Griffin, C. (eds) (1992) *Empowerment through experiential learning: Explorations of good practice*. London: Kogan Page.

Norman, G. R. (1988) Problem-solving skills, solving problems, and problem-based learning. *Medical Education*, **22**, 279–286.

Novak, J. D. and Gowin, D. B. (1984) *Learning How to Learn*. Cambridge: Cambridge University Press.

Pearson, A. (1992) *Nursing at Burford: A Story of Change*. Harrow: Scutari.

Pembrey, S. (1980) *The Ward Sister – Key to Nursing*. London: Royal College of Nursing.

Rew, L. and Barrow, E. M. (1987) Intuition: A neglected hallmark of nursing knowledge. *Advances in Nursing Science*, **10**, 49–62.

Robb, A. J. P. and Murray, R. (1992) Medical humanities in nursing: Thought provoking? *Journal of Advanced Nursing*, **17**, 1182–1187.

Runciman, P. J. (1983) *Ward Sister at Work*. London: Churchill Livingstone.

Sandelowski, M. (1991) Telling stories: Narrative approaches in qualitative research. *IMAGE: Journal of Nursing Scholarship*, **23**, 161–166.

Schön, D. A. (1983) *The Reflective Practitioner: How Professionals Think in Action*. London: Temple Smith.

Schön, D. A. (1987) *Educating the Reflective Practitioner*. London: Jossey-Bass.

Smith, M. J. (1992) Enhancing esthetic knowledge: A teaching strategy. *Advances in Nursing Science*, **14**, 52–59.

Thow, M. and Murray R. (1991) Medical humanities in physiotherapy: Education and practice. *Physiotherapy*, **77**, 733–736.

Titchen, A. (1996) A case study of a patient-centred nurse. In *Essential Practice in Patient-Centred Care* (K. W. M. Fulford, S. Ersser and T. Hope, eds), pp. 182–193. Oxford: Blackwell Science.

Titchen, A. (1998a) Professional craft knowledge in patient-centred nursing and the facilitation of its development. *DPhil thesis*. University of Oxford.

Titchen, A. (1998b) *A conceptual framework for facilitating learning in clinical practice*. Occasional Paper 2, Centre for Professional Education Advancement, Faculty of Health Sciences, The University of Sydney

Titchen, A. and Binnie, A. (1993) A 'double-act': Co-action researcher roles in an acute hospital setting. In *Changing Nursing Practice Through Action Research* (A. Titchen, ed.), pp. 19–28. Oxford: National Institute for Nursing.

Titchen, A. and Binnie, A. (1995) The art of clinical supervision. *Journal of Clinical Nursing*, **4**, 327–334.

Uden, G., Norberg, A., Lindseth, A. and Marhaug, V. (1992) Ethical reasoning in nurses' and physicians' stories about care episodes. *Journal of Advanced Nursing*, **17**, 1028–1034.

25

Teaching clinical reasoning to speech and hearing students

Janet Doyle

In this chapter I hope to convince readers of the need for closer examination of the links and distinctions between the teaching and learning of clinical reasoning, on the one hand, and clinical reasoning as practised by clinicians, on the other. I argue for a better data base on which to draw when assisting students to develop clinical reasoning skills consistent with good clinical practice. I also make a related plea for a greater degree of connection between academic activity and clinical practice. The views expressed here have developed from my experience in the field of speech and hearing sciences, as a practising audiologist and as an educator of student speech pathologists. My colleagues Susan Block, Louise Brown, Georgia Dacakis, Jacinta Douglas, Jenni Oates and Shane Thomas have each assisted significantly with the development of some of the thoughts presented.

For the purposes of this chapter, clinical reasoning is defined as the application of relevant knowledge and skills to the evaluation, diagnosis and rehabilitation of client problems (Jones and Butler, 1991). Hence clinical reasoning is an essential aspect of clinician activity. However, clinical reasoning is only part of what may be termed the clinical decision-making system, in which the major and inter-related components are clinician, client, task and environment (Doyle and Thomas, 1988). This concept of a dynamic system acknowledges the natural complexity of the clinical situation, reminding us of the interactive character of these four components.

Each component is also complex in itself. Clinicians have attributes such as knowledge base,

length, type and variety of clinical experience, style of interpersonal interaction, role perception, perceptions of the problem or task, professional ethos, response to environmental constraints and expectations, and clinical reasoning ability. Clients have a similar range of attributes, including their own perceptions of the problem or task. The task has attributes which include explicitness, complexity, familiarity and relationship to other tasks. The environment has attributes such as the prevailing style of clinician–client interaction, physical and financial resources, stated aims and responsibilities of the facility and its funding sources, and decision-making balance between clinicians and administrators. This environment overlaps with the personal environment of the client and family.

Given this framework, clinical reasoning may be seen as an aspect of the clinician component of the complex natural system which is clinical activity. Clinical reasoning involves formulating and then choosing among various options (Hammond *et al.*, 1980), and exercising judgement which is the cognitive process of evaluating those data (Schwartz and Griffin, 1986). Clinical reasoning results in a decision to behave in a certain way.

Clinical reasoning may be further conceptualized in terms of broad cognitive strategy and in terms of how informational cues are used. General cognitive approaches to judgement, such as the 'exhaustive', 'hypothetico-deductive' and 'pattern recognition' strategies, have been proposed. The hypothetico-deductive approach for example, described by Elstein *et al.* (1978), is thought by many decision researchers and clinical educators to be a highly effective general cognitive strategy. Such strategies are not necessarily used consistently by individuals who employ them, the decision strategy possibly varying with the nature of the problem (Politser, 1981). At a more detailed level, clinical reasoning involves the use of clinical data in the form of a range of informational cues. Decision makers use these cues in various ways. Hence, even given the same general cognitive approach to a clinical problem, individuals may weight informational cues differently.

In the context of this chapter the client base of interest comprises persons with communication disorders. Such disorders include problems with articulation, language, fluency, voice, hearing, cognition, social interaction and certain motor functions such as swallowing. Speech pathologists diagnose and treat a broad range of such communication problems. Audiologists diagnose and treat those persons whose communication difficulties primarily lie with hearing loss.

Clinical practice in speech and hearing sciences

It is useful to review some of the characteristics of clinical practice in the field of communication disorders which impinge on the clinical reasoning process and on our attempts to develop the clinical reasoning skills of students. First, the presenting symptoms of persons with communication problems can be diffuse and can involve complex relationships between component communication skills. The fact that an individual's communication is intimately linked to their particular life setting complicates the picture. Diagnosis and treatment may therefore be concurrent processes, each process contributing to the refinement of the other. Additionally, there may be a need to assess and continually evaluate priorities and goals where multiple aspects of communication are involved. These implications for reasoning and clinical practice need to be considered during the teaching or fostering of students' skills of hypothesis generation and treatment selection. Secondly, although the use of technology in speech pathology practice is increasing and has always been a feature of audiology practice, the prime vehicle of assessment in communication disorders remains communication itself. Speech pathologists and audiologists typically must concurrently observe and interact with the client, as well as observing the interaction to which they contribute. Thirdly, as in

other health science areas, there is a range of potentially suitable approaches to the treatment of many communication problems. For example, fluency problems can be treated with an intensive program, or with longer term, intermittent, individual speech therapy, and may be addressed with relaxation, prolongation, delayed auditory feedback and other techniques (Ham, 1986).

Further, the culture of particular clinical environments may influence treatment choice. In a given clinic, there may be a clinic preference for a particular approach to diagnosis and treatment for various problems. For example, the rationale underlying the management of common vocal disorders may be a traditional symptom-based orientation (e.g. Colton and Casper, 1990) in one clinic, and a more global philosophy (e.g. Aronson, 1990), in another. In some areas of communication therapy, treatment given may be overtly connected to the beliefs and cultural values of clinicians and clients. The area of hearing impairment in children, for example, is known for the vigour with which oral versus manual approaches to communication development and rehabilitation are adopted (Schlesinger, 1986).

Implications for teaching clinical reasoning

Given these and other natural complexities associated with clinical practice in speech and hearing sciences, how is clinical reasoning best taught? The general approach at La Trobe University has been one of encouraging the development of reasoning skills by providing opportunities to observe, discuss, exercise and evaluate clinical reasoning. This fostering approach is consistent with that proposed by Gale (1982) and by Higgs (1990).

We attempt to develop clinical reasoning skills through experiential learning. There are three reasons for this. Firstly, we are not convinced that a purely theoretical coverage of clinical reasoning will result in generalization to clinical practice. Secondly, we want to help students to learn to acknowledge that for many communication disorders, several approaches to diagnosis and treatment may be equally valid. Thirdly, the majority of our teaching staff are themselves practising clinicians and this has led to an educational environment which favours an integrated approach to the development of student skills.

One of our key teaching strategies is the use of simulated patients in classroom learning contexts. The goal of these sessions is to enable students to experience their reasoning role and develop their skill in reasoning in a protected, simulated environment which provides them with feedback on their performance and opportunities for discussion and reflection on their reasoning. Such conscious experience of clinical reasoning in a safe environment is complemented by 300 hours of client contact in a range of clinics during the speech pathology course, with the opportunity to observe and benefit from the clinical reasoning of experienced clinicians.

The need for real-world data

In this chapter my concern is to discuss a fundamental problem which applies across much of health science education. This problem is the lack of a comprehensive data base concerning how clinicians reason in practice, drawn from the everyday practice of qualified clinicians, on which we can draw when discussing the notion of good practice in clinical reasoning and to which we can refer for educational purposes.

Data from the real-world practice of speech pathologists and audiologists have the potential to form an invaluable feedback loop, connecting academic activity and student learning to clinical practice. So how best to gather data to provide the necessary description of clinical reasoning as it occurs in practice? There is good reason to believe that research on clinical reasoning is best conducted in the real world of clinical practice, rather than in the laboratory, or in the university teaching clinic. Although the latter settings offer opportunities to refine the knowledge gained by studies of real-world practice, they cannot be assumed to yield data which generalize to everyday practice of qualified speech pathologists and audiologists. The settings are often simply too different. In general, the external validity of research findings conducted in laboratory settings and those derived purely from the study of hypothetical cases is questionable (Ebbeson and Konecni, 1980; Thomas *et al.*, 1990).

This finding might also apply to the use of simulated patients to study clinical reasoning. Colleagues and I have provided a review of the problem as it pertains to the clinical situation (Thomas *et al.*, 1990). Two main points were made in this review. The first was that the methodology used to study as well as to teach clinical reasoning and decision making in controlled settings may yield data that do not relate well to clinical

behaviour in natural settings. Judgement behaviour in simulated Patient Management Problems, for example, may differ from that in the real clinic (Goran *et al.*, 1973; Page and Fielding, 1980). Therefore, we would assert that it is possible that both student and practising speech pathologists and audiologists might behave differently in laboratory and natural settings.

The second major point made by Thomas *et al.* (1990) was that clinical reasoning in natural settings may be influenced by a range of factors simply not encountered in controlled settings. These factors include sociological influences (Eisenberg, 1979), stress (Bourbonnais and Baumann, 1985; Cleland, 1967; Lippincott, 1979) and time pressures (Doyle, 1989; Meggs and Doyle, 1992). It is important, then, that more research be carried out in natural field settings if we are to develop a good description of the clinical reasoning behaviour of practitioners. Natural field settings contain the complexity of problems as encountered by decision makers (Wigton, 1988). Such field studies are appropriate to the discovery and prediction of decision behaviour (Carroll and Johnson, 1990), allow researchers to select those tasks which are representative of the clinical practice under study, and have the potential to establish the prevalence of heuristics and treatment decisions (Hershey and Baron, 1987).

Not only should we study clinical reasoning in the real clinic, but we should study practising clinicians. To date, many studies of clinical reasoning and decision making have used students instead of, or in addition to, practising clinicians. This practice is not valid if we wish to study what clinicians do when they are no longer students. It is important to avoid confusing the study of student learning with the study of practitioners' clinical reasoning.

A study of practising audiologists' decisions

I will now briefly describe a study of practising audiologists' reasoning and decisions conducted by the author and colleague Shane Thomas. The study addressed a common, and presumably relatively simple, clinical task: whether or not to recommend hearing aid amplification. Subjects were 16 Australian audiologists (eight females and eight males). Assessing client suitability for hearing aid amplification was known to be a normal part of the client practice of each audiologist. Each of the 16 audiologists was asked to study the same set of 80 cases (70 different cases and 10 which were repeated for purposes of assessing reliability) and in each case to note whether they would recommend hearing aid amplification. They were not asked to make any decisions about hearing aid style or electroacoustic characteristics. Each audiologist made his or her recommendations independently, over two sessions.

The cases were designed to be representative of naturally occurring cases. This was achieved by using audiograms from real clients and including information which audiologists were known to seek in consultations with clients (Doyle, 1990). The presentation of each case was in a format typical of audiological data and the task was constructed to be typical of cases encountered by the audiologists in clinical practice.

There were six informational cues embedded in each case. These were the average pure tone loss (Cue 1), the hearing threshold at 2000 Hz (Cue 2), the slope of the hearing loss (Cue 3), speech discrimination ability (Cue 4), the degree of hearing difficulty reported by the client (Cue 5) and the client's attitude towards aiding (Cue 6). We were interested to discover how practicing audiologists utilized these cues to reach the decision, the degree of agreement among audiologists and whether any differences could be explained by different clinical reasoning, even though they were given exactly the same data. The methodological

difficulty remained that audiologist behaviour might be different if faced with real clients, rather than representations of real clients. However, the study had potential to compare the clinical reasoning of individual practising audiologists for the same typical problem.

The results were quite startling. As shown in the left hand column of Table 25.1, the number of cases for which aiding was recommended ranged from 15 to 61. In general there was only a moderate level of agreement ($r = 0.49$) among the 16 audiologists.

To determine how informational cues were used by individual audiologists to reach these obviously different decisions, estimates were calculated, for each audiologist, of the standardized discriminant coefficients (Klecka, 1975) with the six cues as the discriminating variables and the yes/no hearing aid recommendation as the criterion variable. Table 25.1 shows the standardized canonical discriminant function coefficients for each of the six cues, by audiologist. The relative importance of each type of information is indicated by the size of the coefficient. For example, the data for audiologist 4 show that Cue 2 (the client's hearing threshold at 2000 Hz) had a coefficient of 1.03781, much greater than any other cue. Thus, as the value of the 2000 Hz threshold changed, so was the audiologist's opinion about aiding likely to change. Cases in which there was a severe loss of hearing at the 2000 Hz

Table 25.1 Hearing aid decisions and standardized discriminant function coefficients for judgement of cues, by audiologist

	Aiding recommendation		Average pure tone loss	2 KHz threshold	Cues		Client report	Client attitude
	No	Yes			Slope	Speech discrimination		
1	34	36	0.40573	0.39373	0.08212	−0.03289	0.38748	−0.53281
2	17	53	−0.42598	−0.57532	0.02330	0.48327	0.11636	0.41898
3	27	43	0.44732	0.45263	0.09631	0.07485	−0.01130	−0.64250
4	12	58	−0.11984	1.03781	0.06710	−0.5794	0.02834	−0.22561
5	22	48	0.04020	0.83323	0.01949	−0.18647	0.57289	−0.08584
6	21	49	0.19160	0.87474	0.10924	−0.16406	−0.08907	−0.12914
7	11	59	0.05142	0.48066	−0.08496	0.12464	0.88089	−0.34551
8	23	47	0.07032	0.91362	0.05259	−0.33148	−0.08500	−0.22129
9	9	61	−0.09846	0.93606	0.01689	0.03107	0.59053	0.16070
10	24	46	0.21373	−0.58749	−0.01680	0.02001	−0.16698	0.87141
11	15	55	−0.04677	0.97282	0.05971	−0.06532	0.16111	−0.22139
12	55	15	1.48515	−0.84557	−0.28671	−0.10670	0.18838	−0.34628
13	14	56	−0.12367	0.95520	−0.01013	−0.14080	0.35265	−0.35495
14	24	46	−0.32679	0.89558	0.01931	−0.01569	0.37650	−0.69859
15	11	59	0.47770	0.02033	−0.14068	−0.30489	0.55652	−0.60312
16	33	37	0.59132	0.45346	0.17251	0.10975	0.35282	0.06977

frequency would very probably be recommended for aiding, whereas cases in which hearing at 2000 Hz was relatively good would not. In contrast, changes in the values of other cues, such as Cue 5 (the degree of hearing difficulty reported by the client) were not likely to influence audiologist 4's recommendation. Whether the client reported little or great difficulty hearing mattered hardly at all in the clinical reasoning of this particular audiologist.

A classification analysis (Norusis, 1988) showed that the discriminant functions describing audiologists' policies were robust, with a mean correct classification rate of 89.9%. Thus audiologists' different recommendations for the same cases were not the result of any random behaviour, but of highly predictable, yet individualistic, patterns of clinical reasoning.

This demonstration of individualistic decision-making approaches is consistent with general observations of clinical practice. For example, Yeend and Dillon (1992) who found that, at least within NAL Hearing Centres, different audiologists made very different recommendations regarding fitting people with milder losses.

Implications of different clinical approaches for practice and teaching

The fact that individual clinicians may apply clinical reasoning in different ways to particular decision tasks is not surprising, given that outcomes of our intervention are frequently not easy to predict. If decision outcome is likely to be variable and related to a number of interacting factors, it is unlikely that clinicians can readily develop their reasoning based on a knowledge of typical outcomes. In the absence of this knowledge, a range of potentially adequate approaches to the problem develop. Lack of data linking the outcomes of our decisions with the clinical reasoning which resulted in those decisions means that we do not have the ready means of deciding whether one clinical reasoning approach is better than another. This is a significant problem for clinicians such as speech pathologists and audiologists, who deal routinely with questions for which there is no single, obviously correct solution.

What constitutes a good outcome for a particular client? This is by no means an easy question to answer. To continue with the example of hearing aid amplification, the question of what constitutes an adequate or optimal hearing aid fitting has not

been systematically addressed by audiologists. Demorest (1986) considers that because the benefit of hearing aid fitting has not been clearly defined, there can be disagreement about criteria for an adequate solution to the task of providing amplification. In the absence of generally agreed outcome criteria, the task remains ill-defined because it is not clear whether or not a solution has been reached (Miller *et al.*, 1960).

Regardless of the criteria used to judge the adequacy of hearing aid fitting, there is some evidence suggesting that optimal results may not be the norm (Goldstein, 1984; Gray-Thompson and Richards, 1987; Upfold and Smither, 1981; Upfold and Wilson, 1980). Can this situation be linked to variation in clinical reasoning approaches? We cannot know this if we have not yet agreed on what is the benefit to be expected, if we do not do more outcome studies, and if we do not study the clinical reasoning of the practitioners involved.

What does this all mean for educators? Which of the 16 audiologists shown in Table 25.1 has the correct approach to the problem of assessing a client's need and suitability for hearing aid amplification? Is there a single correct approach, or a set of equally correct approaches? Which approach(es) serve(s) as a good model for student audiologists and speech pathologists? How should we use this information to inform our teaching? There is much to be done if we are to first adequately describe what we do, then study the optimality of the decisions resulting from our clinical reasoning and finally feed that information back into our teaching programs.

In summary, we need to describe the clinical reasoning and decisions of practising clinicians (in this case, speech pathologists and audiologists), to examine reasoning and the resultant decisions in terms of optimal client outcomes. Then we can consider what aspects of clinician behaviour are important to foster among student clinicians. In the meantime it is important to provide opportunities, in the clinic and in the classroom, for students to develop cognitive strategies, such as effective hypothesis generation and testing, that are known to be associated, at least in the case of experts, with accurate and efficient decision making.

Acknowledgements

This is a condensed version of the chapter by the same title and author, which appeared in the first edition of this text. Our thanks to Joan Rosenthal who assisted in the revision of this chapter. The table is derived from the first edition.

References

Aronson, A. E. (1990) *Clinical Voice Disorders*, 3rd edn. New York: Thieme.

Bourbonnais, F. F. and Baumann, A. (1985) Stress and rapid decision-making in nursing: An administrative challenge. *Nursing Administration Quarterly*, 9, 85–91.

Carroll, J. S. and Johnson, E. J. (1990) *Decision Research: A Field Guide (Applied Social Research Methods Series, Vol. 22)*. Newbury Park, CA: Sage.

Cleland, V. S. (1967) Effects of stress on thinking. *American Journal of Nursing*, 1, 108–111.

Colton, R. H. and Casper, J. K. (1990) *Understanding Voice Problems: A Physiological Perspective for Diagnosis and Treatment*. Baltimore, MD: Williams & Wilkins.

Demorest, M. E. (1986) Problem solving: Stages, strategies and stumbling blocks. *Journal of the Academy of Rehabilitative Audiology*, 19, 13–26.

Doyle, J. (1989) A survey of Australian audiologists' clinical decision-making. *Australian Journal of Audiology*, 11, 75–88.

Doyle, J. (1990) Talk, Test and Tempt: What Happens in Audiological Consultations. Paper presented to the *9th National Conference of the Audiological Society of Australia*. The Audiological Society of Australia, Thredbo, NSW.

Doyle, J. and Thomas, S. A. (1988) Clinical decision-making in audiology: The case for investigating what we do. *Australian Journal of Audiology*, 10, 45–56.

Ebbeson, E. B. and Konecni, V. J. (1980) On the external validity of decision-making research: What do we know about decisions in the real world? In *Cognitive Processes in Choice and Decision Behaviour* (T. S. Wallsten, ed.), pp. 21–45. Hillsdale, NJ: Lawrence Erlbaum.

Eisenberg, J. M. (1979) Sociologic influences on decision-making by clinicians. *Annals of Internal Medicine*, 90, 957–964.

Elstein, A. S., Shulman, L. S. and Sprafka, S. A. (1978) *Medical Problem Solving: An Analysis of Clinical Reasoning*. Cambridge, MA: Harvard University Press.

Gale, J. (1982) Some cognitive components of the diagnostic thinking process. *British Journal of Educational Psychology*, 52, 64–76.

Goldstein, D. P. (1984) Hearing impairment, hearing aids and audiology. *ASHA*, 26, 24–38.

Goran, M. J., Williamson, J. W. and Gonnella, J. S. (1973) The validity of patient management problems. *Journal of Medical Education*, 48, 171–177.

Gray-Thompson, M. and Richards, S. (1987) A computer program for hearing aid selection: Its trial and development. *Australian Journal of Audiology*, 9, 19–23.

Ham, R. (1986) *Techniques of Stuttering Therapy*. Englewood Cliffs, NJ: Prentice-Hall.

Hammond, K. R., McClelland, G. H. and Mumpower, J. (1980) *Human Judgment and Decision-Making: Theories, Methods, and Procedures*. New York: Praeger.

Hershey, J. C. and Baron, J. (1987) Clinical reasoning and cognitive processes. *Medical Decision Making*, 7, 203–211.

Higgs, J. (1990) Fostering the acquisition of clinical reasoning skills. *New Zealand Journal of Physiotherapy*, 18, 13–17.

Jones, M. A. and Butler, D. S. (1991) Clinical reasoning. In *Mobilisation of the Nervous System* (D. S. Butler, ed.), pp. 91–106. Melbourne: Churchill Livingstone.

Klecka, W. R. (1975) Discriminant analysis. In *Statistical Package for the Social Sciences*, 2nd edn (N. H. Nie, C. H. Hull, J. G. Jenkins, K. Steinbrenner and D. H. Bent, eds), pp. 434–467. New York: McGraw-Hill.

Lippincott, R. C. (1979) Psychological stress factors in decision-making. *Heart and Lung*, 8, 1093–1097.

Meggs, C. and Doyle, J. (1992) Job satisfaction. *Australian Communication Quarterly*, Spring, 12–15.

Miller, G. A., Galanter, E. and Pribram, K. H. (1960) *Plans and the Structure of Behaviour*. New York: Rinehart & Winston.

Norusis, M. J. (1988) *SPSS-X Advanced Statistics Guide*. Chicago: SPSS Inc.

Page, G. G. and Fielding, D. W. (1980) Performance on PMPs and performance in practice: are they related? *Journal of Medical Education*, 55, 529–537.

Politser, P. (1981) Decision strategies and clinical judgment. *Medical Decision Making*, 1, 361–389.

Schlesinger, H. (1986) Total communication in perspective. In *Deafness in Perspective* (D. M. Lutterman, ed.). London: Taylor & Francis.

Schwartz, S. and Griffin, T. (1986) *Medical Thinking: The Psychology of Medical Judgment and Decision-Making*. New York: Springer.

Thomas, S. A., Doyle, J. and Browning, C. (1990) Clinical decision making: What do we know about real world performance? In *Judgment and Decision Making* (W. H. Loke, ed.). Chicago: Scarecrow Press.

Upfold, L. J. and Smither, M. F. (1981) Hearing aid fitting protocol. *British Journal of Audiology*, 115, 181–188.

Upfold, L. J. and Wilson, D. A. (1980) Hearing aid distribution and use in Australia: The Australian Bureau of Statistics 1978 survey. *Australian Journal of Audiology*, 2, 31–36.

Wigton, R. S. (1988) Use of linear models to analyze physicians' decisions. *Medical Decision Making*, 8, 241–252.

Yeend, I. and Dillon, H. (1992) Minimum aidable loss in infants and primary school aged children. Paper presented to the *10th National Conference of the Audiological Society of Australia*. The Audiological Society of Australia, Barossa Valley, South Australia.

26

Teaching clinical decision analysis in physiotherapy

Nancy Watts

Clinical reasoning is a complex and variable process composed of a series of interdependent steps. Each step in the process calls for a somewhat different type of judgemental skill, and each is guided by a complex blend of experience-based intuition and theory-based logic. One way to appreciate the challenges of clinical decision making is to reflect on a few of the many ways it can go wrong.

Some of the most common and serious judgemental errors clinicians make are described in Table 26.1. They have been labelled 'sins' to emphasize that they may be committed not only by novice therapists whose judgemental skills are still being formed but also by highly experienced graduates who clearly know better.

Clinical decision analysis provides a demanding but powerful antidote to such flawed short-cuts in judgement. Developed originally by business planners (Raiffa, 1968) and adapted in recent years for application to health care (Weinstein *et al.*, 1980), decision analysis provides a systematic method for choosing a course of action when the goals of action are important, the costs significant and logical choice difficult because many of the factors that may influence outcomes are unknown or cannot be assessed with certainty.

For a complete analysis six different steps are required: defining the decision problem, defining successful and unsuccessful outcomes, describing several alternative courses of action and their possible consequences, estimating the probability that each possible consequence actually will occur, estimating the costs of alternative approaches, and selecting the strategy that promises the best combination of high effectiveness and low costs.

Table 26.1 Seven deadly sins of clinical decision making

Vagueness	The purpose of evaluation or treatment is unclear. The wisdom of decisions cannot be judged because it is uncertain what they are intended to accomplish or how soon desired results should be achieved.
Narrowness	Alternative methods are seldom considered. If a familiar approach seems effective, little effort is made to identify others that might be even better.
Rigidity	Standardized regimens of evaluation and treatment are routinely used with little regard for important differences in individual patient needs and response. Reactions to treatment are not monitored to detect unexpected results.
Irrationality	Choices are based on habit, convenience, subjective impressions and the charisma of individuals who endorse specific techniques rather than on objective evidence and tested theory.
Wastefulness	Evaluations are extensive, but results have little influence on selection of treatment. Elaborate treatment techniques are used without considering whether less costly methods might be equally effective.
Insensitivity	Personal values and psycho-social concerns of patients and families are ignored. Improvement in physical performance is given higher priority than enhanced quality of life.
Mystery	The process used to arrive at decisions cannot be explained in terms patients and colleagues can understand. Others cannot question or contribute to this process.

Detailed descriptions of these steps and practice exercises to help clinicians learn to perform them have been developed for physicians (Weinstein *et al.*, 1980). Less detailed descriptions show how the method can be applied by physical therapists (Coogler, 1985; Francis 1988; Watts, 1985; Watts, 1989).

Complete decision analyses have much to offer fields such as physical therapy, particularly as tools for applying research to practice and for comparing alternative approaches to treatment in areas of controversy. However, for the individual clinician a complete analysis is too laborious an undertaking to be practical as a means of making the host of different decisions a busy day of practice involves. Fortunately, the component steps of decision analysis still have great utility even if they are used separately or are incorporated into other decision-making approaches. These steps represent practical and logical ways of thinking about patient care and they can be readily incorporated into both the academic and clinical education of students.

Component skills and illustrative teaching methods

Identifying alternatives

Clinical problem solving often is seen as a logical, linear process that leads step-by-step to the right answers for important clinical questions. Such thinking may be called convergent for it pulls together a wide range of information to arrive at a decision about the cause of the patient's problem or the best way to prevent or solve it. Important as it is, however, this type of clinical decision making must be linked with a second, very different, type of thinking in order to be really useful. Referred to by such names as divergent thinking, imagination, creativity, synthesis and lateral thinking this complementary process emphasizes not the selection of the best answer to a question but the richness of the alternatives to be considered before a choice is made. Among the decision-making tasks in which this type of thinking is most important are generating competing diagnostic hypotheses, redesigning treatment for the patient who fails to progress as expected, and finding ways to adapt and improvise treatment without sacrificing effectiveness when time, space, equipment or support services are unsually limited.

Both classroom and clinical teachers can model this component of problem solving in their lectures and conversations with students by pointing out alternative explanations of the problems they discuss and by suggesting a variety of options for intervention. However, the most powerful tool for helping students learn to do this type of thinking for themselves is the question that has more than one 'right' answer. Such questions ask the student to originate ideas and design alternatives by:

- Suggesting alternative explanations: 'What else might account for that?'.
- Predicting diverse possible outcomes: 'Can you think of anything different that might happen?'.
- Proposing varied options for action: 'Is there any other way you might be able to accomplish the same thing?'.

A wealth of references are available for teachers interested in learning more about divergent thinking and its role in practical problem solving. Among the most readable and thought provoking of these are the books by Edward de Bono (1971, 1976, 1978). Abundant ideas on how to formulate questions and manage discussions in order to stimulate student use of specific thinking skills also are provided by the education literature (Christensen *et al.*, 1991; Hyman, 1979; Sanders, 1966; Watts, 1990).

However, success in teaching students to generate alternatives depends on more than an ability to formulate provocative questions. It also often requires patience and flexibility on the part of the teacher in evaluating and responding to student responses. Some of the alternatives they suggest may seem incompletely thought through, naïve or impractical. Others may propose explanations or courses of action with which the instructor is not familiar. Clearly, major errors in reasoning should not go uncorrected. Particularly in working with beginning students, however, minor flaws may need to be ignored, unfamiliar ideas treated with respect and positive feedback be given to what is sound in their suggestions. Premature emphasis on finding the best answer can block student development of confidence and skill in the essential process of identifying alternatives. Helping students master both convergent and divergent thinking requires teachers to have a vision of the purpose of questioning which is broad enough to include both the logical search for right answers and the creative search for new ideas.

Contingency planning

Even the most carefully designed initial plans for

evaluation and treatment often need revision once they are put into effect. As a case evolves new dimensions of the problem may surface, unexpected responses may occur, and the actions of other care-givers may alter what we need to accomplish or are free to attempt. As students learn to identify possible alternatives they also can be encouraged to look ahead, to consider how they will respond if they encounter obstacles, problems . . . or surprising success. This sort of 'What if . . .' thinking is far more complex than simply suggesting alternatives for a single specific decision or response. It involves visualizing a series of inter-related choices which are spread out over time and associated with multiple possible consequences.

The decision-tree diagrams used in decision analysis are one device for keeping track of these alternatives and for comparing them with one another. The format for a decision tree follows several simple conventions. A branching tree is drawn lying on its side with key events shown from left to right across the page in the order in which they are expected to occur. A square indicates each point at which a choice must be made between two or more alternatives for action, and circles show the points at which at least two possible consequences of an action will become known. Lines branching out from these choice and chance points carry short labels describing the options to be considered and consequences that may be seen. Decision trees give us a common language for describing different approaches, and they encourage us to anticipate possible problems and prepare contingency plans for revising care if this proves necessary.

Guiding questions once again play an important part in helping students and recent graduates develop contingency planning skills. In discussions of either real or hypothetical cases the novices are first asked to describe the initial course of action they propose and the results they hope this will produce. Follow-up questions then explore alternative scenarios. As these are developed they can be added to the original plan using a decision tree diagram. For example, one segment of such a discussion with a student preparing to begin post-operative treatment of a patient who has just undergone a total knee replacement might go like this:

● *Instructor*: Let's talk about how you think you'll want to manage this patient between now and the time he goes home. From your examination and review of his chart you know he is a healthy, 58-year-old man whose knee problems were a result of repeated injuries while playing soccer when he was at university. You have identified his main problems as decreased range of motion, poor muscle control of knee extension and pain which limits his active movement. What do you think you'd like to do when you treat him today?

● *Student*: Well, it's just the first day after his surgery and since he doesn't have any discomfort at rest and there are only minimal signs of inflammation, I guess I'd start him off on the level 1 exercise program we were taught at school: quadriceps setting, active assisted motion through the pain-free range and assisted straight leg raising while he's wearing a knee splint. His upper extremities, hip and lung function are very good so he won't need any particular exercises there.

● *Instructor*: OK. Let's record that this way:

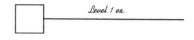

How long would you plan to continue with that? When do you think you might want to move on to something else?

● *Student*: Pretty soon I guess. As soon as he's doing OK with these easy exercises I'd advance him to the level 2 ones.

● *Instructor*: What do you mean by 'doing OK?' Can you be a little more specific about what you want to see him do before you advance to level 2 and tell me how soon you expect he'll reach that point?

● *Student*: Well, the paper on total knee patients we were assigned said that by the second day the patient should have at least 35 degrees of motion with minimal discomfort and be able to do several straight leg lifts without help. If he could do that I'd go on to level 2 the second day.

● *Instructor*: All right, let's show that on the tree this way:

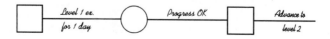

This questioning process is continued until the student's initial plan has been described and diagrammed up to the expected time of discharge from the hospital. Then:

- *Instructor*: That seems like a reasonable plan if your patient responds the way we hope he will. But let's go back and think about what you'll do if things don't turn out quite that way. For example, suppose when you see him the second day your patient complains of severe pain almost as soon as he begins to flex the knee. What would you do then?

Subsequent questions would be designed to help the student identify such contingencies and decide what changes in the original plan may be needed if they occur. As these are added to the decision tree the segment shown earlier might evolve into a branching pattern such as this:

ress have been different from what was expected.

The focus in all of these discussions and tree drawing exercises is on identifying key points at which progress should be assessed, on predicting some of the different ways in which individual patients may respond and on deciding how such differences should influence the course of treatment. Some students will find this easier if they are reminded that the alternatives to be considered usually fall into one of a limited number of generic categories. For example, in considering alternatives for action early in a decision tree the options usually include two or more of the following:

- *Evaluation*: gather further information about the patient or the treatment situation and evaluate it

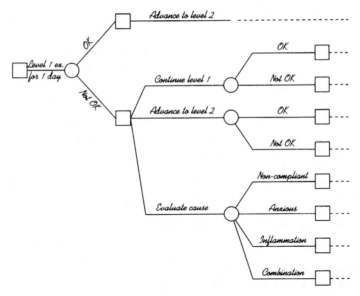

The example shown here is a rather simple one, representative of the way we might use decision trees to teach an inexperienced student. At a more advanced level more complex patients can be chosen for discussion, the student can be given less explicit guidance in identifying important contingencies, and more time can be spent in discussing the rationale for interpretation of different responses and in critiquing proposals for alternative action. A similar approach can be used to reflect on cases that have been treated already. This is particularly worthwhile when these cases have created particular problems or where patterns of progress

- *Intervention*: begin treatment on the basis of the information already available
- *Waiting*: delay action for a specified period of time and then review the situation to decide whether to evaluate, intervene, wait longer or do nothing
- *Do nothing*: in many cases this is combined with providing an explanation to the patient and referring colleague, or making a referral.

In deciding how to follow-up on the patient's initial response, if things go well we might:

- *Continue* what we have been doing without change.

- *Do more* of the same thing to see if that works even better.
- *Do less* to see if we can get the same results more easily.
- *Do something different* to see if it is easier or more effective.

On the other hand, if the initial response is unsatisfactory we might:

- *Keep trying* the same thing a little longer
- *Try harder*: do more of the same thing
- *Try something else* to see if it gets better results
- *Evaluate* WHY the response is not as good as expected
- *Ask for help* while we either stop doing anything further ourselves or continue with one of the other options.

These categories are too general to be adequate as a basis for detailed planning. However, reminding the student of them sometimes helps in identifying specific options that might otherwise be overlooked.

Predicting results and coping with uncertainty

Hypothesis testing is an important component of many logical systems of decision making. However, unless such testing is done with realistic caution it can easily be misleading. The source of this problem lies in the many differences that exist between the scientific laboratory and the clinical world. As Bursztajn and his colleagues point out (Bursztajn *et al.*, 1981), 'for every observed effect the scientist seeks to isolate a specific cause or set of causes, as if it alone can account for the effect'.

However, the clinical world is too chaotic for such simplistic assumptions to hold true on a consistent basis. The clinician has only limited ability to identify, isolate, control and manipulate all the factors that may influence the effects of treatment. Many clinical phenomena have multiple causes and causal relationships may be influenced by a confusing array of individual differences among patients, therapists and treatment situations. Our students need to learn that theories and hypotheses represent at best our educated guesses about what will happen when we use different therapeutic methods. We also can help them learn how to cope with this uncertainty and how to reduce it.

Decision analysis recognizes the uncertainty of clinical expectations by assigning quantitative probability estimates to all chance point branches on a decision tree. These estimates express the clinician's strength of belief that each of the consequences identified as possible at that point actually will occur. For example, in the segment of the decision tree shown earlier the probability of this patient responding badly to the level 1 exercises seems low. Yet this certainly is not impossible. We might then decide to assign a 90% probability to the 'OK' branch after the first circle and only a 10% probability to the branch for 'not OK'. On the other hand, if the patient's initial response is unsatisfactory, the likelihood that simply continuing the same treatment will remedy the situation seems low. At that chance point we might then assign only a 30% probability of an 'OK' response and say there is a 70% chance the response will remain problematic.

Assigning such definite quantitative values to our expectations is an unfamiliar and somewhat intimidating process for many clinicians despite the fact that all clinical choices are based on some type of assessment about the probability of success associated with the treatment alternatives we consider. These estimates usually are expressed by using qualifying terms rather than numbers: 'There's very little risk of a bad side effect here'; 'I think this patient is going to be a problem'; 'This approach usually gets results'. The advantages of quantitative estimates are that they reduce the ambiguity of terms such as 'usually', facilitate comparison of alternative approaches, and confront us forcefully with the need to examine the sources of our beliefs about what to expect. Probability estimates, both quantitative and qualitative, draw on three quite different sources of guidance: the clinician's own experience with similar cases, objective data from directly related clinical research or quality assurance outcome studies and the logical application of less directly related, but still relevant, basic and applied science theory. Students can be helped to make intelligent use of all three sources by using teaching methods such as these:

- Encouraging analysis of opposing points of view and discussion of the strengths, weaknesses, contradictions and unanswered questions that exist in research currently available on a clinical method.
- Emphasizing major factors that may alter, interfere with or enhance the usual pattern of response to each intervention we teach.

- Including a major emphasis in courses on scientific method on topics such as external validity, the use of meta-analysis (Norton and Strube, 1989) and the questions to be answered in research utilization (Stetler and Marram, 1976).
- Arranging for students to take part in quality assurance programs that set minimum acceptable outcome standards for use in auditing the actual results of care.
- Setting aside time during the student's clinical experience for repeated contact with a number of patients who share a similar disorder or complaint and arranging for the student to stay in contact with at least a few patients long enough to see first hand how their progress varies.

Such experiences as these will not teach the student to carry out the interesting statistical analyses of combined probabilities that have attracted such attention in the medical literature on clinical decision analysis. They will, however, foster students' recognition of the uncertainty that surrounds many clinical decisions and help them deal with that uncertainty in a way that can make their future practice more realistic.

Conclusion

The teaching methods outlined in this chapter represent only a tiny sample of the many ways students can be taught to use components of decision analysis methodology in their day-to-day work with patients. The list of decision analysis components discussed is equally incomplete. Among the other steps that deserve equal attention are:

- Analysis of the costs of care.
- Assignment of values or utility ratings to the possible outcomes of a clinical decision.
- Determination of the best strategies for evaluation of patients and critical analysis of how clinical data are used as a basis for practical decisions.
- Comparison of the overall cost-effectiveness of different approaches
- Collaboration with patients to incorporate their preferences and concerns in the decision-making process
- Specifying a basis for evaluating the results of treatment.

None of the component skills of decision analysis can be fully mastered in the time available for entry level education. Graduate clinicians, including those of us responsible for teaching students, will need to continue work on clinical decision making methods throughout our careers. Effective clinical decision making is a difficult job. Fortunately engagement in the process also is contagious. As you do your best to help students learn such component skills as the ones discussed here, you may be pleasantly surprised to find how much you are learning yourself.

References

Bursztajn, H., Feinbloom, R. I., Hamm, R. M. and Brodsky, A. (1981) *Medical Choices, Medical Chances: How Patients, Families, and Physicians can Cope with Uncertainty*. New York: Delacorte Press/Seymour Lawrence.

Christensen, C. R., Garvin, D. A. and Sweet, A. (eds) (1991) *Education for Judgment: The Artistry of Discussion Leadership*. Boston, MA: Harvard Business School Press.

Coogler, C. E. (1985) Clinical decision making among neurologic patients: Spinal cord injury. In *Clinical Decision Making in Physical Therapy* (S. L. Wolf, ed.), pp. 149–170. Philadelphia, PA: F. A. Davis.

de Bono, E. (1971) *The Use of Lateral Thinking*. Harmondsworth: Penguin Books,

de Bono, E. (1976) *Practical Thinking*. Harmondsworth: Penguin Books.

de Bono, E. (1978) *Teaching Thinking*. Harmondsworth: Penguin Books.

Francis, K. (1988) Computer communication: Decision analysis using a spread sheet. *Physical Therapy*, **68**, 1409–1410.

Hyman, R. T. (1979) *Strategic Questioning*. Englewood Cliffs, NJ: Prentice-Hall.

Norton, B. J. and Strube, M. J. (1989) Making decisions based on group designs and meta-analysis. *Physical Therapy*, **69**, 594–600.

Raiffa, H. (1968) *Decision Analysis: Introductory Lectures on Choices under Uncertainty*. Reading, MA: Addison-Wesley.

Sanders, N. (1966) *Classroom Questions, What Kinds?* New York: Harper & Row

Stetler, C. and Marram, G. (1976) Evaluating research findings for applicability in practice. *Nursing Outlook*, **24**, 559–563.

Watts, N. T. (1985) Decision analysis: A tool for improving physical therapy practice and education. In *Clinical Decision Making in Physical Therapy* (S. L. Wolf, ed.), pp. 7–23. Philadelphia, PA: F. A. Davis.

Watts, N. T. (1989) Clinical decision analysis. *Physical Therapy*, **69**, 569–579.

Watts, N. T. (1990) *Handbook of Clinical Teaching*. Edinburgh: Churchill Livingstone.

Weinstein, M. C., Fineberg, H. V., Elstein, A. S., Frazier, H. S., Neuhauser, D., Neutra, R. R. and McNeil, B. J. (1980) *Clinical Decision Analysis*. Philadelphia, PA: Saunders.

27

Facilitating the clinical reasoning of occupational therapy students on fieldwork placement

Susan Ryan

Our understanding of clinical reasoning development is currently being enhanced by world-wide research studies in occupational therapy. Also, different models of fieldwork are presently being proposed, as well as other creative ways to enhance professional thinking, such as practicums, laboratories and studios. More and more current thinking is focusing on the different forms of knowledge required for practice (e.g. Higgs and Titchen, 1995). In addition, more attention is being given to exploring ways of using the existing fieldwork forum more creatively to enhance the clinical reasoning skills of both practising therapists and students. It is recognized that in fieldwork settings there are many experiential learning opportunities which can be used to better advantage. To make best use of these, educators working in these settings need to be knowledgeable about different approaches to learning and clinical reasoning, both of which are highly context dependent. Because clinical reasoning is a process of reflective inquiry involving thinking, reasoning and reflecting, the teaching of clinical reasoning needs to be placed within a reflective framework.

The first section of this chapter examines issues in the profession of occupational therapy and in the nature of fieldwork that have a direct bearing on the facilitation or restriction of clinical reasoning abilities. The second section examines the development of the reasoning process from a student's perspective during the fieldwork experience. The reflective framework recommended for these ideas is the three-stage model proposed by Boud and Walker (1991). This model frames the entire experience, including preparation beforehand, reflection during and discussion after the placement.

Professional issues

Practice in occupational therapy is changing rapidly in most countries. There is a move away from working in short-stay hospital settings towards working in specific community programs such as rest homes, day centres and activity programs, people's homes, doctors' surgeries, community centres, schools, correction centres, and industrial settings. Such environments demand that the therapy program be congruent with the needs of the people in the setting and therapists should be able to explain their reasoning underpinning any program.

In addition to the context changes, the focus of health care is shifting towards prevention rather than predominantly intervention. This movement encourages social and occupational-based ways of working rather than medically focused strategies. Therefore different ideas must be generated, different abilities and skills are needed, and consequently different thinking and reasoning are required. In fact, the whole perception of practice around occupation is being challenged.

Because of these new orientations to practice, old ways of working will be scrutinized and new creative ideas will need to be nourished. Interdependent learning which benefits the experienced therapist as well as the student is needed. Newer, more flexible ways of reasoning will predominate in emerging practice settings. Linear, reductionist ways of reasoning, stemming from the epistemology of cognitive and medical science, increasingly need to be replaced by fluid incremental reasoning strategies as described by Higgs and Jones (1995, p. 6), to suit this new orientation to working.

Mattingly and Fleming (1994) observe that occupational therapists use at least four[1] forms of reasoning in physically-oriented rehabilitation practice: procedural, interactive, conditional and narrative reasoning. This classification is now being challenged by Chapparo (1997) who found that therapists think about more than three things and she states they have potentially a 'five-track mind' They think about (1) the illness, diagnosis and disability, (2) the whole client/carer situation, (3) the therapy context and environment, (4) their own personal beliefs and expectations of therapy, and (5) the degree to which they felt they were able to actualize what was needed to be done. Chapparo's research found that any one of the these tracks had the potential to influence decision making which means that therapists use a multi-dimensional inductive-hypothetical-deductive reasoning style.

All these approaches are also moderated pragmatically according to the setting (Schell and Cervero, 1993). Clinical reasoning studies in other settings, such as mental health, are only now receiving attention (McKay, 1996). By examining these studies carefully the reader can begin to understand the type(s) of clinical reasoning the therapist is using and can begin to question the reasons for these choices. These works also show clearly whether the therapist is using prevention strategies as well as remedial or management interventions.

This diversity of practice has implications for fieldwork because of the different placements a student may experience. Studies in the 1980s in medicine and nursing (Maxim and Dielman, 1987; Patel and Cranton, 1983; Tanner *et al.*, 1987) showed that certain ways of reasoning can be generalized while others are specific to the context. It was found that interpersonal skills, technical skills, attitude to health care, selection of data, history and interview skills, and professional responsibility fell in the category of generalized

---

[1] Fleming identified three tracks in occupational therapy clinical reasoning. Mattingly added a fourth, narrative framing.

skills. In contrast, problem solving, factual knowledge, number and timing of hypotheses, diagnostic accuracy and physical examination were task and context specific. As there are no occupational therapy studies which have examined these factors, this framework informs our education for the present. Educators cannot assume that students will be able to transfer their reasoning abilities from one setting to another and thus a baseline of knowledge needs to be mutually explored from the beginning of each placement. Students may enter even their final placement in a setting for which they have little transferable experience and thus it would be unrealistic to expect them to work at a sophisticated level in all respects. Their specific skills still need to be developed.

While many placements negotiate individual learning contracts, there appears to be a need for a cumulative and reflective record to address experiential learning from previous placements, personal experience and prior areas of work. In this way a fieldwork educator would be able to situate the learning environment within the range of the student's past experiences. Professional bodies in many countries have introduced the concept of a Professional Portfolio for such student records (Alsop, 1995).

Fieldwork issues

Fieldwork education may constitute up to one-third of the total basic education syllabus. The World Federation of Occupational Therapists requires a minimum of 1000 hours of fieldwork in entry level occupational therapy courses and many schools exceed this amount. No one has challenged this specific number of hours or the learning that results from them. Students pass or fail. Now, some universities are asking for placements to be assessed differently and to better reflect higher education requirements (Barnett, 1994), while others use the labour market standards of competency or the industrial framework of capability (Gamble, 1998, personal communication) and yet others have the professional standard of safe practice as the core requirement (Alsop, 1993).

There appear to be differences between the professional needs and higher education standards with regard to fieldwork. Barnett (1994, p. 191) states that 'in higher education ... students come into themselves. The challenge for the educator is to provide an experience in which the student can be released into herself'. Those who think along such lines talk about transformative learning, empowerment and self-realization. These constructs are attributes within adult learning theories used as curricular frameworks in some countries (McAllister *et al.*, 1997). Ways of learning and the forms of assessment need to be congruent with these ideas. Occupational therapy practice needs to look at students' actions, thoughts, reasoning and subsequent reflections, in order to capture the complexity of each situation and the learning that has resulted. This understanding is mirrored in other approaches to fieldwork learning which incorporate active inquiry, actual experience, reflection and continued action in a more constant, cyclical process similar to Kolb's (1984) Learning Cycle. These approaches are outlined below.

The duration and position of fieldwork placements within courses is a critical factor in promoting the development of specific reasoning abilities. With increasing knowledge of the development of reasoning ability, some schools are scrutinizing and re-ordering the pattern of placements (Amort-Larson, 1997; Dickson, 1998). The crucial factors that seem to recur in discussions about fieldwork are (a) the depth of the learning experiences, (b) approaches to integrating knowledge and practice, and (c) provision of time for reflection during placements. Some course content needs to be relinquished to make space for these outcomes to be achieved and a new design of placement is emerging.

In the new design of placement, academic lecturers and fieldwork educators share roles. Sometimes the academic works on site, at other times the fieldwork educator leads sessions at the university. These placements are often set in the new contexts mentioned above, where few occupational therapists work. It has been suggested that these alternative placements having an occupational perspective do not offer 'therapy' as understood in the conventional way. Students often work in pairs or groups at both venues, the university and the placement. Various ways of reasoning and reflecting are employed and the placements often span an academic year or two semesters. They are longer and thinner. The argument for elongation and restructuring of placements is that students will experience working with an organization in depth. They will begin to understand the occupational processes needed to work in a new environment. Fish and Coles (1998, p. 29) describe this situation as follows:

... professional practice is able to be characterized in terms of artistry and ... this view brings with it a range of ways of seeing practice and theory, and uncovers a major obligation for professionals to try to understand better the principles (and not just the actions) on which their practice rests and to recognize fully and be able to articulate the nature of it.

Placement designers (Amort-Larson, 1997; Dickson, 1998) argue that this extension is necessary for a deeper understanding of practice principles, and for developing additional skills such as negotiating, advocating, researching and self-evaluating. These placements are sometimes referred to as role-emerging placements (Alsop and Donald, 1996), where students develop their own way of working and are helped to draw on appropriate knowledge. The principles of these placements are similar to those of the architectural studios described by Schön (1987) where learning is facilitated in a safe environment which allows for experimentation, discussion and reflection.

From clinical reasoning studies, many arguments can be drawn which mitigate against the usual model of fieldwork placement in occupational therapy, where one student works with one therapist usually in one setting. The premise underlying this way of working is that students receive individual attention and have a consistent role model to follow. There are several disadvantages to this system and many formative learning opportunities for developing clinical reasoning abilities are lost. Some of the factors to be considered are:

- The fieldwork educator's primary responsibility is with the client and not the student. Therefore the amount of time spent with the student is limited and actions are primarily concerned with planning procedures and doing formative and summative assessments with the student.
- The crucial relationship between educator and student must be one of trust; if this factor is missing the student has little chance to change the educator's opinion without causing some degree of disruption in the placement.
- The student's knowledge is strongly influenced by the knowledge of one educator and by the content and nature of the program that is offered. Both these factors could limit the learning experience.
- There is little or no peer support or exchange of ideas at the time of the experience.

● Most methods used to promote reasoning and reflection require the student to share feelings. However, because the educator is both educating and assessing, students may feel inhibited about voicing their feelings or concerns to that educator.

For these reasons, different fieldwork arrangements would seem more appropriate. Working in groups of two or four, students may have their learning facilitated by one or several therapists, giving insights into other perspectives. Group visits can be discussed jointly immediately after they have occurred. This way of working allows for self-assessment, peer assessment and collective assessment, which can provide considerable support for both the fieldwork educator and the students. Group work can also help by exposing faulty reasoning processes. Inquiry based learning methods can be encouraged by a professional who withdraws as the students' confidence develops. Planned and structured carefully, the group approach can increase students' depth of understanding, promote self-direction in their learning and reduce the time spent with the supervisor (Molineux, 1998).

Within the usual model of one student working with one therapist, clinical reasoning and reflection can be enhanced by working together in slightly different ways, as suggested in the student-centred text by Alsop and Ryan (1996). Different interaction methods may be adopted developmentally according to the readiness of the student. For instance, advanced students could work alongside educators and the pair could share their reasoning so that the students gain insight into the experienced reasoning processes of the educator. According to Eraut (1994), this sharing rarely happens. It seems extraordinarily difficult for educators to explain their reasoning or share their stories. Certain ways of working have become routines and practical knowledge has become hidden in the depths of tacit or intuitive realms. Titchen (1998) uses the term 'craft knowledge' and has suggested critical ways of questioning which can help unearth this knowledge. As this way of questioning may be perceived by the fieldwork educator to be intrusive, it needs to be agreed upon from the start.

Other interaction strategies include the student shadowing the therapist and undertaking guided observation and discussion. Students have found it helpful to plan an intervention alone and then have the educator check the details before implementation. This freedom allows the student to develop personal working strategies and may also help the educator to learn new approaches to clinical practice and to teaching.

Clinical reasoning: implications for fieldwork education

Traditionally seven phases have been identified in the occupational therapy process: data gathering, assessment, problem identification, therapeutic intervention, problem resolution, closure and evaluation. Some fieldwork education assessment forms echo this logically ordered process, mirroring the medical orientation to practice.

Schön (1987), Higgs (1990), Fish and Coles (1998) and other authors express concern that this linear model of clinical reasoning is too simplified and is not reflective of actual practice. Mattingly and Fleming (1994) contend that experienced therapists constantly revisit and re-evaluate situations even within a single practice session. That is, these therapists are constantly revising their reasoning during their actions, or reflecting in action. Their reasoning is not linear. This highly sophisticated fluid ability to reason runs contrary to logically ordered models of reasoning, recipe formulas, checklists and memorized data.

More recently, courses have begun to design their study around the four ways of reasoning identified by Mattingly and Fleming (1994). While it is an improvement on the traditional linear clinical reasoning model, these four ways of reasoning may be effective in physical rehabilitation but may not apply in other areas of practice. In contrast, inquiry-based learning or other learning methods that focus on a holistic picture from the beginning of the learning activity, assist the student to develop comprehensive reasoning approaches early (Amort-Larson, 1997). Such learning experiences can be designed to move from the simple to the complex so that reasoning integration happens on each occasion. They can iterate and re-iterate knowledge.

Methods that encourage construction of knowledge and the development of understanding, where an individual's conceptual framework serves as the foundation upon which further learning can be built, can be particularly powerful and are likely to be more congruent with the actual complexities of practice. For instance, the educator could use videotapes of practice with concept maps, to promote students' reflection on their knowledge base, their use of knowledge and their clinical reasoning.

In a clinical reasoning study, Ryan (1990) found that qualified but inexperienced therapists extracted only 27% of key data from referral forms compared to experienced therapists. The inexperienced therapists needed to be in the actual situation with the client before they could form images or make decisions. These findings suggest that students need help with interpreting written material and with forming images of the person with the disability prior to meeting them. It could also be concluded that students would benefit from more time spent in informal contact with the client group. For example, students could engage in actively listening to a conversation and writing it down afterwards in as much detail as possible, to develop their communication and interpersonal skills as well as their skills in obtaining, critiquing and using patient information.

Self-directed learning or group exercises with incomplete handouts could facilitate the extraction and formation of prospective reasoning. Images of the client may be heightened by viewing videotapes of that client prior to the actual meeting.

Similarly, investigating the life story of the person with whom they are working by talking to their friends and family will enhance an interactive image and will contribute to the narrative history (McKay and Ryan, 1995; Ryan and McKay, 1999). This work will assist in the formation of a more accurate conditional image of the client.

The development of expertise

Another way of understanding the development of reasoning comes from models which describe the development of expertise in practice. The most notable include models which derive from cognitive development (Perry, 1979), skill acquisition models such as that of Dreyfus and Dreyfus (1986) and the behavioural development model of occupational therapy competence (Frum and Opacich, 1987). Understanding such models will enable fieldwork educators to facilitate clinical reasoning development in their students and to enhance their own reasoning. There are critics of constructs of developmental stages such as Fish and Coles (1998), who argue that once again reasoning is being too much reduced, and that knowledge

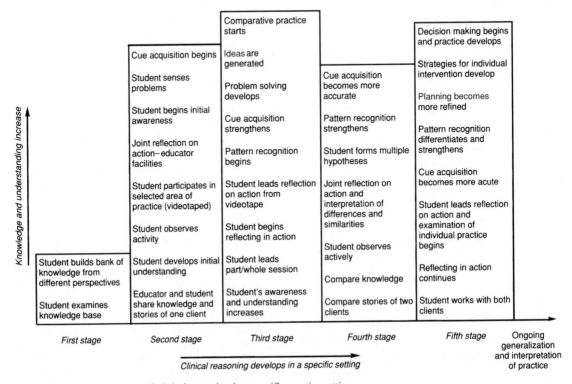

Figure 27.1 The development of clinical reasoning in a specific practice setting

should be built up and appreciated as a whole in an organic way, its shape growing from within rather than being linear and staged.

Within the interpretation of clinical reasoning as a dynamic process with reasoning at each point folding back onto previous levels of understanding, a model of clinical reasoning development is provided (see Figure 27.1). In this process each client encounter builds up a bank of knowledge and experience which enhances understanding. This figure illustrates a progression of learning tasks which can be followed during fieldwork to enhance reasoning skills. It has been developed from my experience of working with students in the fieldwork setting. The horizontal axis marks the development of insights into specific understandings. Each step augments the previous one. In each column the activities build upon each other and use an overlapping technique that folds back onto previous knowledge.

The diagram depicts the development of contextual learning of specific reasoning which needs to occur each time a student enters a different practice setting or engages with a different client population. The learning process starts with the student examining his or her knowledge base which will be different for each person. The educator should not assume the student's starting point and may check some of the espoused knowledge to see if it is indeed at a useful level. This is the reason why learning contracts need to be mutually agreed upon and not be one sided. As awareness of practice increases so does the ability to recognize cues, to sense problems and to begin to solve them. Reflecting-on-action from videotapes leads gradually to the ability to begin the process of reflecting-in-action during practice. The educator can facilitate the formation of ideas quite quickly by telling comparable stories. Reasoning is developed in a dynamic, complex and cumulative way which is particular to each person. Educators who use videotapes throughout the placement as their means of reflective learning can show the first and last recorded tape to the student to illustrate how his or her experience has developed. These videotapes can also be used as a means of assessment.

The key to facilitating reasoning rests with educators, both academic and fieldwork. Apart from being up-to-date with knowledge of the field they need to try creative and innovative ways of organizing learning experiences and obtaining feedback from students (e.g. through action research) so that modules can be fine-tuned.

According to Dickson (personal communication, July 1998) it is essential to have clarity of purpose regarding each particular fieldwork experience, so that both the means and the ends are quite clear and the rhetoric and assignments reflect these goals. Each experience has the potential to focus on a principle of practice. This should be a holistic process, like studying occupation, rather than fragmented, like studying just one way of reasoning which is not situated within a complete picture. In fieldwork education, whichever learning model is followed, there is potential for the full gamut of reasoning experiences.

References

Alsop, A. (1993) The developmental model of skill acquisition in fieldwork. *British Journal of Occupational Therapy*, **56**, 7–12.

Alsop, A. (1995) The professional portfolio – Purpose, process and practice. Part 2: Producing a portfolio from experiential learning. *British Journal of Occupational Therapy*, **58**, 337–340.

Alsop, A. and Donald, M. (1996) Taking stock and taking chances: Creating new opportunities for fieldwork education. *British Journal of Occupational Therapy*, **59**, 498–502.

Alsop, A. and Ryan, S. (1996) *Making the Most of Fieldwork Education: A Practical Approach.* London: Chapman & Hall.

Amort-Larson, G. (1997) Linking theory and practice in occupational therapy education: Is an Inquiry Based Learning module the key? Paper presented at the *Hong Kong International Occupational Therapy Congress*, 22–26 March.

Barnett, R. (1994) *The Limits of Competence: Knowledge, Higher Education and Society.* Buckingham: The Society for Research into Higher Education and Open University Press.

Boud, D. and Walker, D. (1991) In the midst of experience: Developing a model to aid learners and facilitators. Paper presented at the *National Conference on Experiential Learning, Empowerment Through Experiential Learning: Exploring Good Practice*, University of Surrey, 16–18 July.

Chapparo, C. (1997) Influences on clinical reasoning in occupational therapy. *PhD thesis.* Macquarie University, Australia.

Dickson, R. (1998) *Fieldwork 2 Course Outline.* Dunedin: Otago Polytechnic Occupational Therapy Department.

Dreyfus, H. and Dreyfus, S. (1986) *Mind over Machine: The Power of Human Intuition and Expertise in the Era of the Computer.* New York: Free Press.

Eraut, M. (1994) *Developing Professional Knowledge and Competence.* London: Falmer Press.

Fish, D. and Coles, C. (1998) *Developing Professional Judgement in Health Care; Learning Through the Critical Appreciation of Practice.* Oxford: Butterworth-Heinemann.

Frum, D. and Opacich, K. (1987) *Supervision: Development of Therapeutic Competence.* Baltimore, MD: The American Occupational Therapy Association.

Higgs, J. (1990) Fostering the acquisition of clinical reasoning skills. *New Zealand Journal of Physiotherapy,* **18,** 13–17.

Higgs, J. and Jones, M. (1995) Clinical reasoning. In *Clinical Reasoning in the Health Professions* (J. Higgs and M. Jones, eds), pp. 3–23. Oxford: Butterworth-Heinemann.

Higgs, J. and Titchen, A. (1995) The nature, generation and verification of knowledge. *Physiotherapy,* **81,** 521–530.

Kolb, D. (1984) *Experiential Learning: Experience as the Source of Learning and Development.* Englewood Cliffs, NJ: Prentice-Hall.

Mattingly, C. and Fleming, M. H. (1994) *Clinical Reasoning: Forms of Inquiry in a Therapeutic Practice.* Philadelphia, PA: F. A. Davis.

Maxim, B. and Dielman, T. (1987) Dimensionality, internal consistency and interrater reliability of clinical performance ratings. *Medical Education,* **21,** 130–137.

McAllister, L., Lincoln, M., McLeod, S. and Maloney, D. (1997) *Facilitating Learning in Clinical Settings.* Cheltenham: Stanley Thornes.

McKay, E. (1996) 'It was the look on her face!' Throwing light on the clinical reasoning processes of an occupational therapist working in an acute mental health setting. *Master's dissertation.* University of East London, UK.

McKay, E. and Ryan, S. (1995) Clinical reasoning through story telling: Examining a student's case story on fieldwork placement. *British Journal of Occupational Therapy,* **58,** 239–244.

Molineux, M. (1998) An innovative approach to fieldwork education: Results of a pilot study. Paper presented at the *12th International Congress of the World Federation of Occupational Therapists,* Montreal, 31 May–5 June.

Patel, V. and Cranton, P. (1983) Transfer of student learning in medical education. *Journal of Medical Education,* **58,** 126–135.

Perry, W. (1979) *Forms of Intellectual and Ethical Development in the College Years.* New York: Holt, Rinehart & Winston.

Ryan, S. (1990) Clinical reasoning: A descriptive study comparing novice and experienced occupational therapists. *Master's dissertation.* Columbia University, New York.

Ryan, S. and McKay, E. (eds) (1999) *Thinking and Reasoning in Therapy: Narratives from Practice.* Cheltenham: Stanley Thornes.

Schell, B. and Cervero, R. (1993) Clinical reasoning in occupational therapy: An integrative review. *American Journal of Occupational Therapy,* **47,** 605–610.

Schön, D. (1987) *Educating the Reflective Practitioner.* San Francisco: Jossey-Bass.

Tanner, C., Padrick, K., Westfall, U. and Putzier, D. (1987) Diagnostic reasoning strategies of nurses and nursing students. *Nursing Research,* **36,** 358–363.

Titchen, A. (1998) *A conceptual framework for facilitating learning in clinical practice.* Occasional Paper No. 2. Centre for Professional Advancement, The University of Sydney.

28

Teaching clinical reasoning in nursing education

Sheila Corcoran-Perry and Suzanne Narayan

Clinical reasoning has been integral to nursing education for decades in both academic and staff development programs. Beginning in the early 1960s, clinical reasoning was taught as 'the nursing process'. This general process involved linear steps of assessing patient needs, planning and implementing nursing care to meet the identified needs, and evaluating outcomes. Research on nurses' clinical reasoning conducted since the late 1970s has revealed the inadequacy of 'nursing process' as a representation of how nurses actually reason and make clinical judgements (Corcoran, 1986; Tanner, 1987; Tanner *et al.*, 1987). The findings have demonstrated that nurses use a wide range of analytical processes as they encounter patient situations that are characterized by complexity, uncertainty and instability. Therefore, the teaching of clinical reasoning has changed from focusing on a single, linear process to developing a variety of clinical-reasoning skills.

Nurses use clinical reasoning to make both autonomous and collaborative, interdisciplinary judgements about patient care. The scope of nursing practice includes diagnosing and treating human responses to actual or potential health problems (American Nurses' Association, 1980). As participants in the health care team, nurses also engage in collaborative judgements regarding the diagnosis and treatment of patients' disease conditions. Given the complexity of clinical reasoning in nursing and the range of health care issues involved, nurse educators use many instructional methods to help learners develop the necessary reasoning skills and knowledge base.

In this chapter, we describe five instructional strategies that are used in nursing education to teach aspects of clinical reasoning. They are analogy, iterative hypothesis testing, interactive model, 'thinking aloud' and reflection-about-action. Some of these strategies emphasize cognitive processes, while others emphasize knowledge organization. Still others stress both process and knowledge.

Analogy

An analogy is defined as 'a resemblance in some particulars between things otherwise unlike, i.e. a similarity' (Jorgensen, 1980, p. 2). It is a simple but powerful linguistic tool for developing both creative and critical thinking abilities. Often analogies are used to make the unfamiliar familiar, or to make the familiar unfamiliar (Alexander *et al.*, 1987). Nursing educators often use analogies to simplify the mental image of a task, or to view a situation from another perspective (Elsberry and Sorensen, 1986). For example, when students are struggling to understand the circulatory system, an instructor might have students imagine that it is a closed system of tubing (blood vessels) with a pump (the heart) to circulate fluid (blood).

The *synectic* model of teaching is a formal instructional approach that incorporates analogies. It has five phases: (1) describe the present situation or problem; (2) present and describe an analogy for the situation; (3) describe the similarities between the analogy and the situation; (4) describe the differences between the analogy and the situation; and (5) re-explore the original situation on its own terms (Joyce *et al.*, 1992).

A nursing faculty member used this model to help nursing students develop a simple but powerful mental representation (Corcoran and Tanner, 1988). In a medical-surgical setting, the teacher often heard students describe patients in terms of their diseases. To counter these reductionistic perspectives and to develop a sense of patients as whole indivisible persons, the teacher began with Phase 1 in which she acknowledged the difficulty many people have grasping the concept of holism. In Phase 2, the teacher presented an analogy, setting out jars of baking ingredients, which the students identified. The teacher mixed these ingredients in a bowl. The next question was, 'Can I retrieve any of the individual ingredients?' to which the answer was 'No'. Next the teacher revealed a cake, asking the students to describe the analogy. This phase helped students gain insight into the meaning of the term 'whole'. They came to view the whole of a cake as something greater than and different from the sum of its ingredients. In Phase 3, the teacher asked the students to describe the similarities between the cake and a whole person. In Phase 4, the teacher asked the students to focus on the differences between a cake and a person. Phases 3 and 4 involved the students' critical thinking abilities as they analysed the similarities and differences between the cake analogy and the concept of a person. In Phase 5, the teacher and students re-examined the concept of holism. They explored the language that would represent a view of persons as holistic beings.

Analogies promote both creative and critical thinking, two processes central to clinical reasoning. Creative thinking abilities are relevant to hypothesis generation during the diagnostic reasoning process, as well as to the generation of possible interventions. For example, analogies can help one visualize multiple interpretations of cues or causes of presenting symptoms. Similarly, analogies can promote both multiple and innovative ways for treating a given condition or situation. The critical thinking abilities promoted by the use of analogies are relevant to hypothesis and treatment evaluation. For example, the generated alternatives and/or treatments must be compared and contrasted for potential effectiveness and efficiency. Therefore, an analogy can be exploited as a conceptual tool for teaching aspects of clinical reasoning.

Iterative hypothesis testing

Recent research in nursing and in medicine provides evidence that clinicians use an iterative (repetitive) hypothesis testing approach in their diagnostic reasoning (Elstein *et al.*, 1978; 1990; Tanner *et al.*, 1987). The findings show that clinicians form diagnostic hypotheses based on minimal clinical data, activate hypotheses very early in the process and use the activated hypotheses as a context for gathering additional relevant data to confirm or eliminate hypotheses. This repetitious approach enables the decision maker to cope with the limits of short-term memory because only a few diagnostic hypotheses are kept in working memory at one time. Each hypothesis represents a cluster of cues, a single *chunk*. Such chunks place less demands on working memory than do many pieces of unrelated data. One can then rule in or rule out single hypotheses. Clinicians can use the hypothesized diagnosis to collect additional data to either support or reject the hypothesized diagnosis. Or they can compare two or three hypotheses at a time. Also, the diagnostic hypotheses help the decision maker distinguish relevant from irrelevant data, since the classifications of most medical and nursing diagnoses include defining characteristics or critical symptoms. These characteristics or symptoms become the relevant data to collect. Kassirer (1983) proposed a comparable strategy called iterative hypothesis testing for enhancing clinical reasoning. It consists of three phases: asking questions to gather data about a patient, justifying the data sought and interpreting the data to describe the influence of new information on clinical reasoning.

A nursing staff development instructor used iterative hypothesis testing with a group of telephone triage nurses who wanted to improve their diagnostic reasoning skills. They acknowledged that the goal of triage is proper disposition of patients who call the clinic, i.e. referral of the patient to an appropriate health care provider at an appropriate time and place (Corcoran-Perry and Bungert, 1992). However, they did not feel confident about their approach to triage. One of the nurses, Jim, described a patient, Samuel Morris, who called the clinic indicating that he was feeling unwell and had pain. A member of the group began data collection by asking for the history information on Mr Morris' care plan, indicating that she did not know Mr Morris and wanted some background that might allow her to help him more efficiently and effectively. Jim stated that the care plan indicated a history of degenerative joint disease, hypertension and obesity. The nurse who requested the data interpreted the new information. She reported that it made her think of several possible sources of pain, including joint pain associated with his degenerative disease. Another member of the group indicated that she would ask Mr Morris where his pain was. Her justification was that she associated pain with four classic categories of description: location, duration, intensity and distress. Jim quoted Mr Morris' response, 'It feels like it is right under my breastbone'. The nurse who asked for the data interpreted this response by indicating that it made her think immediately of a myocardial infarction (MI). Substernal pain did not seem connected to his degenerative joint condition. The next nurse asked about duration of pain, with the justification that she was pursuing the primary descriptors of pain, as well as classic symptoms of MI. Jim provided the information that Mr Morris' pain had occurred on and off for the past 2 days. It hurt when he took a deep breath. The nurse interpreted that this new information did not fit the classic symptoms of MI and made her think that perhaps he had a recent mechanical injury to his chest. The questioning, justifying and interpreting continued as the nurses pursued the pain descriptors and tested the competing hypotheses. They learned that Mr Morris could not recall a recent activity that might cause injury, but that his chest felt 'tight', and that he experienced sweating and feelings of indigestion. Concluding that he might be experiencing a life-threatening condition, the group chose to have Mr Morris brought to the emergency room (ER) by ambulance for immediate medical attention. Jim reported that Mr Morris had been brought into the ER and had, in fact, suffered an MI. As the group re-examined their reasoning processes, they became more aware of their previously unconscious use of hypothesis generation and testing. They indicated that Mr Morris' situation helped them refine their knowledge of MI symptoms in elderly persons. They now realized that elderly persons might not experience the sudden, sharp and intense pain often described by younger persons with MI. As illustrated, iterative hypothesis testing can be used to enhance diagnostic reasoning. It is helpful for discriminating among specific competing hypotheses and for clarifying the defining characteristics which differentiate them.

Interactive model

The interactive model is a strategy that is designed to teach new knowledge by building on and refining previous learning (Eggen and Kauchak, 1988). The model stresses the interactions between and among the learner and new content, what is already known and what is to be learned, text-book knowledge and that gained through practical experience. The conceptual foundation of the interactive model is schema theory (Rumelhart, 1977; Rumelhart and Norman, 1981). Schemata are mental structures that organize knowledge and guide the way we perceive and categorize information from the world around us. Rumelhart and others suggest that people try to make sense of what they encounter based on prior knowledge and experience. Schemata serve as a way to store this information as elaborated networks of interconnected ideas. Schemata are not static. They are active processes that are constantly being re-evaluated for fit and usefulness. When learning occurs schemata are tuned and refined to accommodate new knowledge.

The interactive model includes three components: advance organizers, progressive differentiation and integrative reconciliation (Ausubel, 1963). The following example illustrates the use of the interactive model to teach the concept of peripheral oedema. The instructor began by presenting an advance organizer, a blueprint or framework that previews the material to be learned and connects it to information already familiar to the student. Advance organizers link new information to an existing schema and provide a way to refine the old schema or create a new one. The advance organizer presented was a brief statement about the concept of oedema. The instructor then used the process of progressive differentiation to help the students examine the relationships within the new content on peripheral oedema and to link the new content to their previous knowledge about the general concept of oedema. She differentiated peripheral oedema into several types. Then she distinguished each type according to usual cause, nature, pigmentation, ulceration, foot involvement and other relevant characteristics. The example shows how the ideas in the refined schema of peripheral oedema are related to previous ideas in an organized way. This linking of concepts provides a basis to encode the information and to store it in long-term memory. Students' refinement of a schema is not just passive learning of the instructor's schema. Instead, students are actively engaged in forming new relationships among ideas, connecting this new content to previous knowledge and building upon their own existing schema. Finally, the instructor applied integrative reconciliation, the third component of the inter-active model, in which students are actively engaged in recognizing similarities and differ-ences, exploring the relationships between con-cepts, and making inferences about underlying causes or other critical features.

Learning through the interactive model pro-motes what Higgs (1992) calls deep learning, i.e. learning for understanding and meaning rather than rote learning of facts and principles. Use of this teaching strategy strengthens the content and organization of the knowledge that the nurse uses during clinical reasoning. Furthermore, the inter-active model also fosters essential skills that underlie clinical reasoning, including cue and pattern recognition and hypothetico-deductive reasoning.

'Thinking aloud'

Thinking aloud is a teaching strategy that is helpful in developing nurses' knowledge and clinical reasoning processes. Originally, thinking aloud was used as a data collection method in research on the cognitive processes people use to solve prob-lems or make decisions. Corcoran and colleagues (1988) suggested that since this method had proved effective in revealing the requisite factual knowl-edge and its structural organization, and the cognitive processes used by research subjects during clinical reasoning, the strategy would also be beneficial in teaching clinical reasoning skills. In this strategy, the nurse is given a particular clinical situation (either real or simulated) and asked to think aloud while making a decision. The thinking aloud verbalizations may be tape-recor-ded and later transcribed. Analysis of the tran-scripts reveals the cues to which the nurse attends, the hypotheses or inferences generated and the nursing actions proposed.

This strategy was employed using a transcript of a cardiovascular clinical specialist thinking aloud about a simulated patient case. The clinical special-ist shared this transcript with new nurses being oriented to a cardiovascular step-down unit. The situation involved a man who had been transferred from a coronary care unit (CCU) to a step-down unit 4 days after experiencing a myocardial infarction. His wife was quite concerned about the transfer. Together the clinical specialist and the new nurses analysed the transcript for the cues to which the specialist attended, her interpretations of cues, the hypotheses generated and the nursing actions proposed. With a more advanced level of nurses, the clinical specialist might examine the transcript for the ways in which cues are com-bined, evidence of ruling hypotheses in or out and the rationale for nursing actions.

The thinking aloud method can be adapted and used to enhance clinical reasoning skills in many situations. Instructors may find it a useful strategy in teaching students in clinical settings. For example, an instructor might ask a student to think aloud as nursing care is planned. The instructor supports and reinforces the student's appropriate use of knowledge and clinical reasoning processes and helps the student become aware of lack of knowledge or errors in reasoning.

Experienced nurses may use the thinking aloud method to enhance their clinical reasoning skills. They could share thinking aloud verbalizations with each other as they make diagnostic or treatment decisions for patients who are partic-ularly challenging or difficult. Thinking aloud may reveal underlying causes of errors in clinical reasoning. Such errors may be revealed through feedback from peers or experts during thinking aloud sessions or by the nurse's enhanced ability to justify clinical inferences and correct his/her own errors in reasoning.

Reflection-about-action

Reflection-about-action is a strategy for promoting deliberation about one's practice within the context of particular clinical situations (Harris, 1993; Schön, 1987). Reflection-about-action occurs when one contemplates prior clinical situations, especially situations that were puzzling, trouble-some or particularly interesting (Harris, 1993). Since the reflections occur after a particular event, the knowledge gained usually cannot make a difference to the event at hand. However, the new knowledge can influence future clinical reasoning in similar situations.

The theoretical underpinnings for this strategy come from the work of Benner (1984), Schön (1983, 1987) and Harris (1993). All effectively argue for a new epistemology of professional practice. This epistemology conceptualizes pro-fessional knowledge as being gained from actual experience in clinical situations. One does not simply apply theoretical knowledge to a clinical situation. Instead, one gains this type of knowledge through the experience of making decisions about clinical situations, particularly situations characterized by complexity, uniqueness, uncertainty, instability and/or conflicting values (Harris, 1993). Clinical reasoning in such situations cannot rely simply on acontextual facts, rules and/or procedures that were learned in a classroom or from the literature. Instead, much of the required knowledge and the clinical reasoning processes are developed in the experience of practice. However, experience in the usual sense is not adequate. One develops this type of knowledge and skill not from simply *doing* something, but from reflecting on clinical judgements made, feelings generated and actions taken within the context of particular situations.

While the clinical setting traditionally has been used as a learning laboratory in nursing education, this site has been considered the place where students develop skill in applying what they already know. It has been assumed that the theoretical knowledge gained in the classroom provides the foundation on which clinical practice is based. However, Benner's (1984) work and that of Schön (1983, 1987) has caused many nursing educators to rethink the purposes for using the clinical setting as a site for learning. Instead of conceptualizing clinical activities as opportunities for students to simply *apply* theoretical knowledge, these educators view such activities as a means for students to develop new and different types of knowledge. This knowledge is integrated with the theoretical knowledge that students bring to their clinical activities and incorporated into their clinical reasoning about particular patient situations.

Reflection-about-action is a strategy that promotes pondering about a particular situation in relation to the environment in which it occurs, as well as the feelings experienced, the judgements made and the actions taken. Consequently, the theoretical and professional knowledge and the reasoning processes implicit in clinical practice can be delineated, elaborated, criticized and transformed for future practice (Harris, 1993). Schön (1987) suggested that clinicians (whether students or professionals) reflect together on practice, using specific examples in the form of cases or demonstrations.

The following example illustrates how reflection-about-action was used in a senior nursing student's elective clinical experience. The student observed and worked with an expert hospice nurse mentor as she cared for several patients who were experiencing severe pain. At the end of each clinical session, the student and mentor reflected together on how they made clinical decisions about the recurrent, troublesome problem of pain control for particular patients. During these reflections-about-action, the mentor referred to aspects of each patient's condition that she thought contributed to the experience of pain. She attended to multiple, diverse cues and related them to her diagnostic conclusion about the patient's level of pain. The student had noted the same patient concerns, but interpreted them as being separate issues. She recognized the cues and generated separate diagnostic hypotheses about each. However, upon hearing the mentor's reflections, the student realized that she had not considered other aspects of the patient's situation as being interdependent and pain related. As a result of this dialogue, the student gained a greater appreciation for the complex nature of pain as a human experience. As the mentor went on to describe her selection of particular drugs and their dosages to control a woman's pain, the student asked about the 'rules' that the mentor used. When the mentor indicated that she had few rules because each case was unique, the student commented, 'But you made statements that sounded like rules or guidelines. And they were statements that I hadn't read in my textbooks or in the studies that I reviewed about pain control'. When the mentor asked the student what rules she heard, the student said, 'Well, you said things like 'Keep it chemically simple', 'It is better to increase the dosage than to increase the frequency of an analgesic' and 'This woman is likely to have constipation as a side effect of the analgesic; I should start a laxative to prevent or at least control that'. The mentor was surprised to hear these statements, not realizing that she had made them. Then she shared with the student particular clinical situations earlier in her practice that had made these informal rules (heuristics) meaningful to her.

This illustration exemplifies how reflection-about-action can be an important strategy for enhancing the clinical reasoning of both nursing experts and nursing students. Taking time to ponder particular clinical experiences enables one to gain new insights, to integrate theoretical and professional knowledge with feelings, actions and outcomes, and to use the experience as a basis for clinical decision making in future practice. In this sense, experience is not simply the passage of time, but rather a source of new knowledge, a challenge to clinical reasoning skill, and an opportunity to transform one's practice. As Schön (1987) pointed out, reflection is critical for both experienced practitioners' and novices' development, renewal and self-correction.

Conclusion

The teaching of clinical reasoning has changed from focusing on a single, linear process to developing a variety of clinical-reasoning skills and a broad, well-organized knowledge base. In this chapter we selected five strategies that nursing educators use to teach diverse clinical-reasoning skills. There are many other strategies that have been used to enhance nurses' clinical-reasoning skills, including computer assisted instruction, use of decision analysis, and simulated laboratories for teaching and testing clinical reasoning. Two excellent resources for other educational strategies to promote development of general reasoning skills are *Models of Teaching* by Joyce *et al.* (1992) and *Strategies for Teachers: Teaching Content and Thinking Skills* by Eggen and Kauchak (1988). It is important for educators to develop a repertoire of strategies, beginning with one or two and adding others over time.

Acknowledgements

This is a condensed version of the chapter by the same title and author, which appeared in the first edition of this text. Our thanks to Joan Rosenthal who assisted in the revision of this chapter.

References

Alexander, P., White, C., Haensly, P. and Crimmins-Jeanes, M. (1987) Training in analogical reasoning. *American Educational Research Journal*, **24**, 387–404.

American Nurses' Association (1980) *Nursing: A Social Policy Statement*. Kansas City, MO: American Nurses' Association.

Ausubel, D. (1963) *The Psychology of Meaningful Verbal Learning*. New York: Grune & Stratton.

Benner, P. (1984) *From Novice to Expert: Excellence in Clinical Nursing Practice*. Menlo Park, CA: Addison-Wesley.

Corcoran, S. (1986) Task complexity and nursing expertise as factors in decision making. *Nursing Research*, **35**, 107–112.

Corcoran, S., Narayan, S. and Moreland, H. (1988) 'Thinking aloud' as a strategy to improve clinical decision making. *Heart and Lung*, **17**, 463–468.

Corcoran, S. and Tanner, C. (1988) Implications of clinical judgement research for teaching. In *Curriculum Revolution: Mandate for Change* (National League for Nursing, ed.), pp. 159–176. New York: National League for Nursing.

Corcoran-Perry, S. and Bungert, B. (1992) Enhancing orthopaedic nurses' clinical decision making. *Orthopaedic Nursing*, **11**, 64–70.

Eggen, P. and Kauchak, D. (1988) *Strategies for Teachers: Teaching Content and Thinking Skills*, 2nd edn. Englewood Cliffs, NJ: Prentice-Hall.

Elsberry, N. and Sorensen, M. (1986) Using analogies in patient teaching. *American Journal of Nursing*, **86**, 1171–1172.

Elstein, A., Shulman, L. and Sprafka, S. (1978) *Medical Problem Solving*. Cambridge, MA: Harvard University Press.

Elstein, A., Shulman, L. and Sprafka, S. (1990) Medical problem solving: A ten-year retrospective. *Evaluation and the Health Professions*, **13**, 5–36.

Harris, I. (1993) New expectations for professional competence. In *Educating Professionals: Responding to New Expectations for Competence and Accountability* (L. Curry, and J. Wergin, eds), pp. 17–52. San Francisco: Jossey-Bass.

Higgs, J. (1992) Developing clinical reasoning competencies. *Physiotherapy*, **78**, 575–581.

Jorgensen, S. (1980) *Using Analogies to Develop Conceptual Abilities*. Washington, DC: US Department of Health, Education and Welfare, National Institute of Education. ERIC ED 192 820.

Joyce, B., Weil, M. and Showers, B. (1992) *Models of Teaching*, 4th edn. Boston, MA: Allyn & Bacon.

Kassirer, J. (1983) Sounding board: Teaching clinical medicine by iterative hypothesis testing. *New England Journal of Medicine*, **309**, 921–924.

Rumelhart, D. (1977) *Introduction to Human Information Processing*. New York: Wiley

Rumelhart, D. and Norman, D. (1981) Analogical processes in learning. In *Cognitive Skills and Their Acquisition* (J. R. Anderson, ed.), pp. 335–359. Hillsdale, NJ: Lawrence Erlbaum.

Schön, D. (1983) *The Reflective Practitioner*. New York: Basic Books.

Schön, D. (1987) *Educating the Reflective Practitioner*. San Francisco: Jossey-Bass.

Tanner, C. (1987) Teaching clinical judgement. *Annual Review of Nursing Research*, **5**, 153–173.

Tanner, C., Padrick, K., Westfall, U. and Putzier, D. (1987) Diagnostic reasoning strategies of nurses and nursing students. *Nursing Research*, **36**, 358–363.

29

Teaching clinical reasoning across cultures

Elizabeth Henley and Robyn Twible

Many countries today demonstrate cultural, ethnic and linguistic diversity, especially the developed countries such as Australia and the USA where a substantial part of the population are migrants or children of migrants. Some developing countries, such as India, have historically been composed of diverse cultures.

In a multicultural society the provision of health care involves many different interactions among people whose needs and views on what constitutes health care may be vastly different from each other and from those of the service provider. These differences can pose problems for both the provider and the recipient if care is not taken to facilitate the processes involved in health care. An important aspect of facilitating effective multicultural interaction is consideration of the extent of similarity between people's cultures. When people from different backgrounds come together in a clinical interaction, that interaction is influenced by many cultures, and the overlap of knowledge and influence between the participants will vary from one situation to another (Fitzgerald, 1992). In some cases, the amount of commonality will be great; in others, especially if the participants come from cultures with very different medical systems, the overlap will be much less. The less overlap there is among participants' cultures, the more challenging it will be for the therapist to effect a successful outcome within the cultural interaction.

Therapy interactions provide the setting for many different forms of complex multicultural interactions. Therefore it is advisable for students in the health sciences to learn how to perform clinical reasoning within cultural contexts. This chapter deals with teaching of clinical reasoning across cultures within the context of therapy education.

Definition of culture

As in all clinical reasoning situations, it is critical to put practice and models of practice into context. It is important, therefore, to determine a working definition of *culture* and what it constitutes. Culture is a complex concept; it is not the 'kind of superficial, cookbook, rule ordered system of etiquette that some . . . seem to think it is' (Avruch and Black, 1991, p. 28). Everyone has a 'culture' which influences all aspects of daily life. It should not be seen as something external to a person, rather it is an integral part of each person. Culture is more than tradition; it is dynamic, evolving continuously.

Another important factor to recognize is that the diversity within cultures is often as great as the diversity across cultures. Therefore, therapists must be careful to avoid the trap of cultural stereotyping when dealing with clients from cultures other than their own. Each person must be viewed from an individual perspective and an open, sensitive reasoning process can be used to facilitate the client–therapist interaction. As Fitzgerald *et al.* (1995, p. 6) point out, the influences of culture on each individual will vary from one situation to the next; people do not necessarily 'understand all aspects of their culture in the same way'.

Before exploring the clinical-reasoning process and the concept of culture, it is important that health professionals understand the distinction between culture and concepts of ethnicity and race. *Race* refers to the biological characteristics of people, involving genetics, anatomical and structural differences (Fitzgerald *et al.*, 1995; Riggar *et al.*, 1993). *Ethnicity* is distinct from race in that ethnicity describes those characteristics of a group of people that provide the group with common markers or a sense of belonging. These markers may include linguistic, behavioural or environmental factors (Fitzgerald, 1991). *Culture*, on the other hand, is

> . . . an abstract concept that refers to learned, shared patterns of perceiving and adapting to the world which are reflected in the learned, shared beliefs, values, attitudes and behaviours characteristic of a society or population. (Fitzgerald et al., 1995, p. 6)

Culture and health

The need for health professions to address issues of culture is widely discussed in the literature (Dyck, 1989; French, 1992; Krefting, 1991). Most of the discussion of culture comes from the fields of occupational therapy, rehabilitation counselling and medical anthropology (Dyck, 1989; Kinebanian and Stomph, 1992; Lightfoot, 1985; Meadows, 1991). A workshop manual (Fitzgerald *et al.*, 1995) exploring cultural diversity for occupational therapists contains an extensive bibliography of over 150 articles dealing with issues of culture in rehabilitation. While many of those articles provide no insight into the interaction between therapists' own culture and that of their clients, others emphasize that health professionals must not only be sensitive to cultural issues but must also implement relevant appropriate services. Kinebanian and Stomph (1992), for example, describe the dilemmas of occupational therapists in the Netherlands dealing with immigrant clients. Such problems are common throughout the western world. These authors provide guidelines to help therapists discover their biases and adapt their services for an increasing number of clients from different cultures.

Krefting (1991) highlighted the issues of culture related to physiotherapy and occupational therapy, and discussed the benefits of incorporating cultural competency into clinical practice. Cultural awareness and knowledge may then appropriately guide therapists towards modifying therapy interventions in ways which are sensitive to client needs. Fitzgerald (1992) further suggests that a lack of knowledge is often not the issue or problem, as knowledge can be gained through education. Rather, the issue/problem lies in a lack of acknowledgement of alternative beliefs and lack of awareness of cultural differences. Fitzgerald (1992, p. 38) points out that 'in every clinical interaction there are at least three cultures and medical systems involved: (a) the personal or familiar culture to the provider, (b) the culture of the client or patient and (c) the culture of the primary medical system'.

A study recently undertaken by Robison (1996) highlighted some of the deficits that exist among physiotherapists in their management of clients from another culture. His findings may also be of value to other health professionals. Issues in inter-cultural interactions are related to the values of the therapists as well as the values of the clients, a fact that many therapists did not recognize. The therapists who recognized these differences were able to modify interactions appropriately. Interestingly, it was found that therapists from migrant backgrounds did not necessarily score higher on Robison's cultural competency index than those from non-migrant backgrounds. Generally, therapists with a poor understanding of their own value system created problems from both the client's and therapist's perspective. These negative experiences produced negative stereotyping and bias towards people from different cultural backgrounds. Not surprisingly, communication difficulties were the most significant problem in inter-cultural interactions. In addition, the therapists who expressed assimilationist or ethnocentric attitudes often lacked an understanding of the components of the human condition. The therapists who expressed dispassionate attitudes tended to display a fear or hesitancy towards treating people from different cultural backgrounds.

In summary, cultural differences in inter-cultural interactions have the potential to create confusion and even conflict. Unsuccessful interactions may be characterized by a lack of satisfaction with the interaction from both the therapist and the client. Cultural values play a significant role in influencing the reactions, beliefs and even outcomes of therapy (Robison, 1996). Successful inter-cultural interactions are characterized by mutual satisfaction, effective communication and positive therapy outcomes (Meadows, 1991).

Educational considerations

Education about cultural issues needs to be embedded throughout the curriculum and needs to permeate all aspects of the educational process. 'No one exposure alone will be adequate to ensure learner growth in terms of increased cultural awareness' (Carpio and Majumdar, 1992, p. 6). It is the type and method of education that is the crucial factor in improving competency (Carpio and Majumdar, 1992; Robison, 1996). Numerous authors have analysed cultural competency in the context of various health professions (Dillard *et al.*, 1992; Fitzgerald *et al.*, 1996; Kinebanian and Stomph, 1992; Walker, 1991).

Today, all education programs should prepare therapists to work in multicultural environments, and a primary objective of educators should be to develop cultural competency in their students and graduates. It is evident from the definition below that cultural competency is an essential ingredient of effective clinical reasoning in inter-cultural contexts. When culture is interpreted broadly and we begin to speak of the differing cultures of women and men, of youth and age as well as the cultures of different society groups, then cultural considerations lie at the core of all clinical reasoning applications.

Cultural competency can be defined as

> ... the ability of individuals to see beyond the boundaries of their own cultural interpretations, to be able to maintain objectivity when faced with individuals from cultures different from their own and be able to interpret and understand behaviours and intentions of people from other cultures non-judgementally and without bias. (Walker, 1991, p. 6)

Robison (1996) states that the first step in developing cultural competency is recognizing and understanding the basic human condition. From this starting point, students must develop a compassion for their fellow human beings and a cultural attitude. Therefore, educators must strive to produce therapists with knowledge-seeking behaviours who are willing to explore their clients' *stories* or *histories*. This information cannot simply be encapsulated into lectures and tutorials. The literature suggests that a variety of methods to achieve this goal should be incorporated across the curriculum.

Consideration must also be given to the cultural competencies of the education providers, for they are the ones who will undoubtedly exert influence over the learning of their students. Faculty who are culturally aware are most likely to incorporate cultural content in their teaching activities and to model culturally appropriate behaviours. It is important that all educators, not just those who specialize in cultural issues, incorporate cultural awareness into their teaching.

Cultural reasoning

Cultural awareness, knowledge acquisition, and use of knowledge about cultures are critical elements of effective clinical reasoning; opportunities for student learning related to these elements need to permeate the curriculum. Table 29.1 illustrates the inter-relationships between clinical reasoning and cultural competency. Parallels exist in these processes in the tasks of awareness/sensing, knowledge acquisition and the use of this knowledge in reasoning and decision-making as a guide for behaviour.

Enhancing self-monitoring skills is considered to be a favourable way of enhancing clinical reasoning (Carnevali, 1995; Refshauge and Higgs, 1995). One way of facilitating the process of conscious reflection is to systematically apply a series of questions or an organizational framework to thinking activities. For example, students are encouraged to identify key words found in the client's history, identify what they know about those key words, identify gaps in their knowledge and the additional knowledge they must acquire before they make judgements about generation of hypotheses. (See Bridge and Twible, 1997, p. 171 for an example.)

Students should be taught to consider culture routinely throughout their interactions with clients (i.e. during assessment, intervention and evaluation). One strategy is to link culture to the existing clinical reasoning teaching so that it pervades all aspects of the curriculum and is incorporated into all case study analyses undertaken. For example, factors which need to be considered include social/cultural background of the client, the beliefs and values in the person's culture (and how these differ from the provider's beliefs and values), as well as the limitations of the provider and the environment in which the service is being provided (Fitzgerald *et al.*, 1995, pp. 23–25).

In reasoning situations, novice learners often make errors because cues are missed and/or underpinning knowledge is absent. A means of checking current knowledge and understanding is essential, because clinical intervention should be

Table 29.1 Key principles to consider in acquiring cultural knowledge

---

● Gather culturally relevant information
    the published literature
    cultural informants or brokers
    clients, family members and other community members of the cultural group
● Validate that information in light of the presenting situation to avoid cultural stereotyping
● Consider the impact of therapy domains of concern and concepts, for example:
    personal space
    communication issues and language, especially expression of an language of emotions, cultural protocols
    time and space
    gender roles
    beliefs and practises associated with health, illness, disability and healing
● Examine your own beliefs, values and attitudes
● Appreciate that interactions are part of a dynamic reciprocal process
● Find a common base from which to work
● Determine the goals from the perspective of all participants
● Select interventions that consider cultural restrictions or taboos, common practices and available resources
● Engage in continual assessment of the level and appropriateness of cultural knowledge
● Substitute joys and challenges for problems and frustrations

---

based upon an informed judgement concerning the client's condition or potential dysfunction (Bridge and Twible, 1997). In inter-cultural interactions cues may be missed because the therapist does not pick up the cultural prompt (i.e. an indication that consideration of culture is particularly important) or the therapist does not have culture-specific knowledge related to the particular client.

The clinical-reasoning literature has identified that the two most difficult areas for novices as 'issue/problem sensing' and 'issue/problem validation or intervening' (Neistadt, 1992; Rogers and Holm, 1991). In the cultural competency literature authors (e.g. Fitzgerald, 1991; Fitzgerald *et al.*, 1996; Robison, 1996) speak of 'awareness competency' and 'knowledge competency', which may be seen as corresponding to issue/problem sensing and issue/problem validation (see Figure 29.1). The intervening step of knowledge acquisition or cultural knowledge acquisition poses few problems for students. Students' difficulties lie firstly with recognizing the need to acquire the knowledge and secondly with applying that knowledge effectively in clinical decision making as part of the therapy process. Therefore in curricula it is imperative to address both cultural awareness and the application of cultural knowledge, in order to promote effective *cultural reasoning*.

Cultural awareness or issue/problem sensing

Issue/problem sensing requires attending to incoming data and reflecting on its meaning. Development of the ability to notice and attend to cues appropriately in the clinical situation is crucial. As Neistadt (1992) points out, the original image of the client is formed automatically as incoming data from the referral and practice setting are processed. This processing happens in relation to current values and beliefs, and includes predictions extrapolated from theory (Bridge and Twible, 1997).

The critical factors in *cultural awareness* are acknowledgement of alternative beliefs and awareness of cultural differences. Development of this knowledge and awareness needs to be fostered in students. Robison (1996) states that the first step in developing cultural awareness and hence cultural competency is recognizing and understanding the person or the human condition; who people are, what their problems are, how they reached this point.

Most people have beliefs about the cause of an illness, what kind of illness it is, the natural course which the illness will take and how it should be treated. Some explanations are common to groups of people and may be seen as having a cultural basis. The sources we draw upon to inform us about our state of health and to explain it to others are classed as popular, professional and traditional (Kleinman, 1980). Based upon these sources of ideas and information, different explanatory models are formed to describe or explain illness and disability. The models used by health practitioners (i.e. professional models) are frequently different from those of their clients (i.e. lay models). It is often difficult to match the therapist's perception of a particular illness and/or disability with the

Table 29.2 Inter-relationship between clinical reasoning and cultural competency terminology

Clinical reasoning	Cultural competency
Issue/problem sensing or noticing	Cultural awareness
Knowledge acquisition	Cultural knowledge acquisition
Making clinical decisions (e.g. issue.problem validation, treatment choices) as the basis for clinical intervention	Making cultural decisions as the basis for behaviour

client's understanding of experience of it. The disparity is likely to be even greater when the client and the health professional come from different cultural backgrounds. Thus any clinical interaction can involve perspectives from multiple cultures and several systems within each culture.

Narrative reasoning and history-taking exercises are an integral part of the therapist–client interaction. It is during history taking that the therapist actively listens to the client's story and establishes a relationship with the client. When therapists incorporate information from the affective and knowledge domains from the client's story into future clinical decisions they set the scene for a client-centred approach to service provision. Examples of case stories can be incorporated into undergraduate tutorial sessions through role plays and use of critical incident methodology (Fitzgerald *et al.*, 1995, pp. 30–35). Cultural influences should routinely be considered within clinical narratives, since cultural awareness enables the therapist to identify what knowledge needs to be acquired.

Knowledge acquisition

Students usually know how to acquire knowledge from available literature if they perceive that their current clinical knowledge base is lacking. For cultural information there are two other important sources: (a) cultural informants or brokers, and (b) clients and family members and other community members of the cultural group.

Fitzgerald *et al.* (1995) provide valuable guidance to assist in the development of cultural knowledge. They outline key principles to consider in acquiring cultural knowledge, frameworks for exploring cultural issues relevant to individual practitioners and the client population, and suggested guidelines for developing department policy for the treatment of clients from culturally diverse backgrounds (refer to Table 29.2). The therapist assimilates all available sources of knowledge, and

validates the information for the current clinical situation. Invariably, the more valid/relevant the level of knowledge invoked the greater the confidence the therapist will have in that knowledge and the smaller the degree of uncertainty (see Figure 29.1).

Using cultural knowledge appropriately or issue/problem validation

Cultural knowledge can be used to determine appropriate mode(s) of communication and form(s) of assessment of the client using observation of their performance of functional activities and physical examination. In addition, cultural knowledge informs the student as he/she develops working hypotheses, validates assessment findings, and selects and implements a management program having considered the implications, assessed the risks and determined the expected outcomes. The focus in issue/problem validation is on the examination of discrepancies between the original clinical image and the real and gradually unfolding clinical scenario (Bridge and Twible, 1997), and this validation process incorporates the application of cultural knowledge.

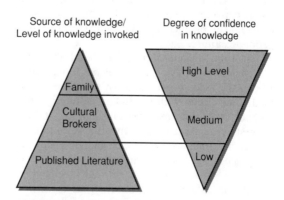

Figure 29.1 Hierarchy of knowledge sources for cultural decision making

Reasoning strategies to facilitate cultural competency

Workshops have been recognized as useful means of providing awareness training, since they challenge the values and biases of therapists and students (Fitzgerald *et al.*, 1996). Such workshops often use critical incident methodology (Brislin *et al.*, 1986; Brislin and Yoshida, 1994) and explanatory models (Kleinman, 1980) as reflective frameworks to identify cultural issues and to understand clients' perceptions of health, illness and service delivery.

A case study: 'The Indian experience'

During the past 4 years we have engaged in a fieldwork program which provides a good example of the implementation of cultural reasoning. This program involves inter-disciplinary student fieldwork placements in community-based rehabilitation (CBR) projects in rural and remote villages in southern India. A principal goal of the program was to facilitate students' understanding of the place of cultural understanding in clinical practice and to develop their cultural competency.

In the preparatory phase students participated in a series of workshops and other activities designed to enhance their cultural competency. During the program a variety of activities further fostered students' cultural awareness and their capacity to engage in 'cultural reasoning'. These activities ranged from the life experiences involved in travelling to remote areas of a country quite different from their own, living in unfamiliar environments and interacting with people whose lives were culturally dissimilar to their own. In addition, the students learned a great deal about performing the tasks of clinical reasoning and clinical practice in the context of the local people's culture.

When the students were interviewed after their placements, it was apparent that the Indian fieldwork experience highlighted for them the impact of the interaction with the Indian culture on their cultural competencies. Though Lightfoot (1985) suggests that experience with diverse cultures is important, findings from our Indian fieldwork experiences suggest that it may be the *type* of experience that results in an enhancement in aspects of cultural competency. That is, people can be exposed to cultural differences, but exposure does not necessarily improve one's cultural

competency (Robison, 1996). A cultural interaction that allows the therapist to experience different cultures positively arises from the therapist having developed skills in cultural awareness and acknowledgement of alternative beliefs.

Students reflected that in order to provide effective therapy, they had to seek knowledge specific to Indian culture and consider the cultural factors that would have an impact on therapy. Examples of such factors included feeding activities which occurred exclusively with use of the right hand, the procedure for toileting which involved squatting, and the impact that the clothing the students wore had on the level of respect gained from the staff and villagers. The students reported that personal values and assumptions were often in conflict with Indian values concerning health care. For instance, based on their own cultural priorities the students espoused independence in activities of daily living for Indian children, but that was not valued by Indian families. The students were initially unaware of this cultural norm and identified the dependence they observed as detrimental to the development of the child. They therefore first encouraged Indian therapists and parents to actively encourage children to do as much as possible for themselves. However, they noticed that this suggestion was not received as a reasonable therapeutic intervention and upon questioning the Indian CBR workers (cultural brokers) the students were informed that it is a cultural norm of Indian parenting to assist their child fully with many activities of daily living until the age of 5, at which time they are allowed to become more independent. In order to achieve a successful therapy outcome, students had to accept that their attitudes towards independence were not culturally appropriate.

Conclusion

The varied situations in which graduates work underline the importance of understanding the unique nature of culture both as a concept and as part of the reality of all of the participants involved in the processes of clinical reasoning and clinical practice. It is important to recognize that each individual presents differently and that assumptions cannot be applied to all people associated with a particular group. Clinical competencies, communication skills, cultural strategies, a culturally aware attitude and compassion are significant factors identified as common across all inter-cultural clinical interactions whether at home or abroad.

When empowered with competent practices, a cultural attitude and a sense of compassion, therapists can successfully interact with people from any cultural background in any country, whether it be outback Australia or an urban hospital. For globally competent therapists, the context is not an obstacle. (Robison, 1996, p. 141)

References

Avruch, K. and Black, P. W. (1991) The culture question and conflict resolution. *Peace and Change*, **16**, 22–45.

Brislin, R. W., Cushner, K., Cherrie, C. and Yong, M. (1986) *Intercultural Interactions: A Practical Guide*. Newbury Park, CA: Sage.

Brislin, R. W. and Yoshida, T. (1994) *Improving Intercultural Interactions: Modules for Cross-Cultural Training Programs*. Thousand Oaks, CA: Sage.

Bridge, C. and Twible, R. L. (1997) Clinical reasoning: Informed decision making in practice. In *Occupational Therapy: Enabling Function and Well-being*, 2nd edn (C. Christiansen and C. Baum, eds), pp. 158–179. Thorofare, NJ: Slack.

Carnevali, D. L. (1995) Self-monitoring of clinical reasoning behaviours: Promoting professional growth. In *Clinical Reasoning for the Health Professions* (J. Higgs and M. Jones, eds), pp. 179–190. Oxford: Butterworth-Heinemann.

Carpio, B. A. and Majumdar, B. (1992) Experiential learning: An approach to transcultural education for nursing. *Journal of Transcultural Nursing*, **4**, 4–11.

Dillard, M., Anconian, L., Flores, O., Lai, L., MacRae, A. and Shakir, M. (1992) Culturally competent occupational therapy in diversely populated mental health settings. *American Journal of Occupational Therapy*, **46**, 721–726.

Dyck, I. (1989) The immigrant client: Issues in developing culturally sensitive practice. *Canadian Journal of Occupational Therapy*, December, 248–255.

Fitzgerald, M. H. (1991) The dilemma – Race? Ethnicity? Culture? *The Rehabilitation Journal*, **7**(2), 5–6.

Fitzgerald, M. H. (1992) Multicultural clinical interactions. *Journal of Rehabilitation*, April/May/June, 1–5.

Fitzgerald, M. H., Mullavey-O'Byrne, C., Clemson, L. and Williamson, P. (1996) *Enhancing Cultural Competency: Training Manual*. Sydney: Transcultural Mental Health Centre of NSW.

Fitzgerald, M. H., Mullavey-O'Byrne, C., Twible, R. L. and Kinebanian, A. (1995) *Exploring Cultural Diversity: A Workshop Manual for Occupational Therapists*. School of Occupational Therapy, The University of Sydney.

French, S. (1992) Health care in a multi-ethnic society. *Physiotherapy*, **78**, 174–179.

Kinebanian, A. and Stomph, M. (1992) Cross cultural occupational therapy: A critical reflection. *American Journal of Occupational Therapy*, **46**, 751–757.

Kleinman, A. (1980) *Patients and Healers in the Context of Culture*. Berkeley, CA: University of California Press.

Krefting, L. (1991) The culture concept in the everyday practice of occupational and physical therapy. *Physical and Occupational Therapy in Pediatrics*, **11**(4), 1–16.

Lightfoot, S. C. (1985) The undergraduate: Culture shock in the health context. *Australian Occupational Therapy Journal*, **32**, 118–121.

Meadows, J. L. (1991) Multicultural communication. *Physical and Occupational Therapy in Pediatrics: The Quarterly Journal of Developmental Therapy*, **11**(4), 31–42.

Neistadt, M. E. (1992) The classroom as a clinic: Applications for a method of teaching clinical reasoning. *American Journal of Occupational Therapy*, **46**, 814–819.

Refshauge, K. and Higgs, J. (1995) Teaching clinical reasoning in health science curricula. In *Clinical Reasoning for the Health Professions* (J. Higgs and M. Jones, eds), pp. 105–116. Oxford: Butterworth-Heinemann.

Riggar, T. F., Eckert, J. M. and Crimando, W. (1993) Cultural diversity in rehabilitation: Management strategies for implementing organizational pluralism. *Journal of Rehabilitation Administration*, **17**(2), 53–61.

Robison, S. (1996) Exposure and Education: The Impact on the Cultural Competency of Physiotherapists. *Honours thesis*. School of Physiotherapy, The University of Sydney.

Rogers, J. C. and Holm, M. B. (1991) Occupational therapy diagnostic reasoning: A component of clinical reasoning. *American Journal of Occupational Therapy*, **45**(11), 1045–1053.

Walker, M. L. (1991) Rehabilitation service delivery to individuals with disabilities: A question of cultural competence. *OSERS News in Print*, 6–11.

30

Using simulated patients to teach clinical reasoning

Helen Edwards, Bill McGuiness and Miranda Rose

In this chapter we describe how and why we have used simulated patients[1] in clinical education. The account focuses on the reality for teachers and students of using simulated patients, and on the processes required to make a simulated patient program work. Simulated patients are not intended to replace the experience gained in working with 'real patients'. They are seen as an optimal preclinical experience, where students have the chance to develop clinical reasoning skills at a deep level before having to deal with the complexity and unpredictability of the real world.

Simulated patients were introduced into the medical education literature in a detailed format by Barrows (1971). In Barrows terms a simulated patient is a healthy person who has been trained to portray the historical, physical and emotional features of an actual patient. This definition incorporates the essential characteristics of simulated patients. They are based on actual case histories, not an amalgam or 'ideal' case developed for teaching or assessment purposes. Lay people are trained to portray all aspects of a real case: historical, physical, social and emotional. After training, the simulated patients are checked for accuracy by an experienced clinician before being used with students. Once trained, simulated patients are used in a structured way in student education, most commonly as a bridge into working in clinics, or in assessment.

Simulated patients have been used to teach and assess a wide variety of clinical skills including interviewing and counselling, data gathering, performing a physical examination, conducting psychosocial assessment, and developing skills in clinical reasoning and decision making. Simulated patients are commonly used in assessment of both individuals and groups. Our rationale for developing simulated patients in the 1980s was to improve aspects of students' clinical education, in particular to prepare students for clinical settings and to reduce the variability and lack of control in clinical teaching. We adhere closely to the Barrows model. Other users modify the original concept, often altering the case, training or presentation to suit their philosophy or circumstances.

The use of simulated patients is supported in the literature. Evidence points to the reliability, value and efficacy of using simulated patients. Gordon *et al.* (1988) reported that experienced clinicians could not differentiate between real and simulated patients during history taking or physical examination. Students relate well to simulated patients (Sanson-Fisher and Poole, 1980). In a well-documented paper, Vu *et al.* (1992) described the development and application of simulated patients over 6 years in a comprehensive assessment program at Southern Illinois School of Medicine. During that time they found that they increased the feasibility, validity, reliability and utility of performance based examinations using simulated patients. Ainsworth *et al.* (1991) used simulated patients in all years of the medical course at the University of Texas. Simulated patients were employed for teaching and assessment, in

[1] The term 'simulated patient' has been gradually replaced, in the USA in particular, by 'standardized patient' to emphasize the scientific basis and application of this teaching approach. In this chapter we use 'simulated patient' throughout.

introduction to patient evaluation, history taking and physical examination skills, introduction to clinical medicine, integrating clinical skills, clinical clerkship, demonstration of competence, senior assessment and during the postgraduate medicine residency.

While papers such as these convince us of the reliability, validity and usefulness of simulated patients, it must be emphasized that simulated patients are not considered a replacement for real patients. Rather, they are an educational tool used to develop and refine students' clinical skills, as they progress to becoming practising clinicians.

Reasons for using simulated patients

The most important reason for teachers to use simulated patients is to manage and control the clinical learning environment. Considerations include programming, level of content, environment, ethics and safety, economy and reproducibility. The process of 'time out' and feedback from patients improves the educational experience for students.

Manipulating programs

Using simulated patients enables clinical teachers to program student–patient interactions to suit the curriculum. That is, teachers can select a particular type of case, nominate the time to study that case, and be reasonably assured that the interaction will actually occur at that time and with the designated case. The teacher can pre-determine the level of clinical reasoning involved in the learning activity. In real clinics, plans are frequently disrupted by reality (e.g. the patient has disappeared to the X-ray department!). Using simulated patients results in efficient use of teachers' and students' time.

Manipulating the level of content

Teachers working with simulated patients can be quite specific about the type of encounter offered to students. This is achieved by manipulating the type and complexity of disorder to be studied, the level of interpersonal skill required for a successful interaction, the complexity of the therapeutic/assessment task, the duration of the encounter and whether the student deals with a part or the whole of a treatment or assessment session.

Novice students can be given a theoretically less complex disorder in their early encounters with clinical reasoning, in order to build confidence. We can match levels of theory acquisition to practice. We can organize practice of specific skills, such as interviewing, without overwhelming students by the complexity of patients' disorders. We may wish to specifically challenge our students' interpersonal skills, e.g. offering them an encounter that will test their ability to keep a patient motivated.

Using simulated patients allows teachers to be prescriptive and to use educational theory to select the particular encounter which best suits the students' learning needs and the teachers' planning. By manipulating variables we can teach clinical reasoning in appropriately small chunks, at a pace that matches students' learning and level of experience. We still expect students to cope with and adapt to the unexpected and to be flexible in the clinical setting, but with simulated patients, we control when and how our students have to be flexible.

Manipulating the environment

Simulated encounters allow control over the type of environment in which encounters take place. Thus at certain times we may wish the student to have to deal with noisy, distracting or threatening environments and at other times we may wish to have the environment as conducive as possible to a successful encounter. We can create hospital-like environments, outpatient clinics, home-based situations, etc., to best meet the learning goal. By comparison, in the real clinical setting, the teacher has to deal with whatever happens to be present.

Other advantages – ethics and safety, economy and reproducibility

The use of simulated patients simplifies some aspects of ethics and safety in clinical practice. Since simulated patients do not really have the conditions for which they are being assessed or treated, they can be used for long sessions or exposed to many repetitions of the same procedure, neither of which would be ethical or practical with a real patient. There is also a reduced risk that the simulated patient can actually be harmed by the students.

It is possible to have a number of students working with the one simulated patient, an economic use of time which may reduce expenditure. Teachers can have greater confidence that every student working with a particular simulated patient is receiving the same kind of clinical experience.

Simulated patients are trained to accurately reproduce their symptoms, case histories and psychosocial backgrounds across different encounters. They are therefore predictable and consistent over time. Real patients are far from this!

Time out

Using *time out* in working with simulated patients is of great benefit when teaching clinical reasoning. The student (or teacher) can call 'time out' at any point during an encounter with a simulated patient to break from the interaction and seek assistance/feedback/reassurance from peers or the facilitator. During time out the simulated patient freezes, staying in role but not interacting with the student until 'time in' is called. At that point the encounter resumes as though there had been no break in the interaction. Time out is used for discussion, group input, problem solving and reviewing performance. Students are often able to reason creatively about the current situation, resume with new strategies and then complete a more successful encounter, thereby furthering their confidence.

There is also the possibility for the student of trialling various interventions, calling time out, receiving some feedback or having time to reflect and then retrialling with a different approach. These time outs are a rich source of opportunity for development of clinical reasoning. This is because the details are fresh in the student's mind, there is space to reflect and there is the chance to resume immediately and try again, rather than having to wait until the next real patient encounter (and perhaps develop some performance or anticipation anxiety in the meantime).

Feedback from patients

At the completion of the encounter, simulated patients can 'de-role' and return as themselves, to give feedback to students on any aspect of the encounter. Students are encouraged to seek specific feedback about their performance, making use of a rich opportunity for further development of clinical reasoning. As issues about the encounter arise, the facilitator or other students may refer to examples from clinical work or theory to assist the student in devising a maximally effective encounter.

Educational focus

The focus in using simulated patients is educational. This contrasts with the mix of education and service delivery which occurs with real patients. In an encounter with a simulated patient the student can be encouraged and permitted to experiment. Students can make mistakes and learn from them without endangering the patient. There are few opportunities for students to experiment in the 'real' clinic and yet this can be an important learning process for students. It helps them to develop deep approaches to learning and to discover their individual style of working, rather than simply adopting that of their clinical teachers.

Example 1 – Simulated patients in use

The following section provides an example of the use of simulated patients with students. This example reflects the planning, reality and dynamic nature of teaching using this method. The descriptions are deliberately presented in the teacher's words, to highlight the teacher's experience in using simulated patients.

Background

One of the difficulties faced by speech pathology students when first attempting to diagnose a communication disorder of neurological origin is the enormous amount of information about their clients that they have to observe and process. Benner (1984) suggests that skilled practitioners use a filtering and 'clinical chunking' process, where they see patterns rather than numerous individual symptoms/behaviours. Novice practitioners are less able to see clinical patterns. They observe and mentally record many individual pieces of information before attempting to make sense of it and see some patterns. In a teaching/learning session it is helpful to be able to present just a part of the overall neurological problem, so that students can begin to see some patterns.

The simulated patient

The simulated patient portrayed is a 36-year-old unemployed mother of two, on a single parent pension. The patient sustained a cerebrovascular accident some 3 months ago and a diagnostic computed tomography scan revealed a large area of decreased attenuation in her left fronto-parietal region. She presents with a dense right upper limb hemiparesis and resolving Broca's type aphasia and is currently an inpatient in a fast stream rehabilitation centre.

The students

The group comprised 20 speech pathology students in the third year of their four year undergraduate program. They were completing their theoretical studies of neurological disorders and were about to enter an off-campus clinical placement in this area.

The learning task

The students' task was to accurately diagnose the communication disorder of the simulated patient while maintaining rapport and attending to any patient queries. The students were given the case history the previous week, and asked to practise relevant testing materials and bring them to the session. The tests, which were divided among four groups of five students, dealt with general interview and conversational sample, auditory comprehension testing, verbal expression testing, and reading, writing and computational testing. Each group had 15–20 minutes to complete its section.

The exercise

From the teacher's viewpoint the session occurred as follows. (The teacher is designated as 'I', the patient as 'Joan'.)

Time in. (Group 1) Joan presents with a flat affect and gives short telegrammatic responses to the students' questions. They find it difficult to get a sample of her speech, and call 'time out' and come behind the one-way screen. *Time out.* Jill: 'She seems so depressed, I can't get her to talk. What should I do?'. I ask for suggestions from the group. There is much talk about the need to motivate Joan, to explain why we need the speech sample, to find out if there is something bothering her, to ask if she needs to talk to someone and to ask if we can help her in some other way. Jill and Sarah take heart and return. *Time in.* Sarah: 'Joan, we need to get an example of you talking so we can see what things we could help you with in therapy, but you seem a bit down today. Is there something troubling you?' Joan (painfully and slowly): 'Well . . . my son, bad, in trouble . . . not stop him . . . speech no good . . . not listen'. The students are off now and although Joan struggles, she wants to communicate. The interview finishes after 20 minutes and we all regroup behind the one way mirror. *Time out.* 'So what have we observed about Joan and does that knowledge suggest we should alter

our testing plans?', I ask the group. There is much discussion about what we already know about Joan and redundancy in testing.

Time in. Group 2 begin the auditory comprehension testing and all goes well until they reach some higher level items, where Joan begins to look flustered and confused. The students push on and Joan becomes more agitated until she breaks down and pushes the testing items off the table. The students did not seem to see it coming and are shocked at her response. *Time out.* 'What's the matter with her? What's she crying about?' implore the pair. More discussion about Joan's responses over the past few minutes, about failure, about the nature of these test items and her probable lack of pre-morbid exposure to such vocabulary/concepts. The group suggests ways to keep her motivated and to meet her need for reassurance. They decide that it is not worth upsetting her just to complete this section of the test which is not giving us much information anyway. We talk about the information we have thus far about her auditory comprehension, and make plans for the specific areas we need to investigate and how to go about getting this for next week. The pair plan to go back and suggest finishing after giving her a task in which we are confident that she will succeed, and telling her about the need for some more small, specific tasks for next time. They also plan to give her a brief summary of what they have observed to date and to ask her whether she has noticed these things affecting her everyday conversation.

Time in. The last two groups follow on. *Time out.* These groups have several trips behind the mirror for time out discussions, during which clinical reasoning is active. Students have the benefit of time, lack of pressure without the client present, and peers to add ideas. My role is to steer their thinking/logic and to avoid faulty reasoning or incorrect facts. I am also a resource person who can confirm students' observations and interpretations or direct them to reading/materials to further their knowledge.

Feedback. After the sessions, Joan de-roles and comes to give the group feedback on how it was to be assessed, to fail, to not understand the purpose of the testing and to have deficits so plainly demonstrated. She also gives reinforcement to the students about their interaction styles, their obvious concern for her well-being and their empathy. The students talk about optimal ways of indicating errors in client responses without making the client feel inadequate, their difficulty in continuing testing when clients are failing. They ask questions about how they could have worded things so that Joan best understood what they were doing.

Reflection/Review. This is the opportunity to summarize the facts we have gathered, to check for their comprehension, to discuss interpretation of the behaviours and patterns observed, and to plan for the next encounter with this patient.

Discussion of this example and how it facilitated clinical reasoning

This example illustrates the richness in learning to be derived from using simulated patients in teaching clinical reasoning. The students were able to observe client behaviour and during time out, verbalize these observations and check them against their teacher's and peers' observations. They had time to reason out the current situation, generate strategies for change and receive feedback about their reasoning before trialling new approaches. The example shows how work with a simulated patient can be a powerful way for students to become aware of and learn to critique their own reasoning. Students could test different approaches or ideas with the simulated patient, receive feedback from their peers and the teacher, and then correct or retrial their approach. In addition, students were able to match their observations to a theoretical management model, and discuss how the model accounted for some behaviours and failed to account for others.

The use of a real patient in this example would not have given the students the freedom to make mistakes, to change their management approach or to learn from their mistakes in such an effective manner. Neither could we have comfortably had the time out from a real patient situation, to allow for the much needed mental processing space or for self-evaluation and development of reasoning abilities. Most importantly, the feedback from the simulated patient adds a true verification of the level of success of the strategies employed. We have found that students appear to place more value on the direct feedback from the simulated patient than on the teacher's account of how it was for the simulated patient.

Example 2 – simulated patients in use

The following section provides a second example of the use of simulated patients with students. In this case, the learning experience is conducted with a large group of students. It is presented as the reflections of the teacher who designed and conducted the activity.

Background preparation

The process of history taking is central to effective diagnosis and clinical management of clients. While the primary aim of history taking is to collect client data, it also involves clinical reasoning. That is, the clinician relies on effective reasoning and decision making during the history-taking phase to help guide the process, to test the reliability of the data collected and to pay attention to the needs of the client (e.g. to arrange a break in the process if it becomes distressing). This example focuses on reasoning during history taking. Interactions with clients are central to developing effectiveness of clinical reasoning and successful clinical management of clients. Students need to learn how to reason during client interactions, and how to make use of the data they obtain for diagnostic and management decisions.

We have found that students often experience anxiety when confronted with planning and implementing client interactions in the clinical setting. This exercise aimed to prepare year one nursing students for history taking through practice with simulated patients. It occurred one week before the students' first clinical fieldwork experience.

The exercise allowed students to practise history taking and reasoning in the simulated environment without the client suffering any consequences from student mistakes. It was also intended that feedback from the simulated patient, teacher and peers would help develop students' data collection and reasoning abilities. The specific task was for students in small groups to take the client's history, and to explore the reasons behind timing and technique in collecting client information of an intimate nature.

Organising the learning activity

To enable 250 students to participate, four simulated patients were used over a 2-day period. The case studies provided a mix of common client scenarios, each combined with a variety of social problems. They included depression, cerebrovascular accident, head injury and arthritis. One teacher was assigned to two simulated patients to introduce the students, monitor the interaction and call time out where appropriate. Students, divided into groups of four, were allocated 20 minutes to conduct the interview.

To help students develop an appreciation of the variety of emotional responses they might experience and the variety of decisions they might need to make during initial interactions with clients, the students were not told that the patients were simulated. They believed that a group of patients with a variety of chronic illnesses had agreed to an interview with the students. During the interview students were asked to assess the patients' reactions to the level of information (general and intimate) obtained, and to document their reasons for the time and techniques they selected to elicit intimate information. Students documented these findings in a journal, together with their feelings.

The majority of students were obviously nervous when entering the interaction. Some repeated in intricate detail the verbal patient description which was provided by the teacher immediately prior to the interaction. Others sought reassurance that the teacher would be close by if required. The students were introduced to the patients and the interaction began.

The power of the simulated patients to generate the emotions commonly experienced during nurse–client interactions was continually evident. Helen, rehabilitating from a closed head injury with an adynamic affect, proved to be the most difficult for the students. Helen's lack of non-verbal feedback increased the students' unease. There were often long periods of silence accompanied by nervous glances between students and teachers. The prolonged periods of silence not only caused unease for the students, but I too found myself considering interjections to help the conversation from time to time. It required a constant effort to remind myself that the focus for this was experiential learning, and that the confusion and unease the students experienced was a necessary motivator to encourage them to explore their reasoning, feelings and behaviour. Many of the students assigned to Helen were unable to elicit more than basic information.

Other simulated patients exhibiting 'normal' responses helped the students feel more at ease. Students elicited more useful data and a greater amount of intimate information from conversations with these patients. In fact, so personal was the information given by Sheila, a woman caring for her sick husband at home, as well as running the family business, that it brought a tear to some students' eyes. Another group of students were convinced that they could actually see the knee swelling described by Patsy (another simulator), even though the knee was normal.

Once it was obvious that a lull had developed in the conversation with a 'patient', usually approximately 20 minutes into the exercise, time out was called and the patient was asked to de-role. This event, was for me, the most dramatic. Some students began to laugh, stating that they felt like they were on 'Candid Camera'. Others became angry, saying that they felt 'cheated'. One student said that she felt that she could no longer trust me and that she would not be able to be sure that patients she encountered in her clinical rotation were real. Fortunately the angry students were in the minority, with most students experiencing relief that the patients were simulated.

The sense of relief following the disclosure provided a comfortable platform for the students to discuss their performance and reasoning. Students who had gathered little intimate information related that they had had difficulty deciding when to seek this information because of the absence of appropriate cues. The simulator and teacher helped the students explore other possible indicators and techniques for gathering this information. Students who had been more successful were able to describe the reasons for their timing and use of techniques for data collection. Client cues, student comfort level, age and sex of the client, and severity of the presenting symptoms were commonly identified by this group as factors contributing to their successful reasoning and performance.

The students' written feedback was used to expand upon the feedback discussions. The majority of students were able to identify key elements to be considered when deciding when and how to explore client information of a more personal nature. Students also discussed how they had performed in relation to these elements and how they would make improvements. Some students stated that they had not recognized the complexity of this type of clinical decision until completing and analysing this simulated patient session. This observation provides an insight into an important advantage of the use of simulated patients over actual clinical practice. Simulated learning experiences more frequently and more readily promote reflection on learning experiences. Such reflection encourages students to turn their experiences into learning.

In our exercise, students' feelings also became the focus for reflection. Students identified a sense of empathy with their clients and compassion for them, even after they had learned that the clients were simulators. The anxiety witnessed by the monitoring teachers was also mentioned in the students' journals. Many questioned their abilities to carry out the interaction prior to the exercise, but later reported that they felt more comfortable about performing this task in the future. All students stated that they found the exercise to be of benefit, including students who had felt angered by the deception.

Evaluation

We believe that the aim of enabling students to develop their reasoning and interaction skills with patients, buffered by the security of simulation, was met in this exercise. The interaction provided the vehicle and motivation for students to analyse their reasoning and interactions, and it provided some positive feedback about their existing skills. Subsequent journal entries from students' clinical rotations demonstrated an increased awareness of their own and their colleagues' reasoning and interpersonal behaviour. The client histories collected by the students also demonstrated that desirable learning had occurred, including students' enhanced ability to decide when and how to elicit relevant information. With the benefits of hindsight I would have informed the students that the patients were simulated. The literature recommends this, asserting that once the interaction begins the student forgets that the patient is simulated. This was an assertion that I chose to ignore, believing that the experience would be more meaningful and effective if the students thought the patients were real. The anger expressed by some students indicated that this course of action could be detrimental. In fact, the assertion that simulation is forgotten was supported during this exercise. Even though some students had been told by their peers that the patients were simulators, it made little difference to the outcome. One student, for instance, stated in her journal, 'I felt silly at first because she wasn't a real patient, but after a while I forgot as she was very believable'. Apart from its learning value, this exercise demonstrates how simulated patients can be used in a cost-effective manner with large groups of students. Students were able to explore their reasoning and behaviour in a secure environment, and were better prepared for the demands of the real clinical world.

Making simulated patients work for you

The decision to incorporate simulated patients in a teaching program entails commitment at a number of levels. Our experience of more than 10 years of using simulated patients suggests that four areas are particularly crucial to successful use of simulated patients: the teacher's approach, quality control, financial arrangements and organizational commitment.

Teachers must be committed to using simulated patients properly. Simulated patients are not like a book which can be borrowed just when needed. They need to be 'looked after' and treated respectfully and humanely, with consideration for the arduousness of their role. Teachers must be clear about how they wish to use a simulated patient in their teaching and what is appropriate training and debriefing for such a teaching session. Students also need to be adequately prepared, to act in an appropriate manner and to take the teaching session seriously. Our experience has been that students quickly forget the 'artificial' nature of the encounter and participate in a 'real' way with the simulated patients.

Simulated patients are used with students at different year levels in a number of courses and settings. A system of quality control is necessary to ensure that simulated patients are trained and used appropriately, and in particular that they perform consistently across time and across different situations. Our quality control strategies include careful selection of the people to become simulators, careful consideration of possible cases for simulation, systematic training involving a clinician, checking sessions with 'outsiders' as part of training, a user's manual for teachers, feedback sheets from teachers after each session, debriefing between teachers in meetings, and an annual meeting between teaching staff and simulators.

As our simulated patients scheme has become devolved from faculty to department level to meet financial pressures and to comply with the 'user pays' philosophy which is increasingly common in higher education, we have found the task of ensuring quality becoming increasingly difficult. At the same time, this difficulty has made us more acutely aware of the need to have quality control measures built into the system.

Using simulated patients is a labour intensive and expensive operation. To fit into the traditional university financial system and thus avoid some financial problems we have had in the past, we use the Tutor pay scale for our simulators, and pay for training at the same rate as actual simulation. By comparison, other organizations use different rates depending how simulated patients are used (e.g. prolonged sessions, giving extensive feedback, particularly taxing roles or undergoing invasive procedures). It is necessary to budget for the use of simulated patients, and while it may be cheaper than operating in the 'real' clinic there can be resistance to adding another expense to the teaching curriculum.

The final prerequisite for successful implementation is organizational commitment. It is essential, because the infrastructure required to run a successful simulated patients program is more than an individual or even a small group of staff can expect to provide successfully. A successful simulated patients program depends on having a bank of appropriately trained simulators. This requires deciding on cases to be simulated, recruiting and training patients, and organizing and monitoring their use. We have found it best to designate one person as the main focus of the scheme, who can interact with individual simulators throughout their recruitment, training and use. Devolving responsibility to several people in smaller units loses this focus.

Conclusion

Using simulated patients to teach clinical decision making is a particularly rich and flexible teaching approach which allows students to develop skills in a safe, structured environment. With appropriate organizational structure, teachers can use simulated patients to help students become aware of how they behave in interacting with clients, and how and why they make clinical decisions. These skills can be directly transferred into the 'real' clinical setting.

References

Ainsworth, M. A., Rogers, L. P., Markus, J. F., Dorsey, N. K., Blackwell, T. A. and Petrusa, E. R. (1991) Standardized patient encounters: A method for teaching and evaluation. *Journal of the American Medical Association*, **266**, 1390–1396.

Barrows, H. S. (1971) *The Simulated Patient*. Springfield, IL: Charles Thomas.

Benner, P. (1984) *From Novice to Expert: Excellence and Power in Clinical Nursing Practice*. Menlo Park, CA: Addison-Wesley.

Gordon, J., Sanson-Fisher, R. and Saunders, N. A. (1988) Identification of simulated patients by interns in a casualty setting. *Medical Education*, **22**, 533–538.

Sanson-Fisher, R. W. and Poole, A. D. (1980) Simulated patients and the assessment of medical students' interpersonal skills. *Medical Education*, **14**, 249–253.

Vu, N. V., Barrows, H., Marcy, M. L., Verhulst, S. J., Colliver, J. A. and Travis, T. (1992) Six years of comprehensive, clinical, performance-based assessment using standardized patients at the Southern Illinois University School of Medicine. *Academic Medicine*, **67**, 42–50.

31

Teaching clinical reasoning in clinical education: Orthoptics

Linda McKenzie

Orthoptists are allied health personnel who work in the area of applied ocular physiology as part of eye health care and rehabilitation teams. Orthoptists are trained in the assessment and treatment of patients who have defects of eye movement or binocular vision and the loss or reduction of visual function that accompanies such disorders. The overall aim of the orthoptics course is to produce competent clinicians who are able to manage effectively the clinical problems presented to them in practice. Therefore, the development of competence in clinical reasoning is a necessary part of the orthoptist's education. This chapter presents a problem-based learning program which addresses this issue.

The educational program for orthoptists at La Trobe University is a 3-year Bachelor of Applied Science degree. Problem-based learning was introduced into the orthoptics course in 1981 to promote the integration of the theoretical and clinical aspects of the course and to facilitate the development of the students' clinical reasoning skills. The problem-based program in the orthoptics course includes the core subjects Orthoptics I, II and III, in years 1–3 of the course, respectively.

Clinical reasoning and problem-based learning

Clinical reasoning has been defined as 'the skills necessary to evaluate and manage patient problems effectively, efficiently and humanely' (Barrows and Tamblyn, 1979). The process of clinical reasoning has been described as one of hypothesis generation and testing (Barrows and Feltovich, 1987; Barrows and Tamblyn, 1979). This process includes formulation of an initial concept of the problem from the patient's presentation and from other cues, initial data collection and problem distillation, generation of diagnostic and management hypotheses, implementation of an inquiry strategy and clinical investigation, problem synthesis and formulation of diagnostic and management decisions. These steps are followed by patient management and evaluation of management.

It is well established that problem-based learning offers one of the best methods for developing clinical-reasoning skills (Barrows, 1985; Barrows and Tamblyn, 1979; Norman, 1988). In problem-based learning the student is presented with a clinical problem to solve in a simulated situation. This problem acts as a stimulus to the development of reasoning skills and to the acquisition of clinical knowledge and experience by the student. Using a simulated clinical experience has the advantage that students gain knowledge and skills in a setting where common clinical pressures such as time restrictions, patient welfare priorities and responsibility for clinical decisions are lessened.

Cox (1987) states that 'teaching . . . should be designed to provide the usable knowledge and skills that the students can apply to health problems . . . in an applied science, students must learn how to apply that science, in addition to knowing the concepts and principles of the science'. The use of clinical problems as the framework of a curriculum allows students to apply their existing knowledge and clinical experience to the management of clinical problems. Their simulated experience in solving the clinical problem replicates the process which occurs during clinical practice.

Problem-based learning encourages the achievement of various educational objectives (Barrows, 1985). These include:

- Development of clinical reasoning skills.
- Integration of information into a cohesive learning unit.
- Consolidation, application and integration of theoretical and clinical knowledge.
- Development of self-directed learning skills, and the motivation to become self-initiating and self-evaluating learners.
- Development of critical thinking.
- Ability to function as an individual within a group setting, and development of independence, collaboration and co-operation in a functioning team.
- Development of communication skills.
- Development of appropriate attitudes and values through discussion of social, ethical and medico-legal issues.

Problem-based learning promotes 'deep' learning, in which students seek to gain an understanding of the subject and are motivated by an interest in the subject. It is a desirable approach for students in the health sciences because it promotes effective learning and parallels the behaviour expected of competent clinicians. That is, competent clinicians are expected to seek meaning and demonstrate internal motivation both in their everyday clinical reasoning and patient management activities and in their life-long professional development.

It appears that although individual students may have a preferred learning style, their approaches to learning are also influenced by the teaching they receive and the learning environment (Newble and Clarke, 1986). Problem-based, self-directed learning approaches encourage deep learning by promoting a deeper understanding than is possible through rote learning. Deep learning is promoted by stimulating interest and motivation to learn and by providing a framework for students to apply their learning to a clinical problem.

Problem-based learning in the Orthoptics program

In the Orthoptics program at La Trobe University the method of problem-based learning used varies over the 3 years of the course, becoming more student-directed as students progress. In the taxonomy of problem-based learning methods developed by Barrows (1986), the method used in both the first and second years of the course would be labelled the *case method*.

The case method involves the presentation of a case vignette for discussion. This method encourages student-directed learning, supported by teacher-direction in the amount and sequencing of information to be learned. Students are challenged to develop their knowledge and collect patient data in order to decide the cause of the problem. Using this knowledge and data students then practise hypothesis generation, information analysis and decision making.

The case method has some potential limitations. In particular, the amount of clinical reasoning that occurs can be limited to some extent if the patient information is presented as a complete case, in comparison to the clinical setting where the student or clinician would have to deal with incomplete presenting information. Because inquiry skills are not highly challenged if the information is presented as an organized unit, the method used in our course involves presenting the case vignette on a step-by-step basis. This promotes the use and development of inquiry skills without expecting students early in the course to employ the full extent of free inquiry that an experienced clinician would use in actual clinical practice with a real case.

As the students progress in the course the problem-based learning format moves towards the method designated in Barrows' (1986) taxonomy as 'problem-based' and 'closed-loop problem-based' learning. These use sequential management problems or patient management problems. In this situation the students develop their knowledge, apply it to patient diagnosis and management, and evaluate previous decisions. Using this method, students are challenged in all steps of clinical reasoning; the learning process is strongly student-directed, with the teacher being a facilitator.

This progression in the extent of student direction in learning and in the clinical reasoning demands placed on students is supported by both Barrows (1986) and Norman (1988). The latter suggests that the presentation of prototypical problems in the early years assists the students to understand basic mechanisms and concepts, and that the use of more complex problems subsequently aids the development of clinical diagnosis skills and the discovery of discriminating features.

The time allocated to problem-based learning varies from two 1 hour sessions per week in first year to one 3 hour session per week in third year. These sessions are run with the entire year groups, i.e. up to 30 students in first year, and between 16 and 24 in second and third years.

The first- and second-year programs

The first- and second-year programs mostly use a case method, where the patient details are presented by case notes, photograph or video. Group discussion then evolves around such general questions as 'What do I know about this?', 'What appears to be the problem?' and 'What do I need to learn about this?'. Such questions relate primarily to the hypothesis generation stage and the recall and application of previous knowledge. They also enable students to refine their knowledge needs into learning goals under direction from the tutor who helps them to sequence their learning tasks and identify the amount of content to be learned.

The cases presented are simple, with the aim of stimulating the learning and application of particular basic concepts such as anatomy, physiological mechanisms, optical principles, disorders of the systems and the clinical consequences of diagnosis and management. Consequently the learning needs are largely predictable and on completion of the discussion period during which the students define their learning needs, they are provided with a set of learning goals for the problem.

These learning goals are given to assist students and to act as a study guide as described by Laidlaw and Harden (1990). Each learning goal provides an introduction to an area of content and a framework for the learning task, emphasizing the important concepts, directing students to the most appropriate reading and adding further information as necessary. The study guide assists in defining knowledge necessary for the problem and distinguishing it from extra knowledge that is available, but not necessary. This is valuable for beginning clinicians since it assists in setting limits on the expected level of knowledge to be acquired (Cox, 1987; Laidlaw and Harden, 1990). Such limits are of concern to the student, especially at the beginning of the course when they cannot differentiate between necessary and unnecessary information, and are faced with the rather daunting task of gaining an entirely new body of knowledge. One of the major aims at this stage is to help students understand key concepts and their application and avoid an over-emphasis on particular details.

After the students have individually collected the information set out in their learning guides they return to the group with the knowledge gained. At this stage discussion involves the clarification of this new knowledge, further discussion of the problem and elaboration or rejection of diagnostic hypotheses.

The content is designed to clarify the major physiological process under discussion and the effects of disorders of this process, in relation to the case being studied. In terms of the clinical-reasoning process, the class is now at the stage of formulating the problem. At this level an actual diagnosis may not be made, but some statement concerning the nature of the problem, based on a synthesis of the information collected, and a statement of the underlying cause or process, is encouraged. In addition the class would generate some management hypotheses. During the discussion the tutor directs questions to allow the students to identify and demonstrate their areas of confidence and ascertain areas which may require assistance in relation to the problem objectives.

The whole class discussion sessions are supported by further small group learning sessions such as tutorials and seminars. At the completion of some problem units the students are given a self-assessment problem which allows them to test the application of their knowledge on another clinical problem, and to question their knowledge of the underlying concepts and their ability to generate hypotheses, to formulate a diagnosis and to propose a management plan.

The third-year program

In the third year, the program is presented in the free-inquiry format of patient management problems (McKenzie, 1987). The student group proceeds through a patient problem. At any stage it is both an individual and group process where students have their own ideas, but may be challenged by other students. Where a diagnostic or management decision must be made, it is a group decision.

Problem discussion sessions

The problems in the third year commence with the initial or presenting information of the patient as it would occur in a clinical setting. This information is provided by the tutor and may be in the form of a referral letter, a tape (audio or video) of a patient interview, a hospital record summary, a photograph or simply the appointment booking by the patient. Presenting information is analysed to decide on the important data and to formulate the students' initial concept of the patient's problem. This process leads to the generation of working hypotheses, and to a decision concerning further information required about the patient, i.e. the inquiry strategy.

At this stage students may seek details of the patient's history or relevant medical, ophthalmic and orthoptic assessment results from the tutor. The information may be given either verbally, as handout charts or overhead projections as relevant, investigative procedures and their efficiency.

If results of a requested test are not on the information sheet then this is stated by the tutor, promoting a critical evaluation of the investigative procedure. After the group has decided that sufficient investigation of the patient has taken place, the group discusses diagnostic hypotheses. These may be confirmed or negated by the group and a preliminary diagnostic decision made. Through participation in this process students develop an important skill, the ability to make an initial diagnostic decision for an unfamiliar problem based on what may seem to be incomplete data, or despite what might appear to be conflicting data.

The problem also requires management decisions, involving discussion of treatment options and a group decision for the preferred management option. The management plan should include a plan for treatment at this first visit, long-term management including prognosis and a general outline of the proposed treatment procedures. Having made an initial diagnostic and management decision the group then decides on when it will 'review' the patient. At the next visit the students are told the procedures that were actually performed which may or may not coincide with their management decisions. This leads to a critical evaluation of the treatment hypothetically performed in comparison with the treatment the group had chosen. If the patient has a general medical condition the discussion will include consideration of the management procedures performed by other health personnel and the reciprocal relationship of the ocular status to other aspects of the patient's management. Awareness is also raised of the behavioural, social, economic, ethical and medico-legal aspects of patient management. As discussion of the problem continues, critical evaluation of the management becomes a major area for discussion.

The process is ongoing and cyclical, involving continual data and information collection, analysis, synthesis and decision making. The students experience the need to learn, the process of applying knowledge to clinical cases and situations, and the process of critically analysing and synthesizing theoretical and clinical information in order to make clinical decisions.

This procedure continues throughout the patient management problem. The problems are set over a typical clinical time span which may be anything from a few months to several years. Discussion of each problem normally takes place over 2 weeks. During the problem discussion any topics the students consider they do not understand are written on a learning needs list. At the completion of the first session the students allocate these topics to be researched either individually or as a group before the next session. At the beginning of the next session they report back to the group, discussing the topics in relation to the patient problem, and evaluating the decisions that they had previously made in the light of their new knowledge. This skill of evaluating the effectiveness of their learning and re-applying the knowledge to the problem is an important extension of the problem-based learning process (Barrows, 1986). For each problem the group elects one student to be a scribe, recording the group discussion, so that data are available from one week to the next. This allows students to participate fully in the group discussion, since a photocopy is given to each student.

Seminar

A seminar is conducted at the completion of each problem, providing feedback on the students' management decisions, presenting alternative methods of investigation and treatment, and allowing further discussion and clarification of areas of difficulty in the problem. This seminar serves to highlight the areas of differential diagnosis and alternative management strategies in a discussion setting which allows presentation of the tutor's views and the opinions of others. It contrasts with the problem discussion sessions when the students are not given feedback during their reasoning process, to avoid disruption of their decision-making process and to facilitate discovery learning.

The seminar is conducted by a different staff member from the group tutor and is held approximately 2 weeks after completion of the current problem. During this time another problem is commenced. The 2 weeks' delay allows the lecturer time to read the group reports and the students to further study the topic. The seminars encourage students to organize their learning and apply the knowledge to other examples, thereby enhancing retention and recall (Barrows, 1985).

Problem design and choice of problems

The patient management problems have been chosen after consideration of essential subject areas to be covered and problems that will be encountered in practice, as advocated by Cox (1987). To ensure adequate coverage of all the areas necessary for clinical and theoretical competence, the problems used during the year are plotted on a matrix with particular disorders, signs or symptoms cross-referenced against investigative or treatment procedures, administrative and ethical procedures, general medical conditions, different age groups and other factors such as rehabilitation or hospitalization. The choice of problems then allows study of examples of the most common conditions and some examples of the less frequently occurring problems. This facilitates the development of the skills required to investigate and treat most conditions which present in the clinical situation.

The problems are taken from actual case histories of patients and are chosen for various reasons. Generally cases are selected because of a complicating feature or treatment procedure that sets them apart from what students regard as 'classical text book patients', thus stimulating wide discussion. Because the patient management problems are actual patient histories, they include information concerning the choice and results of particular treatment procedures. A resource file is compiled for each problem and consists of articles or information relevant to the problem. It is available to the students after the completion of the problem. This encourages the students to research their own material, rather than following teacher-prepared objectives. It is primarily used as a guide for further reading.

The role of the tutor

'The skill of the tutor is to make learning student-centred instead of teaching-centred; facilitating learning instead of dispensing knowledge' (Barrows, 1985). The tutor provides the patient information on request from the group and is there to aid students in determining what they need to know.

The tutor initially must establish a good working climate and assess and facilitate group dynamics. Students are encouraged to both give and receive constructive criticism of their viewpoints.

The tutor's role is continually active. Non-directive comments and questions may be required to challenge the students to elaborate and justify their views, to encourage all students to give their opinion and to encourage the group to reach consensus. In addition, the tutor encourages individuals and the group to recognize their own learning needs, and to take appropriate actions and use relevant resources to fulfil these needs.

Tutors face the difficult task of not giving in to the temptation of providing the 'answers' during the group discussion. Instead, they need to accept the challenging role of guiding the students to their own achievements. It is important that the students not be given feedback during the process as to the right or wrong decisions, actions or thoughts but that they be allowed to reason through each step (Barrows and Feltovich, 1987). School staff and clinicians may be used by the students as resource persons to discuss the patient problems, giving of their knowledge and experience to the students. However, this advice is restricted to outside the problem discussion sessions which should be student-centred.

Assessment

The type of assessment used throughout the orthoptics subjects is of the type described as modified essay questions (MEQs) (Feletti and Engel, 1980). This method of assessment allows students to demonstrate their competence by applying their knowledge to a series of patient problems. It allows assessment of the students' ability to formulate diagnostic hypotheses, plan investigative procedures, diagnose, make appropriate management and treatment decisions, and evaluate clinical results. The student may be requested to complete such tasks as generating hypotheses based on a patient presentation, listing further information that they would require in order to diagnose a problem, interpreting clinical data, suggesting a diagnosis, formulating a management plan or writing a report. For each of these tasks the students may be requested to give reasons for their answers, explain the physiological and pathological mechanisms and justify their decisions.

In first and second years, the MEQs are in a standard examination format where the entire paper can be viewed. Each question consists of the presentation of some case details followed by a series of questions. The first- and second-year papers consist entirely of short cases.

In the third year the assessment is by booklet-type MEQs consisting of ongoing patient management problems, as described by Feletti and Engel (1980). This format simulates the chronological nature of clinical decision making, where the students must complete each question independently and are unable to preview the coming questions or return to change previously answered questions. In using this type of assessment it is necessary to provide the student with some guidelines as to the suggested time to be spent on each section because they are unable to gain an overview of the paper as is common during reading time at the commencement of the examination.

Conclusion

As a staff member involved in both lecture and problem-based programs, I find that more staff time is required initially in the preparation of the problems, compared to the preparation of a lecture. This time is spent in designing problems, ensuring that all necessary content areas are covered by the selected problems, searching for appropriate references, setting learning goals, preparing handouts and organizing all supporting resources.

I would emphasize the constant need to encourage the students through the first stages, as they may take time to adjust to this method. Their greatest concern is related to their confidence, being unsure of the amount of detail and knowledge that is required of them. In the year the problem-based learning program was introduced, many hours of staff time were spent with individual students discussing their difficulties and reading and confirming their notes. However, this workload decreased in subsequent years as both the teachers' and students' confidence in the method developed.

This is a powerful teaching/learning method. The teacher's role as a 'facilitator of learning' is very different from that involved in presenting a lecture of summarized information. It involves facilitating a discussion, initially to raise an awareness of the students' learning needs and subsequently to discuss material previously studied by the students, and aiding the students in the final steps of understanding and applying that knowledge to the clinical problem. It is both an effective and enjoyable method of learning, and satisfaction can be achieved through the deeper and more informed student discussion which occurs as the students' knowledge base increases. The use of problem-based learning allows the students to learn within the context of a clinical problem, to gain an organized body of knowledge and to practise consciously their clinical reasoning skills.

Acknowledgements

This is a condensed version of the chapter by the same title and author, which appeared in the first edition of this text. Our thanks to Joan Rosenthal who assisted in the revision of this chapter.

References

Barrows, H. S. (1985) *How to Design a Problem-Based Curriculum for the Pre-Clinical Years*. New York: Springer.

Barrows, H. S. (1986) A taxonomy of problem-based learning methods. *Medical Education*, **20**, 481–486.

Barrows, H. S. and Feltovich, P. J. (1987) The clinical reasoning process. *Medical Education*, **21**, 86–91.

Barrows, H. S. and Tamblyn, R. M. (1979) *Problem-Based Learning in Health Sciences Education*. Atlanta, GA: National Medical Audiovisual Centre, National Library of Medicine.

Cox, K. (1987) Knowledge which cannot be used is useless. *Medical Teacher*, **9**, 145–154.

Feletti, G. I. and Engel, C. E. (1980) The modified essay question for testing problem-solving skills. *Medical Journal of Australia*, **1**, 79–80.

Laidlaw, J. M. and Harden, R. M. (1990) What is . . . a study guide? *Medical Teacher*, **12**, 7–12.

McKenzie, L. (1987) Problem-based learning in the final year of orthoptics. *HERDSA News*, **9**, 3–4.

Newble, D. I., and Clarke, R. M. (1986) The approaches to learning of students in a traditional and in an innovative problem-based medical school. *Medical Education*, **20**, 267–273.

Norman, G. R. (1988) Problem-solving skills, solving problems and problem-based learning. *Medical Education*, **22**, 279–286.

32

Teaching clinical reasoning to nurses during clinical education

Gail Hart and Yoni Ryan

Nurses have a critical role within the health care sector. In acute care institutions they provide a 24 hour service to individuals with life-threatening illnesses. In long-term health care institutions and in the community they provide ongoing care and continuity for a wide range of clients. While many other health care professionals contribute to health care services in all settings, the clinical decision making skills of nurses provide baseline data that inform all members of the team (Field, 1987).

In order to ensure that nurses are well prepared for their central role in the delivery of health care services they must develop effective clinical reasoning skills. Such skills are best tried and tested in the real-world experience of clinical practice. The clinical setting, however, is a complex learning environment that lacks the order and control of a classroom. Students are bombarded with unfamiliar stimuli, their role is unclear, and they have difficulty identifying learning opportunities and applying problem-solving skills they have developed in other areas of study (White and Ewan, 1991).

The principles of adult learning offer direction to assist in the development of clinical reasoning skills. The key for nurse educators is to create a supportive and collegial learning environment which fosters adult learning. This involves acknowledging and building upon the learners' clinical experiences and creating opportunities for learners to reflect on their learning, to share their experience with peers and to engage in critical discussions and debate on clinical reasoning in practice.

Learning by doing

Learning by doing is an important concept in a practical profession such as nursing. The phrase 'learning by doing' has sometimes been used to suggest that the only way of learning the practice of nursing is by rehearsing skills within a clinical setting. When used to express this perspective, the phrase is more accurately described as 'learning by doing (knowing how)'. Here the practitioner has observed and repeated a skill or procedure until it can be performed efficiently and demonstrated to others. Hospital-based nurse education programs provided the opportunity for such practice but did not ensure an understanding of the underlying principles. The application of theory and the transfer of principles to practice require a further step and a new phrase 'learning by doing (understanding why)'. At this level the practitioner is also able to explain 'why', to suggest further general applications and to outline how a specific skill or procedure relates to a wider body of knowledge. Such understanding necessitates a strong theoretical base for nursing practice.

Beyond understanding is an additional step in clinical reasoning, 'learning by doing (adapting)'. Some practitioners move beyond the practical application of theory to practice by reflecting on their own practice and by adapting their approach. In effect, their practice becomes reflection-in-action and theoretical knowledge is generated from the practical situation (Jarvis, 1987).

Benner (1984) has outlined the development from novice to expert nurse and has differentiated five levels in terms of the approach of nurses to clinical decision making. According to Benner, both the novice and the competent nurse make judgements on the basis of a set of rules acquired in a context-free situation. Students, recent graduates and even experienced nurses entering a new area will painstakingly follow a skills-oriented procedure step-by-step, without being sensitive to patient cues or data that suggest the need for a modified or alternative intervention. In contrast, expert nurses working in a familiar environment intuitively assess the situation in a holistic way and only later reflect on the process to identify the principles underlying their decision. Field (1987) has observed, however, that many expert practitioners are unable to explain the basis for their action. They 'know how' but they lack the ability to provide a theoretical rationale for their decisions.

If many of the most expert practitioners are unable to justify clinical decisions and interventions according to a conceptual model or theory it is unlikely that the chasm separating theory and practice will be easily bridged.

Clinicians as preceptors

The concerns identified above have important implications for the effectiveness of preceptor programs. The term *preceptor* is used to describe 'a unit-based nurse who carries out one-to-one teaching of new employees or nursing students, in addition to his/her regular unit duties' (Shamian and Inhaber, 1985).

Preceptors have been widely used to assist recent graduates to make the transition from university to the workplace and in the supervision of nursing students during clinical placements. Both of these situations are critical periods in the development of graduate and student nurses' confidence in applying their skills in critical thinking to the clinical problems they encounter in practice. They are unlikely to meet this challenge successfully without support, encouragement and example from more experienced colleagues.

The role of preceptor is a challenging one, particularly since the widespread introduction of tertiary-educated nurses into the workforce, which has created role ambiguity and role confusion, not only for recent graduates but also for those experienced nurses with the responsibility of guiding recent graduates' beginning practice. Yet many nurses identified as preceptors are either unable or unwilling to demonstrate and encourage clinical reasoning. They are often not adequately prepared or rewarded for their role (Young *et al.*, 1989). Some guidance for preceptor training programs is now available (e.g. Brammer and Zelmer, 1996; White and Ewan, 1991), but further research into the optimization of conditions for promoting individual and professional growth is necessary, particularly in understanding how to maximize the use of the clinical learning environment and how to utilize adult learning theory. The following sections deal with these areas.

The clinical learning environment

The experiences which nursing students gain in the clinical setting offer the best opportunity to integrate skills learned in practice and in the university laboratory with theory learned in the classroom. It is the responsibility of the clinical educator to enable such integration to occur. Unlike teaching in the laboratory or classroom, however, clinical education takes place in a complex setting, much of which is beyond the control of the teacher.

Most research related to clinical education has focused on teacher behaviours from the perspective of students (Ripley, 1986; Windsor, 1987), although Morgan and Knox (1987) have also contrasted the perspectives of faculty staff and students. Despite the research interest in identifying effective clinical teaching behaviours, Karuhije (1986) found that few clinical teachers were adequately prepared for their role. Wong and Wong (1987) drew attention to the lack of preparation available for most clinical instructors and the low prestige associated with clinical teaching in nursing. Thus, while the clinical setting offers an ideal opportunity to test and revise clinical reasoning skills, the clinical educator's role in fostering the development of clinical reasoning may well be limited.

Hart (1992) surveyed 516 registered nurses to investigate the attributes that characterized a positive clinical learning environment. This research supported the significance of the social context of learning for nurses working in the clinical setting. Hart emphasized the value of a collaborative approach between administration and education for the development of effective strategies to support formal and informal opportunities for staff to develop a collegial work environment.

Adult learning theory

As indicated above, a significant constraint on the facilitation of student learning is lack of preparation for the clinical teaching role, including an understanding of the nature of learning. The focus of this discussion is on adult learning theory, since there is a fundamental link between expectations of autonomous decision making and responsibility for one's actions, which both adult learning and clinical reasoning place on the individual. To facilitate the development of clinical reasoning skills, educators are well advised to acknowledge and enhance students' strengths as adult learners and to capitalize on the immediacy of practice as a powerful motivator for student learning and a trigger for clinical reasoning.

Until the late 1960s there was little systematic research in adult learning. This allowed two options for the development of a field of study. Knowledge could either be generated from practice (grounded theory) or borrowed from relevant fields of study and synthesized to suit the special purposes of adult learning. This second approach was enunciated in the 1970s by Knowles (1990), to develop his andragogical model for adult learning. This model borrows from clinical psychology, developmental psychology, sociology, social psychology and philosophy, and is predicated on the following assumptions (Knowles, 1990, pp. 57–63)

- *Adults have a need to know.* Adults are concerned about the benefits that will accrue from applying new knowledge, and are intrinsically motivated to improve their working environment.
- *The learner's self concept influences his or her approach to learning.* Adults have a self concept as responsible decision makers and are capable of self-directed activity. Unfortunately many adults have been conditioned by earlier educational experiences to behave as passive recipients. There is a need to create learning opportunities that facilitate the students' transition from dependent learners to self-directed learners.
- *The learner's past experience plays a role in his or her learning.* Adults bring a rich resource of life experience to any learning situation. Experiential techniques that tap this experience through group discussion, simulation, problem solving, case methods and peer support techniques optimize learning.

- *Adults have a readiness to learn.* Adults demonstrate readiness to learn in response to developmental tasks. For example, new employees will usually demonstrate a readiness to learn those things that they need to know in order to cope effectively with their new responsibilities.
- *Adult learning is task-oriented or problem-centred.* Adults are motivated to learn to the extent that they perceive it will help them deal with and resolve real life problems. Learning is most effective when new knowledge, skills and attitudes are presented in a context which closely approximates reality.
- *Internal motivation is a major factor in adult learning.* The most powerful motivators for adults are internal pressures such as the desire for increased job satisfaction, self-esteem and quality of life. Tough (1979) found that a motivation to grow and develop was intrinsic to adults but could be blocked by barriers such as a negative self-concept as a learner, inaccessibility of opportunities or resources, time constraints and programs that violate principles of adult learning.

Knowles (1990) outlines the contribution that behaviourist, cognitive, personality and humanistic theorists have made in acknowledging the significance of the human and interpersonal climate of the learning environment. Behavioural psychologists stress the importance of recognizing and rewarding motivation to learn and apply new knowledge, skills and attitudes. Cognitive theorists emphasize clarity of roles, open communication and constructive feedback about performance. An environment that tolerates and even welcomes mistakes as evidence of risk taking and learning is also encouraged. Personality theorists stress the significance of a 'mentally healthful' climate that respects individual and cultural differences and moderates stress levels. Humanistic psychologists suggest that collaboration rather than competition should be fostered in order to promote group loyalty, supportive peer interaction and a democratic approach to decision making. Social learning theorists such as Bandura (1971) also stress the significance of modelling within a professional environment as a powerful motivation in personal development, and Cross (1981, p. 228) argues that 'learning will flourish if nourishing, encouraging environments are provided'. Finally, the concept of organizational climate is central to Knowles' model of andragogy.

Adult learning theory has far-reaching implications for the working and learning environment of nurses. The design of learning programs and environments based on the above assumptions can facilitate learning.

Implementing a listening–dialogue–action sequence in clinical education

Paulo Freire (1970) argues that the social context of education is never neutral. Individuals carry with them a lifetime of experience which shapes their perspective and influences their interactions with others. Freire (1983) proposes a listening–dialogue–action sequence to encompass the principles of active learner participation and to acknowledge the social context of education. As individuals and groups test out their analyses within practice they set in place a recurring spiral of action–reflection–action. This framework of listening, dialogue and action is used below to illustrate opportunities for developing clinical reasoning skills within the clinical setting.

Listening (reflection)

Clinical reasoning begins with the identification of a problem or issue encountered in practice. It requires a sensitivity evidenced by a willingness to listen or attend to one's own thoughts and feelings as well as those of others. Attending or listening provides a means of exploring experience in order to lead to new understanding and appreciation. This strong link between the learning experience and the reflective activity which follows is inherent in the concept of the reflective practitioner (Kemmis, 1985; Schön, 1983).

To strengthen this link from practice to theory, practitioners need opportunities to reflect on practice and develop an approach to practice that is actually reflection-in-action (Jarvis, 1987). One is often prompted to attend, listen or reflect when one experiences an uneasiness or inner discomfort about a situation or practice. Boud *et al.* (1985) emphasize the value of creating time for reflection as a means of enhancing learning from experience. They advocate scheduling a debriefing period for a group or allocating specific time for maintaining a personal journal outlining experiences and reactions to them. Hart (1997) also describes the use of practice incidents and peer consultation as reflective techniques which promote professional development within clinical settings.

Reflective journal writing involves practitioners making a written account of critical incidents from their clinical experience. It allows practitioners to reframe problems encountered in day-to-day practice and to develop manageable solutions. By documenting practice on a regular basis the complex and individualized nature of many health care situations is highlighted, and nurses are less likely to develop the selective inattention that Schön (1983) describes as a response to engaging in repetitive and routine practice. They are more likely to be flexible and creative in their approach to problem solving.

Dialogue (peer consultation)

Peer consultation is a process whereby a practitioner confers with a colleague or group of colleagues to seek resolution of a clinical or organizational issue. Within this process group members are valued as equals and peers, expertise and power is shared, active participation is encouraged and there is an atmosphere of openness and respect for differing values; group trust and co-operation are high. Numerous writers have advocated peer consultation and have highlighted the potential benefits:

- Establishment of a non-threatening learning community (Erickson, 1987).
- Decreased work-related anxiety (Pasacreta and Jacobsen, 1989).
- Self-discovery, insight and personal growth on the part of the participants (Bilderback, 1989; Fontes, 1987).
- Increased acceptance, validation and support between group members (Bilderback, 1989; Fontes, 1987).
- Recognition for, and promotion of professional expertise (Bilderback, 1989; Hart, 1990).
- Prompt evaluation of competency (Bilderback, 1989).
- Improved communication and information sharing (Hart, 1990; Pasacreta and Jacobsen, 1989).
- Improved staff morale (Pasacreta and Jacobsen, 1989).
- Improved quality of care (Pasacreta and Jacobsen, 1989).

Peer consultation offers the opportunity for nurses to share their expertise in clinical reasoning. The group context is important because it provides the opportunity for nurses to pool their knowledge and skills to resolve a clinical problem. The main advantages are the active participation of the learner and the contribution of multiple viewpoints to a particular issue. The teacher acts as a facilitator or 'co-learner' rather than an instructor or supervisor.

Action (collaboration)

The process of clinical reasoning is effective if it informs and improves clinical practice. To achieve this outcome it is essential to have administrative support of the decision-making role of nurses and of the implementation of teaching/learning strategies to promote clinical reasoning. Support is particularly required in terms of staffing and the use of staff time. That is, both the development of clinical reasoning skills and implementation of clinical reasoning in nursing practice are resource-intensive in terms of staff time.

Teaching/learning strategies to promote clinical reasoning are many and varied. In this chapter the principal strategies advocated are reflection, peer consultation and thinking aloud. Urden (1989) asserts that professional knowledge is embedded in practice and recommends a range of strategies to support clinical knowledge development, including joint rounds, clinical forums/discussions, peer review and specialty consultation. Each of these strategies incorporates the concepts of collaboration and peer consultation within a group context.

Problem-based learning is another approach which has gained popularity over the last decade in the health sciences. It too utilizes such strategies as collaborative learning, peer consultation, small group work and self-directed learning, couched in a practice setting.

Both Revans (1980) and Knowles (1980) have argued that problem-based learning is effective because (a) the people closest to problems are best suited to solving them and (b) adults learn best when their experience is utilized. Further, Quinn and Smith (1987) have argued that the medical profession has effectively used peer consultation and collaboration to build and maintain a power base.

Exempla

Harman *et al.* (1989) describe a continuing education program to develop clinical decision making skills for experienced nursing staff. A 1-day workshop plus a follow-up teaching session for small groups and individuals was introduced for 900 nurses representing 34 units at Toronto General Hospital. Nurses were encouraged to identify and use peer support to select appropriate nursing diagnoses and develop care plans. The authors suggested that the creation of an atmosphere which promoted the open discussion of common concerns and frustrations about nursing practice and clinical reasoning was important. The support, commitment and involvement of the work unit managers was considered critical to the success of the program. Regular meetings between the managers were organized to provide opportunities to discuss concerns regarding program implementation and receive peer support.

In a collaborative venture between a university school of nursing and a teaching hospital, Farrell and Bramadat (1990) developed two strategies to promote clinical reasoning skills. The first, paradigm case analysis, allows students to 'share in the discussion of real life cases of experienced clinicians' (p. 154). This strategy provides an opportunity for dialogue, fosters openness to criticism and allows participants to trace the decision-making process. Their second strategy, stimulated recall during action, was introduced in recognition of the limitation of retrospective case analysis and in an effort to stimulate reflection-in-action as opposed to reflection-on-action (as per Schön, 1987). Nurses were concurrently observed in practice and questioned about their process of clinical reasoning. Both strategies encouraged clinicians and students to verbalize and document their reasoning.

Maltby and Andrusyszyn (1990) discuss the value of a case-study approach to teaching decision making for post-basic students. The students were divided into small groups to share their collective experience in order to address a broad range of case studies. Students commented favourably that the learning experience increased their awareness of their decision making and encouraged lateral thinking.

An educational game to enhance nurses' emergency decision-making knowledge and skills was developed by Schmitz *et al.* (1991) with attention to the principles of adult learning. It offered the advantage of acquiring and testing knowledge in a safe context and via a team approach rather than in the high-risk environment of an accident and emergency unit. The authors concluded that this learning experience helped 'foster co-operation, communication, cohesiveness and peer learning and support' and that 'the game in a novel, fun and challenging way helps build an underlying collegial framework for nursing practice' (p. 156).

Conclusion

Any strategy to develop and enhance the clinical reasoning skills of students and recent graduates must be sensitive to the workplace culture and encompass both an educational and administrative focus. Many experienced and expert nurses need assistance to move from 'knowing how' to 'understanding why' and then developing the confidence to adapt their practice on the basis of reflection and peer consultation. Providing such opportunities within the workplace and ensuring a responsiveness to suggestions for improved practice demands both an administrative and educational commitment. Only when the workplace culture supports a commitment to professional development and quality will students be confident to use a process of continuous improvement that ensures that theoretical understanding is linked to and underpins clinical 'know-how'. It is also such an environment, a learning community, that will encourage experienced nurses to contribute to the development of both the theory which underpins nursing practice and the process of clinical reasoning in nursing, by utilizing, testing and refining models and conceptual frameworks within their practice.

References

Bandura, A. (1971) *Social Learning Theory.* Merristown, NJ: General Learning Press.

Benner, P. (1984) *From Novice to Expert: Excellence and Power in Clinical Nursing Practice.* Menlo Park, CA: Addison-Wesley.

Bilderback, B. (1989) Surviving the stages of peer consultation. *American Journal of Nursing,* **89**, 113–116.

Boud, D., Keogh, R. and Walker, D. (1985) *Reflection: Turning Experience into Learning.* London: Kogan Page.

Brammer, J. and Zelmer, A. (1996) *Clinical Teaching in the Health Professions.* Geelong, Australia: Deakin University Press.

Cross, K. P. (1981) *Adults as Learners.* San Francisco: Jossey-Bass.

Erickson, G. P. (1987) Peer evaluation as a teaching–learning strategy in baccalaureate education for community health nursing. *Journal of Nursing Education,* **26**, 204–206.

Farrell, P. and Bramadat, I. J. (1990) Paradigm case analysis and stimulated recall: Strategies for developing clinical reasoning skills. *Clinical Nurse Specialist,* **4**, 153–157.

Field, P. A. (1987) The impact of nursing theory on the clinical decision making process. *Journal of Advanced Nursing,* **12**, 563–571.

Fontes, H. C. (1987) Small group work: A strategy to promote active learning. *Journal of Nursing Education,* **26**, 212–214.

Freire, P. (1970) *Pedagogy of the Oppressed.* New York: Herder & Herder.

Freire, P. (1983) *Education for Critical Consciousness.* New York: Continuum Press.

Harman, L., Wabin, D., MacInnis, L., Baird, D., Mattiuzzi, D. and Savage, P. (1989) Developing clinical decision-making skills in staff nurses: An education program. *Journal of Continuing Education in Nursing,* **20**, 102–106.

Hart, G. (1990) Peer consultation and review. *Australian Journal of Advanced Nursing,* **7**, 40–46.

Hart, G. (1992) The clinical learning environment: Nurses' perceptions of professional development in clinical settings. *PhD thesis.* University of New South Wales, Sydney.

Hart, G. (1997) Clinical Teaching Strategies to Encourage Reflective Practice. *International Journal of Practical Experience in Professional Education,* **1**, 53–63.

Jarvis, P. (1987) Lifelong education and its relevance to nursing. *Nurse Education Today,* **7**, 49–55.

Karuhije, H. E. (1986) Educational preparation for clinical teaching: Perceptions of the nurse educator. *Journal of Nursing Education,* **25**, 137–144.

Kemmis, S. (1985) Action research and the politics of reflection. In *Reflection: Turning Experience Into Learning* (D. Boud, R. Keogh and D. Walker, eds), pp. 139–163. London: Kogan Page.

Knowles, M. C. (1980) *The Modern Practice of Adult Education: Andragogy Versus Pedagogy.* New York: Cambridge Books.

Knowles, M. C. (1990) *The Adult Learner: A Neglected Species,* 4th edn. London: Gulf Publishing.

Maltby, H. J. and Andrusyszyn, M. A. (1990) The case study approach of teaching decision-making to post-diploma nurses. *Nurse Education Today,* **10**, 415–419.

Morgan, J. and Knox, J. (1987) Characteristics of 'best' and 'worst' clinical teachers as perceived by university nursing faculty and students. *Journal of Advanced Nursing,* **12**, 331–337.

Pasacreta, J. V. and Jacobsen, P. B. (1989) Addressing the needs for staff support among nurses caring for the AIDS population. *Oncology Nursing Forum,* **16**, 659–663.

Quinn, C. A. and Smith, M. D. (1987) *The Professional Commitment: Issues and Ethics in Nursing.* New York: Saunders.

Revans, R. E. (1980) *Action Learning: New Techniques for Management.* London: Blond & Briggs.

Ripley, D. M. (1986) Invitational teaching behaviors in the associate degree clinical setting. *Journal of Nursing Education,* **25**, 240–246.

Schmitz, B. D., MacLean, S. L. and Schidler, H. M. (1991) An emergency pursuit game: A method for teaching emergency decision making skills. *The Journal of Continuing Education in Nursing,* **22**, 152–158.

Schön, D. (1983) *The Reflective Practitioner.* London: Temple Smith.

Schön, D. (1987) *Educating The Reflective Practitioner: Toward a New Design for Teaching and Learning in the Professions.* San Francisco: Jossey-Bass.

Shamian, J. and Inhaber, R. (1985) The concept and practice of preceptorship in contemporary nursing: A review of pertinent literature. *International Journal of Nursing Studies*, **22**, 79–88.

Tough, A. (1979) *The Adult Learning Project*. Toronto, Ontario: Ontario Institute for Studies in Education.

Urden, L. D. (1989) Knowledge development in clinical practice. *The Journal of Continuing Education in Nursing*, **20**, 18–22.

White, R. and Ewan, C. (1991) *Clinical Teaching in Nursing*. London: Chapman & Hall.

Windsor, A. (1987) Nursing students' perceptions of clinical experience. *Journal of Nursing Education*, **26**, 150–154.

Wong, J. and Wong, S. (1987) Towards effective clinical teaching nursing. *Journal of Advanced Nursing*, **12**, 505–513.

Young, S., Theriault, M. S. and Collins, D. (1989) The nurse preceptor: Preparation and needs. *Journal of Nursing Staff Development*, **5**, 127–131.

33

Peer coaching to generate clinical-reasoning skills

Richard Ladyshewsky, Robert Baker and Mark Jones

Novice practitioners, or health professionals who lack clinical experience in general, often have more limited clinical-reasoning skills than experienced clinicians. They commonly have a reduced ability to judge the relevance and importance of particular clinical tasks, particularly when contrasted to expert performance (Oldmeadow, 1996). Novices also tend to make reasoning errors when attempting to make clinical decisions. Such errors stem from a knowledge base that is being restructured, moving from a predominance of biomedical knowledge to more clinically meaningful patterns (Boshuizen and Schmidt, 1995; Carnevali, 1995). Boshuizen and Schmidt (1992) term this tendency to make frequent errors an 'intermediate effect'.

The education of novices (students or inexperienced graduates) clearly needs to address the development of their clinical-reasoning abilities. In this paper we will discuss the use of peer-centred learning in clinical education as a method to facilitate the development of clinical reasoning in novice practitioners. Support for peer-centred learning as a means of promoting clinical-reasoning skills development is widely reported in the literature (Barker-Schwartz, 1991; Boshuizen and Schmidt, 1992; Boshuizen and Schmidt, 1995; Graham, 1996; Higgs, 1992; Refshauge and Higgs, 1995; Regehr and Norman, 1996; Schell and Cervero, 1993; Terry and Higgs, 1993).

Learning from peers

Learning from peers is sometimes referred to as co-operative learning. Co-operative learning, however, is a broad educational strategy that encapsulates many forms of peer-centred learning. For example, Johnson *et al.* (Johnson and Johnson, 1978, 1987; Johnson *et al.*, 1981) use the term co-operative learning to describe principles of group learning, i.e. learning which is enhanced by group interdependence and individual accountability.

The literature on peer learning/teaching and the definitions that emanate from this work are abundant. Gerace and Sibilano (1984), for example, define peer teaching as a collaboration between two people of equal rank working together to solve a problem. Riggio *et al.* (1994) use the term reciprocal peer tutoring, whereby students alternatively play the role of tutor and tutee. Lincoln and McAllister (1993) examine the concept of peer learning in detail and raise an important differentiation between process and procedure. Peer learning is the process and is related to the outcomes of the collaborative learning experience. In contrast, peer tutoring, peer teaching, peer review and peer evaluation are specific procedures which allow peer learning to occur. The procedure that is discussed in this chapter to describe the peer learning experience, is reciprocal peer coaching (RPC). It is an educational procedure in which peers coach one another through clinical experiences. The coaching activities centre around demonstration, observation, collaborative practice, feedback/discussion and problem solving.

Modes of learning and RPC

Experience-based learning

The influence of past and present clinical experience is a significant part of the novice practitioner's learning. Clinical experiences are used to restructure biomedical knowledge into more meaningful clinical patterns, which ultimately guide practice (Boshuizen and Schmidt, 1995; Carnevali, 1995). Hence, the quality and influence of experience and the learning that follows is central to clinical competence.

The importance of experiential learning and the impact of experience on the cognitive structure of the learner is described in detail by numerous authors (e.g. Barker-Schwartz, 1991; Boud, 1988; Brown *et al.*, 1989; Graham, 1996, Kolb, 1984). Boud (1993) argues that learners construct newer forms of knowledge and understanding using their previous experiences as a template. These experiences are not only influenced by the novice practitioner's underlying knowledge base, they are influenced by the social and cultural context of the learning situation as well. Brown *et al.* (1989) describe learning which encompasses both the physical and social contexts, as situated learning. Learning in these real-life situations allows concepts to evolve because the situation and the negotiations/discussions that occur with others recast the information into a more densely textured form (Graham, 1996).

Boud (1988, 1993) has challenged educators to place more emphasis on how students learn from complex experiences. Based on constructivist learning theory which states that learners construct their own unique forms of knowledge, it can be argued that more attention needs to be paid to learning from experience (Boud, 1993; Brown *et al.*, 1989). Strategically engaging the learner in the actual learning experience, therefore, is one method of enhancing learning.

Quite often, during the course of a clinical education experience, a novice practitioner is exposed to a wide variety of patients and problems. Hopefully, some of this experience is translated into learning and the novice practitioner's competence is improved. More often than not, however, novice practitioners do not gain as much as they

could have from the patient management experience, particularly if they have poor self-reflection or self-evaluation skills. In light of this situation, strategies which actively engage the learner in the experience are important if one is to maximize learning outcomes.

Boud (1988) describes a strategic approach to learning from experience as a series of three stages which is generalizable to any learning experience. The first stage involves 'returning to the experience' so that the learner can recapture as many parts of the experience as possible. The second stage involves 'attending to feelings' and involves reflecting on the feelings that arose during the experience. Recognizing these feelings helps the learner to understand how these feelings influence their specific interpretations and general understanding. The third stage involves 're-evaluating the experience', where the new experience is related to prior experiences and new knowledge is re-organized using a variety of cognitive and metacognitive strategies such as association, integration, validation and appropriation (Boud, 1988). *Association* involves connecting ideas and feelings which are part of the original experience, to existing knowledge. *Integration* involves processing these associations to see if there are patterns or linkages to other ideas. *Validation* tests the internal consistency of these emerging concepts in relation to existing beliefs and knowledge, and *appropriation* involves making this new knowledge an integral part of how one acts or feels.

The influence of experiential learning and the use of discussion to enhance cognitive processing is also seen in the theoretical perspectives of other educational theorists. Belenky *et al.* (1986) describe two concepts: connected knowing; and separate knowing. While both forms of knowing are important, connected knowing is a preferred educational orientation because it includes the sharing of common experiences and discussion of the feelings that inform ideas. Separate knowing is an orientation to learning that is characterized by impersonal and objective reasoning, commonly referred to as critical thinking. Barker-Schwartz (1991) argues that learning activities that involve discussion of experiences and illustrate theory in practice, will promote connected knowing. RPC, which promotes observation of theory in practice, collaborative practice, feedback/discussion and problem solving, can be used to promote this connection.

This perspective on connected knowing is also supported in principle by Boshuizen and Schmidt, 1992 and Carr *et al.* (see Chapter 21). These authors see the integration of general and situated (in context) knowledge emanating from reflection and discussion. By exploring the connections between these two knowledge domains, e.g. through collaborative discussions with a peer, encapsulation of biomedical knowledge into more relevant and robust clinical forms can take place. Carr *et al.* (Chapter 21) also state that by transforming biomedical knowledge into more useful clinical formats, performance in future encounters may be enhanced.

The use of RPC, therefore, appears to provide a rich opportunity for novice practitioners to more actively engage themselves in the learning experience. By preparing novices to engage in strategic and reflective clinical discussions with their peers, opportunities for enhancing clinical reasoning and metacognition may occur. Further, the development of more robust clinical knowledge is possible because of the opportunities to refine and restructure knowledge.

Learner-managed learning – Developing learning strategies, using metacognition

Bandura's (1971, 1997) perspectives on social learning theory describes three kinds of reinforcements that influence learning outcomes. The first is direct external reinforcement. Under this form of reinforcement, persons regulate their behaviour on the basis of the consequences they experience directly. The second is vicarious reinforcement. This type of reinforcement occurs by observing the experiences of others and then modifying your own behaviour based upon the consequences you have just observed. Thirdly, self-administered reinforcement involves regulating your own behaviours according to standards. The nature of RPC provides rich opportunities for these three types of reinforcement to occur. For example, feedback from a peer may help the novice to recognize certain consequences of their behaviour or their failure to recognize a standard of behaviour required. All of these reinforcements contribute to the learners' metacognitive learning framework as they provide opportunities for identifying gaps and deficiencies in cognitive strategies and knowledge.

In a review of adult learning theory Mezirow (1981) discusses the three forms of empirical knowledge identified by Habermas (1972), i.e. technical, practical and emancipatory knowledge. Mezirow discusses these three approaches to learning and their influence on the generation of knowledge. He argues that most educational methods emphasize the first two perspectives, which focus on the provision and evaluation of knowledge and skills. While these methods may be appropriate for competency based education, Mezirow feels they ignore the emancipatory perspective. Emancipatory learning '. . . involves an interest in self-knowledge, that is, the knowledge of self-reflection . . . Insights gained through critical self-awareness are emancipatory in the sense that at least one can recognize the correct reasons for his or her problems' (Mezirow, 1981, p. 5). Mezirow argues that metacognition or personal awareness about knowledge enhances cognition.

Emancipatory learning can be promoted by encouraging discussion and dialogue with peers and by participating in, and leading learning groups (Mezirow, 1981). This helps learners to identify real problems involving, for example, power relationships, institutional ideologies that are embedded in myths and their own personal feelings. Mezirow argues that by critiquing these psycho-cultural perspectives, alternative meaning perspectives can be created. This type of emancipatory learning is critical in clinical reasoning, particularly if one considers the importance of personal knowledge in pragmatic/ethical reasoning (Jones, 1997; Neistadt, 1996; Schell and Cervero, 1993). These forms of reasoning involve considering the moral, political and economic dilemmas in clinical practice.

The above discussion illustrates the importance of learning how to learn and the use of metacognition to monitor cognition during learning and clinical reasoning. Metacognitive skills are cognitive skills that are necessary for the management of knowledge and other cognitive skills (Biggs, 1988). Metacognition involves being aware of one's own cognitive processes and controlling them (Higgs and Titchen, 1995). Skills in metacognition have been shown to enhance problem solving and learning (Biggs, 1988; Biggs and Telfer, 1987). Thus, learning programs such as clinical education programs which aim to enhance students' capacity to generate and acquire new knowledge and to enhance their clinical-reasoning abilities need to develop the students' metacognitive skills (Higgs, 1992; Higgs and Jones, 1995; Jones *et al.*, 1995; Lincoln and McAllister, 1993; Terry and Higgs, 1993; Tichenor *et al.*, 1995).

While this independent metacognition and 'reflection-in action' (Schön, 1991) can be used by an individual practitioner, peers can consciously engage in specific discussions at each stage of the experience, thus heightening the cognitive and metacognitive experience (Higgs and Titchen, 1995; Jones, 1995). Reciprocal peer coaching is a particularly useful method to facilitate metacognition because of the joint problem solving activities that take place between peers (Terry and Higgs, 1993). The discussion, problem solving and coaching that take place in RPC heighten the novice practitioner's awareness of knowledge gaps and errors of cognition. This metacognitive activity can lead to enhanced clinical reasoning skill and greater levels of competency (Higgs and Jones, 1995).

RPC in clinical education programs

One of the reasons for encouraging RPC in the clinical education setting is that clinical educators/supervisors may not always be available to assist novice practitioners/students. Time pressures and heavy workloads may make it difficult for the supervisor to explore clinical reasoning frequently in action with the student (Cason *et al.*, 1977; Higgs, 1992). RPC can relieve the supervisor of some of this responsibility, particularly with more straightforward clinical problems (Goldenberg and Iwasiw, 1992). Costello (1989) found that a significant amount of learning occurred between peers as part of the hidden curriculum. Claims by students that they were taught 'most' by other students compared to instructors and ward personnel have also been reported in the literature (Lewin and Leach, 1982).

Even with good supervisor availability, novices may still not ask their superiors for support because of fear of negative appraisal. May and Newman (1980) point out that effective problem solving is most likely to occur in an environment where students are free to test out their thinking skills, explore alternatives and discover approaches that may or may not match other clinician's solutions. In situations, however, where novice performance is subject to continuous evaluation, novices may feel reticent to test out their thinking with their supervisors (Erickson, 1987). Boud (1988) sees learning partnerships as one strategy to overcome this reticence.

Fostering peer discussion in the clinical setting promotes exposure of the learners' thoughts and arguments, and allows for discussion and restructuring of knowledge to take place (Regehr and Norman, 1996). This can be facilitated by having students work with the same patient over the course of a placement and/or having them see other patients with similar or dissimilar diagnoses

(Cohn, 1989; Grant *et al.*, 1988). The discussion that emanates from these experiences should enable students to create stronger relational structures in their knowledge base, leading to better encapsulation of their knowledge and more finely tuned clinical patterns and prototypes (Bordage and Lemieux, 1986). Resnick (1988) contends that the collective problem solving that occurs in RPC leads to insights and solutions that would otherwise not occur as it brings to light misconceptions that have been erroneously directing novice practice.

Several examples of peer-centred learning are described in the health sciences education literature. These learning strategies have been used in the classroom and in the clinical setting with good results. Graham (1996), for example, conducted a qualitative study of ten physical therapy students in an entry-level masters program. One of the key themes to emerge from this study was the value of discussion. Discussion with peers was seen to be a key conceptualisation strategy. Students stated that they would study course content initially, then engage in a discussion with peers to boost their comprehension.

Iwasiw and Goldenberg (1993) studied peer learning among nursing students using a surgical dressing change procedure. They measured the cognitive and psychomotor gains of nursing students taught by peers and those taught by nursing instructors. Cognitive gains were significantly higher for the peer group and psychomotor gains, although not significant, showed greater improvement among the peer group. DeClute and Ladyshewsky (1993) compared the clinical competency scores of physiotherapy students in peer-centred learning placements to those in individual learning placements. Clinical competency scores of the peer group were significantly higher across all performance dimensions.

Remaining studies in the health sciences tend to be more descriptive in nature and examine the social and affective benefits of peer-based learning (Beeken, 1991; Cason *et al.*, 1977; Costello, 1989; De Dea, 1996; Gerace and Sibilano, 1984; Haffner-Zavadak *et al.*, 1995; Kleffner and Dadian, 1997; Ladyshewsky, 1993; Lincoln and McAllister, 1993; Tiberius and Gaiptman, 1985). Some of these additional benefits include: greater patient care productivity; enhanced individual effort among learners; more positive communication; greater inter-collegial support; efficient use of teaching resources particularly when there is a high student:staff ratio; a shift from extrinsic to intrinsic motivation to learn; higher educational achievement; increased opportunities for learning; and greater practice using critical-thinking skills.

Preparation for peer learning

Coaching skills may need to be developed by novice practitioners before engaging in a peer learning experience. Before they can capitalize on the potential benefits of RPC, learners may need to develop skills in leadership, communication, trust building, decision making and conflict management, all important elements of both adult learning and skilled clinical reasoning (Goldenberg and Iwasiw, 1992; Johnson and Johnson, 1987). Lincoln and McAllister (1993) add that teaching of learning theory and practice in peer learning is an essential part of preparation for peer learning. An understanding of how to optimize learning not only enhances students' ability to maximize their own learning experiences and outcomes but also equips them with valuable strategies to promote patient learning: an essential skill for all health professionals. The need to develop these co-operative learning skills in students is particularly important in the health sciences as students may be reticent to support one another given that they have to compete vigorously with one another to enter professional schools (Lynch, 1984). This argument is supported by Sharan (1980) who points out that students accustomed to years of individual competition for grades are not likely to engage in mutual assistance automatically.

For a successful peer learning experience to take place positive interdependence, individual accountability and group processing ability need to be present (Johnson, 1981; Johnson and Johnson, 1978, 1987; Slavin, 1990). Positive interdependence means that there is a co-operative goal structure in place and learners perceive that they can only attain their goals if the other learners with whom they are linked also obtain their goals. In clinical practice, this may mean outlining specific co-operative learning objectives or delineating joint tasks. Students must also be held accountable for their participation, otherwise the learning outcomes of the group are compromised. Further, learners should be given the opportunity to engage in face-to-face group interactions.

RPC – An illustration

In our clinical education program RPC operates as follows: two novices are designated as coaching partners for the duration of a clinical placement. They are given the joint responsibility to evaluate a patient. The novices are encouraged to openly discuss their ideas and plans for the evaluation with one another. Further, they are encouraged to ask open-ended questions of one another such as, 'What are the reasons for doing these tests?', 'What sort of findings will result and what do they mean?', 'If a negative result occurs what alternative hypotheses might be considered?'. Knowledge gaps may also be identified as part of this reciprocal coaching process. In some cases, the novices may be able to assist one another in working through this knowledge gap. In other cases, the pair may need to consult their supervisor or do additional research to bridge this knowledge gap.

Students report positively on these learning experiences. Their comments include:

I learned more than I would have by myself because when you are working together you actually push each other to seek out new information.

I hadn't any experience with gerontology but my friend had worked in a nursing home before so I was able to learn a lot from her.

It was hard to remember everything, but by doing the post-operative procedure together we were able to get through all the information.

You don't feel so isolated so you feel more empowered to ask things.

Conclusion

Actively engaging novice practitioners in their learning and development is a key component of professional education that needs to be reinforced in professional preparation programs. By implementing learning models that encourage novice practitioners to learn alongside their peers, the potential for increasing clinical competence and clinical reasoning skills is enhanced. Peer learning strategies, such as the RPC approach described in this chapter, can enrich the depth of the clinical learning experience and heighten the metacognitive aspects of novice practitioners' learning. These are important educational imperatives for developing high level cognitive outcomes such as concept identification, analysis of problems, judgement and evaluation. The RPC approach to clinical learning, therefore, should be encouraged as a model of professional development for novice practitioners.

References

Bandura, A. (1971) Social Learning Theory. New York: General Learning Press.

Bandura, A. (1997) *Self Efficacy: The Exercise of Control*. New York: Freeman.

Barker-Schwartz, K. (1991) Clinical reasoning and new ideas on intelligence: Implications for teaching and learning. *American Journal of Occupational Therapy*, **45**, 1033–1037.

Beeken, J. (1991) Cooperative learning: Planning for success. *Journal of Ophthalmic Nursing and Technology*, **10**(2), 66–68.

Belenky, M., Clinchy, B., Goldberger, N. and Tarule, J. (1986) *Women's Ways of Knowing*. New York: Basic.

Biggs, J. (1988) The role of metacognition in enhancing learning. *Australian Journal of Education*, **32**, 127–138.

Biggs, J. B. and Telfer, R. (1987) *The Process of Learning*. Sydney: Prentice-Hall.

Bordage, G. and Lemieux, M. (1986) Some cognitive characteristics of medical students with and without diagnostic reasoning difficulties. Paper presented at the *25th Annual Conference of Research in Medical Education*, New Orleans.

Boshuizen, H. and Schmidt, H. (1992) On the role of biomedical knowledge in clinical reasoning by experts, intermediates and novices. *Cognitive Science*, **16**, 153–184.

Boshuizen, H. and Schmidt, H. (1995) The development of clinical reasoning expertise. In *Clinical Reasoning in the Health Professions* (J. Higgs and M. Jones, eds), pp. 24–32. Oxford: Butterworth-Heinemann.

Boud, D. (1988) How to help students learn from experience. In *The Medical Teacher* (K. Cox and C. Ewan, eds), 2nd edn, pp. 68–73. London: Churchill Livingstone.

Boud, D. (1993) Experience as the base for learning. *Higher Education Research and Development*, **12**, 33–44.

Brown, J., Collins, A. and Duguid, P. (1989) Situated cognition and the culture of learning. *Educational Researcher*, **18**, 32–42.

Carnevali, D. (1995) Self-monitoring of clinical reasoning behaviours: Promoting professional growth. In *Clinical Reasoning in the Health Professions* (J. Higgs and M. Jones, eds), pp. 179–190. Oxford: Butterworth-Heinemann.

Cason, C., Cason, G. and Bartnik, D. (1977) Peer instruction in professional nurse education: A qualitative case study. *Journal of Nursing Education*, **16**, 10–22.

Cohn, E. (1989) Fieldwork education: Shaping a foundation for clinical reasoning. *American Journal of Occupational Therapy*, **43**, 240–244.

Costello, J. (1989) Learning from each other: Peer teaching and learning in student nurse training. *Nurse Education Today*, **9**, 203–206.

DeClute, J. and Ladyshewsky, R. (1993) Enhancing clinical competence using a collaborative clinical education model. *Physical Therapy*, **73**, 683–689.

De Dea, L. (1996) The process, design, and implementation of an alternative, collaborative approach to clinical education using the 3:1 supervisory model. Paper presented at the *12th International Congress of the World Confederation for Physical Therapy*, Washington, DC.

Erickson, G. (1987) Peer evaluation as a teaching–learning strategy in baccalaureate education for community health nursing. *Journal of Nursing Education*, **26**, 204–206.

Gerace, L. and Sibilano, H. (1984) Preparing students for peer collaboration: A clinical teaching model. *Journal of Nursing Education*, **23**, 206–209.

Goldenberg, D. and Iwasiw, C. (1992) Reciprocal learning among students in the clinical area. *Nurse Educator*, **17**, 27–29.

Graham, C. (1996) Conceptual learning processes in physical therapy students. *Physical Therapy*, **76**, 856–865.

Grant, R., Jones, M. and Maitland, G. (1988) Clinical decision making in upper quadrant dysfunction. In *Physical Therapy of the Cervical and Thoracic Spine* (R. Grant, ed.), pp. 51–80. New York: Churchill Livingstone.

Habermas, J. (1972) *Knowledge and Human Interest*. London: Heinemann.

Haffner-Zavadak, K., Konecky-Dolnack, C., Polich, S. and Van Volkenburg, M. (1995) Collaborative models. *PT Magazine*, February, 46–54.

Higgs, J. (1992) Developing clinical reasoning competencies. *Physiotherapy*, **78**, 575–581.

Higgs, J. and Jones, M. (1995) Clinical reasoning. In *Clinical Reasoning in the Health Professions* (J. Higgs and M. Jones, eds), pp. 3–23. Oxford: Butterworth-Heinemann.

Higgs, J. and Titchen, A. (1995) Propositional, professional and personal knowledge in clinical reasoning. In *Clinical Reasoning in the Health Professions* (J. Higgs and M. Jones, eds), pp. 129–146. Oxford: Butterworth-Heinemann.

Iwasiw, C. and Goldenberg, D. (1993) Peer teaching among nursing students in the clinical area: effects on student learning. *Journal of Advanced Nursing*, **18**, 659–668.

Johnson, D. (1981) Student–student interaction: The neglected variable in education. *Educational Researcher*, **1**, 5–10.

Johnson, D. and Johnson, R. (1978) Cooperative, competitive, and individualistic learning. *Journal of Research and Development in Education*, **12**, 3–15.

Johnson, D. and Johnson, R. (1987) Research shows the benefits of adult cooperation. *Educational Leadership*, **45**, 27–30.

Johnson, D., Maruyama, G., Johnson, R., Nelson, D. and Skon, L. (1981) Effects of cooperative, competitive, and individualistic goal structures on achievement: A meta-analysis. *Psychological Bulletin*, **89**, 47–62.

Jones, M. (1995) Clinical reasoning and pain. *Manual Therapy*, **1**, 17–24.

Jones, M. (1997) Clinical reasoning: The foundation of clinical practice, Parts 1 and 2. *Australian Physiotherapy Journal*, **43**, 167–170 and 213–217.

Jones, M., Jensen, G. and Rothstein, J. (1995) Clinical reasoning in physiotherapy. In *Clinical Reasoning in the Health Professions* (J. Higgs and M. Jones, eds), pp. 72–87. Oxford: Butterworth-Heinemann.

Kleffner, J. and Dadian, T. (1997) Using collaborative learning in dental education. *Journal of Dental Education*, **61**, 66–72.

Kolb, D. (1984) *Experiential Learning: Experience as the Source of Learning and Development*. Englewood Cliffs, NJ: Prentice-Hall.

Ladyshewsky, R. (1993) Clinical teaching and the 2:1 student-to-clinical instructor ratio. *Journal of Physical Therapy Education*, **7**, 31–35.

Lewin, D. and Leach, J. (1982) Factors influencing the quality of wards as learning environments for student nurses. *International Journal of Nursing Studies*, **19**, 125–137.

Lincoln, M. and McAllister, L. (1993) Peer learning in clinical education. *Medical Teacher*, **15**, 17–25.

Lynch, B. (1984) Cooperative learning in interdisciplinary education for the allied health professions. *Journal of Allied Health*, **13**, 83–93.

May, B. and Newman, J. (1980) Developing competence in problem solving. *Physical Therapy*, **60**, 1140–1145.

Mezirow, J. (1981) A critical theory of adult learning and education. *Adult Education*, **31**, 3–24.

Neistadt, M. (1996) Teaching strategies for the development of clinical reasoning. *American Journal of Occupational Therapy*, **50**, 676–684.

Oldmeadow, L. (1996) Developing clinical competence: A mastery pathway. *Australian Physiotherapy Journal*, **42**, 37–44.

Refshauge, K. and Higgs, J. (1995) Teaching clinical reasoning in health science curricula. In *Clinical Reasoning in the Health Professions* (J. Higgs and M. Jones, eds), pp. 105–116, Oxford: Butterworth-Heinemann.

Regehr, G. and Norman, G. (1996) Issues in cognitive psychology: Implications for professional education. *Academic Medicine*, **71**, 988–1000.

Resnick, L. (1988) Learning in school and out. *Educational Researcher*, **16**, 13–20.

Riggio, R., Whatley, M. and Neale, P. (1994) Effects of student academic ability on cognitive gains using reciprocal peer tutoring. *Journal of Social Behaviour and Psychology*, **9**, 529–542.

Schell, B. and Cervero, R. (1993) Clinical reasoning in occupational therapy: An integrative review. *American Journal of Occupational Therapy*, **47**, 605–610.

Schön, D. (1991) *The Reflective Practitioner: How Professionals Think in Action*. London: Ashgate Publishing.

Sharan, S. (1980) Cooperative learning in small groups: Recent methods and effects on achievement, attitudes, and ethnic relations. *Review of Educational Research*, **50**, 241–271.

Slavin, R. (1990) Research on cooperative learning: Consensus and controversy. *Educational Leadership*, **47**(4), 52–54.

Terry, W. and Higgs, J. (1993) Educational programmes to develop clinical reasoning skills. *Australian Physiotherapy Journal*, **39**, 47–51.

Tiberius, R. and Gaiptman, B. (1985) The supervisor–student ratio: 1:1 versus 1:2. *Canadian Journal of Occupational Therapy*, **52**, 179–183.

Tichenor, C., Davidson, J. and Jensen, G. (1995) Cases as shared inquiry: Model for clinical reasoning. *Journal of Physical Therapy Education*, **9**, 57–62.

34

Teaching clinical reasoning: A case-based approach

Ian Scott

The development of effective clinical-reasoning skills is a fundamental pre-requisite to the making and survival of the modern doctor. Clinical reasoning can be defined as the thinking and decision-making processes required to achieve the goal of optimal patient care in which making a diagnosis is the essential first step. The hypothetico-deductive (or guess and test) model of diagnostic reasoning has been well studied and enumerated since the late 1970s (Barrows and Feltovich, 1987; Elstein *et al.*, 1978; Fraser, 1992; Glass, 1996; Kassirer, 1983).

The tasks of clinical reasoning

Successful and efficient clinical reasoners are those who can readily perform the following tasks when encountering novel clinical problems which experience-based pattern recognition is unable to quickly solve:

(a) Perceive initial key features of the problem and frame it correctly (e.g. conceptualize a clinical presentation as being more likely an acute rather than chronic problem, or a medical rather than surgical problem).
(b) Quickly generate relevant hypotheses which account for some or most (if not all) of the key features.
(c) Use efficient, focused, hypothesis-driven lines of inquiry (including physical examination and preliminary investigations as well as history-taking) in eliciting further information for testing the validity of generated hypotheses.

(d) Interpret elicited data correctly (i.e. accurately weigh the evidence in supporting or refuting specific diagnoses) in relation to known facts about patterns of disease, and make appropriate deductions.
(e) Reformulate and refine existing hypotheses, or generate new ones, in an iterative process led by the disclosure of new and relevant findings.
(f) Eliminate competing hypotheses and verify one or a few hypotheses as the provisional diagnosis and the basis for further clinical action.
(g) Prescribe interventions that, on the basis of the best available scientific knowledge and expert opinion, are likely to confer a significant benefit on the patient.
(h) Explain to patients the rationale behind the diagnostic and management decisions being made, and the extent to which decisions are based on probabilities rather than certainties.
(i) Enable patients to participate in decision making and candidly discuss the benefits and risks of proposed interventions.

A case-based approach to teaching clinical reasoning

Reasoning skill is significantly dependent on prior knowledge and experience of specific clinical problems (content or case specificity) (Elstein *et al.*, 1978). Content specificity negates the notion of a generic set of reasoning skills which, when applied to any clinical problem, can consistently yield the correct solution. However, for those with limited content knowledge, a number of reasoning rules or heuristics (McDonald, 1996) can assist in performing the reasoning tasks already outlined. Using case studies as the medium for learning in which participants are encouraged by tutors to 'think out loud' as a problem unfolds (Kassirer and Kopelman, 1991; Thomas, 1992), students can practise using these heuristics and applying hypo-thetico-deductive methods in resolving real-life clinical problems (see below).

Case studies come in different forms: (i) chronological recounts (presenter to audience) of actual cases, (ii) replay of videotaped interviews between individual students and real or standard-ized patients, or (iii) paper-based or computer-based simulations. Various instructional courses in clinical reasoning have made use of one or more of these methods (Lewkonia *et al.*, 1993; Margolis *et al.*, 1982; Schwartz *et al.*, 1992; Scott, 1995). Common to all is the provision of introductory comments followed by the active gathering and processing of data by students in solving a problem for which subsequent informa-tion is provided only if requested. Such an approach accelerates acquisition of the pattern-rich, situation-specific and readily recallable heu-ristic knowledge of experienced clinicians (Bor-dage and Zacks, 1984). In the hands of skilled, tactful tutors case studies also provide a realistic but non-threatening forum for identifying and remedying reasoning errors and developing intel-lectually self-correcting (or meta-cognitive) skills (Biggs and Telfer, 1987).

Videotapes of student–patient interviews have educational advantages in that the interactive skills of interviewing and examination (Sanders *et al.*, 1997), the tools for gathering primary data upon which decision making is based, can be assessed and their interdependence with reasoning skills emphasized. The stop and replay function of videotapes also allows critical parts of the interview, those pivotal to final conclusions or demonstrating errors in logic or data elicitation, to be interrogated in greater detail. Computerized exercises, whilst less able than videotapes (even with interactive video clips) to replicate the behavioural dimensions of clinical encounters, still show considerable promise in tracking and evaluating the logic and interpretive skills used by students in solving problems (Myers and Dorsey, 1994). Whilst the most valid and reliable means of formally assessing (as opposed to teaching) clinical reasoning skills are yet to be determined (van der Vleuten and Newble, 1995), it is likely that structured analyses of observed

'think out loud' reasoning exercises (Kassirer *et al.*, 1982) may prove, in the first instance, to be the most feasible and useful.

Using case studies to instantiate reasoning heuristics

The following discussion demonstrates how, for each of the key reasoning tasks, case examples can be used to instantiate heuristics and highlight potential reasoning errors related to each task.

Perceiving initial cues

Verbal and non-verbal information obtained early in the clinical encounter (initial cues) determines first impressions about the patient's problems. These in turn influence the choice of initial hypotheses and further inquiries. Initial cues need to be accurately characterized in determining how much they suggest significant pathology (Galen and Gambino, 1975; Wasson *et al.*, 1992). However, symptoms and signs can be characterized differently by different clinicians in different settings (Koran, 1975; Platt and McMath, 1979). The use of precise descriptors and scaling methods (such as objective measures of exercise tolerance in a patient with dyspnoea, or cognitive functioning in a patient with suspected dementia) quantifies illness effects over time and indicates potential seriousness (Feinstein, 1987). Patients may use medical labels (such as 'heart attack' or 'asthma') or express supposedly factual statements (such as 'I had a fit' or 'I suffer kidney failure'), all of which must be validated by using non-leading questions to prompt complete narrative descriptions.

The psychosocial as well as physical limitations imposed by illness are also often under-appreciated by clinicians (Schor *et al.*, 1995) but frequently lie behind the patient's decision to present (Beckman and Frankel, 1984). Whilst reliable in the detection of somatic illness, clinicians often overlook psy-chosocial disorders (Burack and Carpenter, 1983). Active listening, picking up non-verbal cues, and exploring emotionally laden gestures and utter-ances are vital if the true problem is to be fully ascertained and misdiagnosis avoided.

Framing the problem and forming the initial concept

Upon gathering a critical mass of information, a process of categorizing and clustering the data should begin that helps conceptualize the problem (Barrows *et al.*, 1982). Clinical descriptions should be reduced, within the limits of accuracy, to concise medical terms that help frame the problem and trigger plausible hypotheses. Depicting the temporal course of illness as acute or chronic, sudden or gradual, or specifying the extent of a physical syndrome as unilateral or bilateral, proximal or distal, total or partial are some basic examples (Bordage and Lemieux, 1991). At a more advanced level, the findings of weakness, hyper-reflexia, and extensor plantar responses can be more aptly expressed as 'pyramidal tract signs' or 'spastic paresis', phrases that collapse many words into a few and which have syndromic connotations (Benbassat and Schiffmann, 1976). Similarly, complaints of 'vomiting', 'abdominal pain' and 'peritonism' can be grouped as 'acute abdomen', suggesting possible causes such as ruptured viscus or strangulated bowel.

A number of first-principle heuristics can help generate hypotheses if clustering strategies are proving ineffective. First, the basic pathological process can be inferred from the temporal pattern of symptoms and loss of function (Balla *et al.*, 1990). Vascular and mechanical illness will manifest abruptly (over minutes); infectious, inflammatory or metabolic illness will develop over hours to days; neoplastic disease over many weeks to months; and degenerative disease over months to years. Second, the anatomic location of disease can be inferred by the nature of certain symptoms (Fulop, 1985). For example, pleuritic chest pain suggests disease of parietal pleura or chest wall structures. Third, a larger set of possible diagnoses for a given constellation of clinical findings may be suggested by consciously considering four possible conceptual scenarios: (a) acute illness in a previously healthy patient, (b) exacerbation of a chronic illness which is brought on by some new insult, (c) complications or sequelae of a chronic illness (the natural history of disease) and (d) adverse effects resulting from medicines and procedures used to treat underlying illness (Russell, 1985). From the case study-based use of such heuristics, students can more quickly generate ideas that are 'in the right ballpark'.

Generating (or triggering) hypotheses

Hypotheses (or 'hunches' or 'guesses') serve a number of important cognitive functions. First, they limit the number of diagnostic possibilities and thereby reduce the potential scope of inquiry.

Second, they organize information such that deductive inferences can be more readily made (i.e. whether the presence or absence of certain cues supports or refutes a particular hypothesis). Third, the gathering and interpretation of new information becomes more directed and discriminatory in the presence of discrete hypotheses. Fourth, by subsuming many cues under one hypothesis, information processing is rendered more rapid and efficient (Miller, 1956). Given these functions, students should be required when doing case studies to state their hypotheses shortly after receiving the initial cues (key presenting symptoms are often sufficient). The more inclusive the initial hypotheses, the more likely the correct diagnosis will be considered (Barrows *et al.*, 1982) and the more the predictive value of initial cues will come to be appreciated.

For clinical novices, expertise will be limited to lay medical knowledge, classic disease descriptions memorized from textbooks or tutorials, or recent, vividly recalled clinical encounters. Certain diagnoses are thus hypothesized only if cues match the classical picture or if certain cues recall specific past events (Grant and Marsden, 1987). Asking the question 'Yes, but why did you think that?' or 'Yes, but what else could it be?' prompts students to reflect on the reasons for their initial choice of hypotheses.

The array of generated hypotheses will also depend on the student's preferred reasoning approach to any given problem (Kassirer, 1989a): (i) *causal* reasoning (solving a problem from first principles based on an understanding of biology and pathophysiology), (ii) *probabilistic* reasoning (postulating solutions based on an awareness of disease prevalence and risk factors) or (iii) *deterministic* reasoning (choosing solutions on the basis of simple axioms and 'if–then' rules). With case studies students can practise using these reasoning approaches strategically (either singly or in combination) according to their past experience with the problem. In some instances causal reasoning will be the most effective method (Balla *et al.*, 1990); in others probabilistic or deterministic reasoning will be more useful, with causal reasoning being used secondarily to verify biological plausibility of generated hypotheses (Boshuizen and Schmidt, 1992).

Students must also learn to reason effectively within emotionally laden and clinically taxing circumstances, environments difficult to replicate in case-study exercises. The case of a seriously ill patient accompanied by distressed relatives presenting after hours to an isolated hospital exemplifies the need for 'sharp-end' decision making under less than ideal conditions. The leisurely generation (and testing) of hypotheses as abstract activities, whilst not inappropriate initially, should gradually give way to more pragmatic case simulations which impose constraints of limited time and urgency.

Testing and refining hypotheses using focused inquiry strategies

The process of hypothesis testing and refinement (or 'case building') calls for efficient, selective use of hypothesis-based inquiry strategies (questions, items of examination or simple tests) which yield specific information that can reliably discriminate between hypotheses (Barrows and Tamblyn, 1980). These 'search' techniques are preferred to standardized 'scanning' or checklist approaches (such as the time-honoured 'systems review') which consume time and effort in producing distracting data of little real value (Hoffbrand, 1989).

Efficient search strategies focus on findings which help rule in or rule out certain hypotheses on the basis of their known association (or lack of) with particular disease states. *Specific* cues, if present, strongly support a diagnosis. An example: chest pain which is heavy and retrosternal and relieved quickly by anginine is more predictive of a diagnosis of angina than is burning chest pain radiating down the left arm. The latter is a less specific symptom which, whilst capable of being angina, also occurs in other syndromes such as gastro-oesophageal reflux. *Sensitive* cues tend to exclude certain hypotheses if absent but by themselves do not confirm any one disease. An example: the absence of exertional dyspnoea would weigh heavily against the diagnosis of cardiac failure, but if present could be compatible with other possibilities such as emphysema or blood clots in the lung.

A better appreciation of the diagnostic (or *predictive*) value of various symptoms and signs rationalizes the choice of search inquiries (Why do you want to know that?) and helps decide how much elicited findings increase or decrease the likelihood of specific diseases (How do you interpret these findings? What weight are you going to place on them?). A common error is to overemphasize evidence in favour of a particular diagnosis whilst neglecting equally strong contradictory evidence (Kern and Doherty, 1982). Practical Bayesian tools that describe the magnitude of

change in disease probability according to the presence or absence of particular findings (so-called cue weights) are now available (Sox *et al.*, 1988), an example being the system of 'gongs' proposed by Glass (1996).

Reliable hypothesis testing rests on six heuristics: probability (Is it likely based on the law of averages?), utility (Is it a potentially serious diagnosis that one cannot afford to miss?), parsimony (Is it the simplest diagnosis that links the observations together?), adequacy (Does it explain all key features?), coherency (Is it biologically plausible?) and prediction (Does it correctly predict future events?). Probability and utility deserve special mention. Unusual manifestations of common diseases are more common than classic manifestations of rare diseases, which cautions against over-reliance on classic disease descriptions as the basis for diagnosis. Such advice is particularly pertinent to elderly patients with multisystem disease presenting with atypical syndromes. Conversely, students must seek a higher threshold of proof for hypothesized diseases that are uncommon or rare, despite what may appear on the surface to be highly suggestive features. To do otherwise runs the risk of subjecting the majority of such patients to unnecessary anxiety, testing and treatment (Balla *et al.*, 1983; Mold and Stein, 1986).

On the other hand, if a diagnosis is being seriously considered which, whilst uncommon, reflects potentially lethal disease for which curative treatment is possible in the early stages (e.g. a mole undergoing change in colour which most likely denotes seasonal variation but which may reflect early melanomatous transformation), a lower index of suspicion is appropriate, particularly if means exist for definitive diagnosis with minimal risk (in this case excising the mole and obtaining histological diagnosis). Conversely, if there already exist sufficient data for making a diagnosis (no matter how serious) highly probable, the student should understand that obtaining more data which does little to assist prognostication or decide management is wasteful of effort and resources. These probability:utility trade-offs, and the probability thresholds that underpin them, are recurring themes in medicine which students consciously need to address (Moskowitz *et al.*, 1988). Failure to appreciate their importance leads to an excessive reliance on diagnostic tests (the accuracy of which is often poorly understood) in an illusive search for diagnostic certainty. The correct path is developing effective reasoning skills that can rule in likely diagnoses or rule out unlikely ones given a clinically pragmatic quantum of information (Kassirer, 1989b).

In light of new information, which may include investigation results as well as responses to empirical treatment, initial diagnoses undergo revision, refinement and reordering as iterative processes. Hypothesis testing and refinement are best practised within case exercises by withholding key progress findings until students have (i) committed themselves to provisional diagnoses, (ii) decided what further information they require and for what reasons, and (iii) developed rule-in and rule-out criteria for determining which hypotheses should remain as new information is elicited (Wolff *et al.*, 1985). Asking students at strategic points to provide a running synthesis of the problem to date also helps review the logic used in resolving the problem so far. This synthesis should be an hypothesis-referenced, meaningful summary of all relevant information rather than a step-wise, 'dear diary' narrative (Benbassat and Schiffmann, 1976). Competing hypotheses which need to be tested further and persisting deficits in the evidence base for other hypotheses are thus flagged for further consideration.

Determining and communicating a plan of management

Having satisfied the above criteria of validity, hypotheses become the bases for a plan of action. The action may involve investigations (which confirm the diagnosis in cases of serious illness or assist in risk assessment) and/or therapeutic interventions (which provide symptomatic relief, alter the natural history of disease, or the responses to which are of diagnostic value). Students need to appreciate that the use of tests and treatments should be based, as far as possible, on the best available scientific evidence of efficacy combined with good clinical judgement (Evidence-based Medicine Working Group, 1992). This requires skills in formulating clinical questions, searching and critically appraising the literature for answers, and then applying valid and useful results in practice (Sackett *et al.*, 1997). Such skills are best developed using actual case studies that pose important questions and where research evidence can substantially inform management decisions. The principles of clinical epidemiology are useful not only in determining the validity and utility of 'objective' tests and treatments but also of seemingly more subjective items of history-taking and examination (Panju *et al.*, 1998).

Nevertheless, much of clinical practice has not been well researched (Naylor, 1995) and effective decisions must be made in the face of uncertainty. At the same time, patients want to participate in an informed way in decisions about their health, particularly in relation to potential benefits and risks. Inability to engage in such dialogue and to disclose the reasoning behind stated recommendations impairs the student's ability to optimize patient health (Greenfield and Ware, 1995) and avoid patient dissatisfaction (Beckman *et al.*, 1994). Moreover, the ability to acknowledge uncertainty and explain contingency plans (Hewson *et al.*, 1996) helps to reinforce, rather than undermine, professional credibility in the eyes of patients (Gerritey *et al.*, 1990).

Common reasoning errors

Errors in reasoning occur for three principal reasons: (i) faulty perception or elicitation of cues, (ii) incomplete factual knowledge (about a disease process or clinical condition) or (iii) misapplication of known facts to a specific problem. The first deficiency is one of basic clinical skills whilst the second is one of content knowledge. Each is readily identified and acknowledged by both tutor and student in the setting of case studies and corrected by clinical skills teaching and problem-based learning. The third involves incorrect use of heuristics and, whilst familiar to experienced clinicians, its causes and remedies are not so easy to elucidate. A number of common errors have been characterized which need to be recognized and explicitly discussed with students in reasoning exercises (Dawson and Arkes, 1987; Detmer *et al.*, 1978; Kassirer and Kopelman, 1989, 1991; Riegelman, 1991). They include:

● *Forming the wrong initial concept (or mental representation) of the problem (framing error).* This can result from failure to attend to and define critical cues (Benbassat, 1984); stereotyping cues (e.g. translating the non-specific symptom of 'lightheadedness' to the more pathologically specific 'vertigo' in the absence of supporting evidence) or accepting patients' use of medical phrases (such as 'migraine' or 'rheumatism') on face value (Feinstein, 1964); over emphasis on the relevance of previous diagnoses or investigation results; incorrect weighting or clustering of cues (e.g. lumping abdominal pain and diarrhoea to suggest diverticular disease [a surgical frame] rather than diarrhoea and tremor to suggest hyperthyroidism [a medical frame]). Remedies include attention to detail in noting and enumerating initial cues, clustering them in different ways to suggest different frames, and avoiding under- or over-interpretation of cues (Platt and McMath, 1979).

- *Failure to generate plausible hypotheses and adequately test them.* This may result from previously mentioned framing errors; anchoring and confirmation bias (Friedlander and Phillips, 1984) where cues are selectively chosen or interpreted as confirming preconceived ideas (e.g. regarding confusion in a known alcoholic as evidence of yet another episode of intoxication rather than considering occult sepsis); over-reliance on prototypical or 'classic' syndromes as preferred hypotheses (Gruppen *et al.*, 1991); over-interpreting cues which have little disease-related predictive value or indeed represent normal variation (Christensen-Szalaiski and Bushyhead, 1983); overestimating the known prevalence of diseases through too readily invoked rare diagnoses (Balla *et al.*, 1983); ignoring the import of normal or absent findings (e.g. failing to reconsider the diagnosis of pneumonia in a previously healthy patient with no fever) (Beyth-Maron and Fischhoff, 1983); and over-specifying an hypothesis in pathological terms in the absence of supporting evidence (e.g. suggesting a diagnosis of hepatoma rather than chronic liver disease in a patient with isolated hepatomegaly).

- *Inadequate testing and premature acceptance of hypotheses.* This may be driven by psychological biases such as clinician regret (Ayanian and Berwick, 1991). This is the tendency to accept a highly unlikely but prognostically poor diagnosis if in any way one can favourably influence the outcome and thereby avoid a sense of regret for not having done so in the rare event that it turns out to be the correct diagnosis. Such errors can be avoided if students learn to consistently apply some simple cautions: How common is this diagnosis? Why am I sticking with it? What should I look for that may disprove it? Are there other ways of looking at this problem? Practising these rules in the context of case studies prevents fixation on a limited number of hypotheses (Wolff *et al.*, 1985), helps build sophisticated knowledge structures and promotes purposeful use of discriminatory search strategies.

If students reach an impasse in reasoning through a case study, productive lines of thought may be activated by reviewing the logic to see if any of the above reasoning errors are at fault, or employing one or more of the following strategies (Barrows and Pickell, 1991): (a) review and if necessary reconfirm or re-elicit all primary data elicited from either patient or external sources to ensure major cues were not missed or their significance not appreciated; (b) re-organize the data to see if this suggests new hypotheses; (c) re-analyse the problem synthesis to see if what appears to be a single problem may in fact be multiple (e.g. pneumonia and hypotension viewed as the single entity of septicaemia rather than the combination of pneumonia and complicating silent myocardial infarction); and (d) present the problem to a colleague who may suggest new ideas or challenge the validity of elicited findings or stated interpretations.

The role of the tutor in reasoning exercises

The critical role of the tutor in facilitating development of students' reasoning skills cannot be overemphasized. This role can be made more effective if tutors: (a) insist on using a 'thinking out loud' format to problem-solving which makes the reasoning process (of both student and tutor) explicit and transparent; (b) emphasize problem-specific reasoning rather than the recall of unconnected facts or performance of irrelevant routines; (c) keep the reasoning process focused on the problem at hand whilst exploiting opportunities to redress identified gaps in factual knowledge or deficiencies in use of heuristics; (d) deliberately challenge strongly supported hypotheses (playing the devil's advocate) to highlight the need always to consider alternative explanations; (e) adopt a didactic teaching role only when expert knowledge is critical to the resolution of a problem and the opportunity cost to the student of obtaining it from other sources is inordinately high; and (most importantly) (f) provide accurate, specific and constructive feedback to students about their use of reasoning heuristics at opportune times. Tutor effectiveness is further enhanced if the reasoning process is a shared, group activity involving 'hot' problems that neither tutor nor students have previously analysed. Although some tutors may worry about losing credibility in the eyes of students, the latter feel more comfortable about verbalizing tentative thoughts if tutors openly acknowledge their own difficulties in solving a perplexing problem (Benbassat and Cohen, 1982).

Conclusion

Although much is now known about the nature of clinical reasoning, little has been applied in the deliberate teaching of this skill in medical education (Grant, 1989; Kassirer, 1995). Traditionally, expert reasoning has been regarded as an intuitive art, non-specifiable and unteachable, and totally reliant for its development on prolonged trial-and-error experience in real clinical settings. However, using authentic case studies coupled with 'think out loud' formats led by competent tutors, the reasoning process can be deconstructed to reveal the teachable heuristics embedded within it. This approach enables students more quickly to acquire the critical thinking skills and attitudes necessary for making more accurate clinical decisions.

References

Ayanian, J. and Berwick, D. (1991) Do physicians have a bias toward action? *Medical Decision Making*, **11**, 154–158.

Balla, J., Biggs, J., Gibson, M. and Chang, A. (1990) The application of basic science concepts to clinical problem-solving. *Medical Education*, **24**, 137–147.

Balla, J., Elstein, J. and Gates, P. (1983) Effects of prevalence and test diagnosticity upon clinical judgements of probability. *Methods and Information in Medicine*, **22**, 25–28.

Barrows, H. and Feltovich, P. J. (1987) The clinical reasoning process. *Medical Education*, **21**, 86–91.

Barrows, H., Normal, G., Neufeld, Z. and Feightner, J. (1982) The clinical reasoning of randomly selected physicians in general medical practice. *Clinical and Investigative Medicine*, **5**, 49–55.

Barrows, H. S. and Pickell, G. C. (1991) *Developing Clinical Problem-Solving Skills: A Guide to More Effective Diagnosis and Treatment*. New York: Norton Medical Books.

Barrows, H. and Tamblyn, R. (1980) *Problem-Based Learning: An Approach to Medical Education*. New York: Springer.

Beckman, H. and Frankel, R. (1984) The effect of physician behaviour on the collection of data. *Annals of Internal Medicine*, **101**, 692–696.

Beckman, H., Markakis, K., Suchman, A. and Frankel, R. (1994) The doctor–patient relationship and malpractice: Lessons from plaintiff depositions. *Archives of Internal Medicine*, **154**, 1365–1370.

Benbassat, J. (1984) Common errors in the statement of the present illness. *Medical Education*, **18**, 417–422.

Benbassat, J. and Cohen, R. (1982) Clinical instruction and cognitive development of medical students. *Lancet*, **1**, 95–97.

Benbassat, J. and Schiffmann, A. (1976) An approach to teaching the introduction to clinical medicine. *Annals of Internal Medicine*, **84**, 477–481.

Beyth-Maron, R. and Fischhoff, B. (1983) Diagnosticity and pseudodiagnosticity. *Journal of Personality and Social Psychology*, **45**, 1185–1195.

Biggs, J. and Telfer, R. (1987) *The Process of Learning*, 2nd edn. Sydney: Prentice-Hall.

Bordage, G. and Lemieux, M. (1991) Semantic structures and diagnostic thinking of experts and novices. *Academic Medicine*, **56**, S70–72.

Bordage, G. and Zacks, R. (1984) The structure of medical knowledge and the memories of medical students and general practitioners: Categories and prototypes. *Medical Education*. **18**, 406–416.

Boshuizen, H. and Schmidt, H. (1992) On the role of biomedical knowledge in clinical reasoning by experts, intermediates and novices. *Cognitive Science*, **16**, 153–184.

Burack, R. and Carpenter, R. (1983) The predictive value of the presenting complaint. *Journal of Family Practice*, **16**, 749–754.

Christensen-Szalanski, J. and Bushyhead, J. (1983) Physicians' misunderstanding of normal findings. *Medical Decision Making*, **3**, 169–175.

Dawson, N. and Arkes, H. (1987) Systematic errors in medical decision making. *Journal of General Internal Medicine*, **2**, 183–187.

Detmer, D., Fryback, D. and Gassner, K. (1978) Heuristics and biases in medical decision making. *Journal of Medical Education*, **53**, 682–683.

Elstein, A., Shulman, L. and Sprafka, S. (1978) *Medical Problem Solving: Analysis of Clinical Reasoning*. Cambridge, MA: Harvard University Press.

Evidence-Based Medicine Working Group (1992) Evidence-based medicine – A new approach to the teaching and practice of medicine. *Journal of the American Medical Association*, **268**, 2520–2525.

Feinstein, A. (1964) Scientific methodology in clinical practice: IV. Acquisition of clinical data. *Annals of Internal Medicine*, **51**, 1162–1173.

Feinstein, A. (1987) *Clinimetrics*. New Haven, CT: Yale University Press.

Fraser, R. (1992) The diagnostic process. In *Clinical Method: A General Practice Approach*, 2nd edn (R. Fraser, ed.), pp. 35–58. London: Butterworth-Heinemann.

Friedlander, M. and Phillips, S. (1984) Preventing anchoring errors in clinical judgement. *Journal of Consulting and Clinical Psychology*, **52**, 366–371.

Fulop, M. (1985) Teaching differential diagnosis to beginning clinical students. *American Journal of Medicine*, **79**, 745–749.

Galen, R. and Gambino, S. (1975) *Beyond Normality: The Predictive Value and Efficacy of Medical Diagnosis*. New York: Wiley.

Gerritey, M., De Vellis, R. and Earp, J. (1990) Physicians' reactions to uncertainty in patient care. *Medical Care*, **28**, 724–736.

Glass, R. (1996) *Diagnosis: A Brief Introduction*. Melbourne: Oxford University Press.

Grant, J. (1989) Clinical decision making: Rational principles, clinical intuition or clinical thinking. In *Learning in Medical School: A Model for the Clinical Profession* (J. Valler, M. Gibson and A. Chang, eds), pp. 81–100. Hong Kong: Hong Kong University Press.

Grant, J. and Marsden, P. (1987) The structure of memorised knowledge in students and clinicians: An explanation for diagnostic expertise. *Medical Education*, **21**, 92–98.

Greenfield, S. and Ware, J. E., Jr (1995) Exploring patient involvement in care: Effects on outcomes. *Annals of Internal Medicine*, **102**, 520–528.

Gruppen, L., Wolf, S. and Billi, J. (1991) Information gathering and integration and sources of error in diagnostic decision making. *Medical Decision Making*, **11**, 233–239.

Hewson, M. G., Kindy, P. J., Van Kirk, J., Geruris, B. A. and Day, R. P. (1996) Strategies for managing uncertainty and complexity. *Journal of General Internal Medicine*, **11**, 481–485.

Hoffbrand, B. (1989) Away with the system review: A plea for parsimony. *British Medical Journal*, **298**, 817–819.

Kassirer, J. (1983) Teaching clinical medicine by iterative hypothesis testing: Let's preach what we practice. *New England Journal of Medicine*, **309**, 921–923.

Kassirer, J. (1989a) Diagnostic reasoning. *Annals of Internal Medicine*, **110**, 893–900.

Kassirer, J. (1989b) Our stubborn quest for diagnostic certainty: A cause of excessive testing. *New England Journal of Medicine*, **320**, 1489–1491.

Kassirer, J. (1995) Teaching clinical problem-solving: How are we doing? *New England Journal of Medicine*, **332**, 1507–1509.

Kassirer, J. and Kopelman, R. (1989) Cognitive errors in diagnosis: Substantiation, classification and consequences. *American Journal of Medicine*, **86**, 433–441.

Kassirer, J. and Kopelman, R. (1991) *Learning Clinical Reasoning*. Baltimore, MD: Williams & Wilkins.

Kassirer, J. P., Kuipers, B. J. and Goorey, G. A. (1982) Toward a theory of clinical expertise. *American Journal of Medicine*, **73**, 251–259.

Kern, L. and Doherty, M. (1982) 'Pseudodiagnosticity' in an idealised medical problem-solving environment. *Journal of Medical Education*, **57**, 100–104.

Koran, L. (1975) The reliability of clinical methods, data and judgements. *New England Journal of Medicine*, **294**, 642–646; 695–701.

Lewkonia, R., Harasyn, P. and Darwish, H. (1993) Early introduction to medical problem-solving. *Medical Teacher*, **15**, 57–65.

Margolis, C., Varnoon, S. and Barrak, N. (1982) A required course in decision-making in pre-clinical medical students. *Journal of Medical Education*, **57**, 184–190.

McDonald, C. (1996) Medical heuristics: The silent adjudicators of clinical practice. *Annals of Internal Medicine*, **124**, 56–62.

Miller, G. (1956) The magical number seven: Plus or minus two – Some limits on our capacity for processing information. *Psychology Review*, **63**, 81–97.

Mold, J. and Stein, H. (1986) The cascade effect in the clinical care of patients. *New England Journal of Medicine*, **314**, 512–514.

Moskowitz, A., Kuipers, D. and Kassirer, J. (1988) Dealing with uncertainty, risks, and trade-offs in clinical decision – A cognitive approach. *Annals of Internal Medicine*, **108**, 435–449.

Myers, J. and Dorsey J. (1994) Using diagnostic reasoning (DxR) to teach and evaluate clinical reasoning skills. *Academic Medicine*, **59**, 428–429.

Naylor, C. (1995) Gray zones of clinical practice: Some limits to evidence-based medicine. *Lancet*, **345**, 840–842.

Panju, A., Hemmelgarn, B., Nishihawa, J., Cook, D. and Kitching, A. (1998) A critical appraisal of the cardiovascular history and physical examination. In *Evidence-Based Cardiology* (S. Yusuf, J. A. Cairns, A. J. Camm, E. L. Fallen and B. J. Gersh, eds), pp. 24–28. London: BMJ Books.

Platt, F. and McMath, J. (1979) Clinical hypocompetence: The interview. *Annals of Internal Medicine*, **91**, 898–902.

Riegelman, R. (1991) *Minimising Medical Mistakes: The Art of Medical Decision Making*. Boston, MA: Little, Brown.

Russell, I. (1985) Condition diagramming: A new approach to teaching clinical integration. *Medical Education*, **19**, 220–225.

Sackett, D. L., Richardson, W. S., Rosenberg, W. and Haynes, R. B. (1997) *Evidence-Based Medicine: How to Practice and Teach EBM*. London: Churchill-Livingstone.

Sanders, M., Mitchell, C. and Byrne, G. (1997) *Medical Consultation Skills: Behavioural and Interpersonal Dimensions of Health Care*. Melbourne: Addison-Wesley.

Schor, E., Learner, B. and Malsperis, S. (1995) Physicians' assessment of functional health status and wellbeing: The patient's perspective. *Archives of Internal Medicine*, **155**, 309–314.

Schwartz, R., Donnelly, M., Nash, P. and Young, B. (1992) Developing students' cognitive skills in a problem-based surgery clerkship. *Academic Medicine*, **57**, 694–696.

Scott, I. (1995) Clinical reasoning: Exploring teaching and learning. *ANZAME Bulletin*, **22**, 8–30.

Sox, H., Blatt, M., Higgins, M. and Marton, K. (1988) *Medical Decision Making*. Boston, MA: Butterworth-Heinemann.

Thomas, E. (1992) Teaching medicine with cases: Student and teacher opinion. *Medical Education*, **26**, 200–207.

van der Vleuten, C. and Newble, D. (1995) How can we test clinical reasoning? *Lancet*, **345**, 1032–1034.

Wasson, J., Walsh, B., Thompkins, R., Sox, H. and Pantell, R. (1992) *The Common Symptom Guide*, 3rd edn. New York: McGraw-Hill.

Wolff, S., Gruppen, L. and Billi, J. (1985) Differential diagnosis and the competing hypotheses heuristic: A practical approach to judgement under uncertainty and Bayesian probability. *Journal of the American Medical Association*, **253**, 2858–2862.

35

Fostering clinical decision making in critical care nursing

Alastair Burn and Joy Higgs

Nursing in critical care contexts is concerned with the provision of life support, the monitoring of patients with critical illnesses and their responses to therapeutic interventions, and the prevention of complications. It is also concerned with providing patient comfort, whenever possible eliciting the understanding and co-operation of the client, while providing information, understanding and support to the patient's significant others, especially family (McKinley, 1997).

Of all the branches of nursing, critical care nursing has been most closely associated with and influenced by the concerns and characteristics of modern scientific medicine. A consequence has been a focus on meeting the physical needs of the patient, often at the expense of other types of support (e.g. emotional support) (Jacobs, 1990).

Patients admitted to intensive care units (ICUs) frequently require ventilatory and other life support, together with intensive monitoring of physiological functions using a range of technologically advanced equipment. Mechanical ventilators, electrocardiographic monitoring devices, invasive physiological monitoring devices, and electronically controlled infusion units for the administration of fluids and intravenous medications may be among the instrumentation used, alongside more prosaic systems for the collection and recording of body wastes. Thus, as well as competence in dealing with the interpersonal relationships involving patient, family, nursing and medical superiors and colleagues, critical care nurses must also have a range of skills which enable them to monitor and control the operation of a range of equipment.

Clinical decision making in critical care nursing

Decision making is intrinsic to the provision of nursing care. A knowledge of the types of decisions made and of the various factors which influence decision making is important for a proper understanding of nursing practice. This knowledge is particularly evident in critical care nursing, where practitioners may be called upon to demonstrate a high level of independent decision making. A nurse in this environment is faced on a daily basis with the care of seriously ill people. To manage the various activities required to achieve and maintain patient stability, the nursing contribution to the improvement of patient well-being, whether this is of a physiological or psychosocial character, requires sound reasoning and decision-making skills.

Decision making in intensive care may be influenced by the existence of ward protocols, procedure manuals and decision-making practices such as nursing care plans and assessment tools (Bucknall and Thomas, 1996a). While protocols and advanced technology are crucial to critical care, interpersonal relationships play an important role in determining the character of the environment and the clinical decisions which are made within it. Interacting effectively and compassionately with patients and care givers is central to the nursing role.

Another factor influencing nursing decision making in critical care units is the expanded role of critical care nurses which results from the expansion of knowledge and the increasing impact of technological advances, especially in high-dependency environments like intensive care. In these situations, nurses may be required to take decisions quickly, without consulting colleagues or waiting for physicians' orders, because of the negative impact delay may have on patient outcomes (Bucknall and Thomas, 1996b). Thus critical care nurses may be required to make diagnoses which are both medical and nursing in character, and to take appropriate action.

The critical care nurse's principal aim is to provide high quality care to facilitate a positive outcome for patients and their significant others. In so doing, the nurse seeks to avoid costly and sometimes tragic mistakes that can occur as a consequence of faulty reasoning and the errors in decision making which may result (Fonteyn, 1995). However, reasoning and decision making occur in a context where the decision maker is frequently conscious of the fact that the outcome of a decision, even an apparently trivial one, may have serious consequences. This sense of accountability and pressure is more evident in the critical care nursing environment than in other, less acute situations. The critical context of decision making and the high demand for quality in decision making in critical care nursing thus present a special challenge.

Clinical decision making is both a component and an outcome of the process of clinical reasoning. Fonteyn (1995, p. 60) defines clinical reasoning in nursing as:

> ... the cognitive processes and strategies that nurses use to understand the significance of patient data, to identify and diagnose actual or potential patient problems, and to make clinical decisions to assist in problem resolution and to enhance the achievement of positive patient outcomes.

A related term is *clinical judgement*. Tanner (1987, p. 154), describes clinical decision making as 'a series of judgements made by the nurse in interaction with the patient'. In this chapter we ascribe to the term *clinical judgement* the following meaning:

> ... the weighing up of evidence arising in the clinical situation, against an appropriate background knowledge, including that which the practitioner can be expected to know from the literature in the field, as well as her[1] past experience of similar situations, and upon the basis of which she formulates a decision to take an appropriate action.

[1] The female gender pronoun is used throughout for convenience.

Clinical decision making research focusing on critical care nursing

As may have been expected, early investigations in the research literature about the decision making of critical care nurses concerned their ability to make rapid decisions during crisis situations. Baumann and Bourbonnais (1982) examined decision-making abilities of critical care and coronary care nurses at varying levels of expertise. They found that knowledge and experience were the most important factors influencing rapid decision making. In a later study (Bourbonnais and Baumann, 1985) some nurses described how they were able to anticipate emergency situations on the basis of earlier incidents and the majority reported that they considered intuition played a role in decision making.

The importance of intuition was further investigated by Benner. Applying the 'Dreyfus model', an approach derived from a phenomenological perspective, Benner (1984) conducted a series of studies into clinical judgement in nursing. The model (Dreyfus and Dreyfus, 1985) identified that people usually pass through at least five stages of qualitatively different perceptions of the task and/ or mode of decision making as their skill improves. These five stages are novice, advanced beginner, competent, proficient and expert.

In nursing it is claimed that these five stages reflect changes in four aspects of skilled performance (Benner, 1984; Benner *et al.*, 1992; Tanner *et al.*, 1993). The first involves a progression from reliance on abstract principles as a basis for judgement to the use of past concrete experiences. The second is a shift from reliance on analytical, rule-based thinking to intuition. The third is a change in the learner's perception of the patient situation from a view of the situation as a compilation of equally relevant pieces of information to a perception of a complete whole, in which only certain components are relevant to decision making about care at any given time. The fourth is a movement from the position of detached observer, standing outside the situation, to a position of full involvement in the patient situation. According to this model, any nursing student or registered nurse entering a new clinical area is regarded as a novice. The advanced beginner, on the other hand, is able to show 'marginally acceptable performance', having coped with a sufficient number of similar real situations. Competence is typified by the nurse who has been on the job in the same or a similar situation for 2–3 years. The proficient nurse perceives situations as wholes and it is this holistic understanding that improves her decision making. The expert nurse has 'an intuitive grasp of each situation and zeroes in on the accurate region of the problem without wasteful consideration of a large range of unfruitful, alternative diagnoses and solutions' (Benner, 1984, p. 32).

To explore the model in the context of the practice of critical care nursing, Benner *et al.* (1992) conducted individual and group interviews with nurses practising in adult, paediatric and neonatal ICUs from eight hospitals in the US. The nurses gave narrative accounts of exemplars from their practice. From this study the authors derived a concept of the 'clinical world', akin to the Husserlian idea of *Lebenswelt* or 'life-world'. With experience, the nurses' clinical worlds became progressively more differentiated, paralleling the Dreyfus model phases. Each level of practice was characterized by advances in clinical knowledge, a resultant shift in the clinician's grasp of the real world and concomitant changes in clinical-reasoning practices.

Intuition, as implied in Benner's usage, is not guessing but is the result of recognizing similarity and of deep situational involvement (Dreyfus and Dreyfus, 1985). The Dreyfus model suggests that 'better thinking is done intuitively, because experts who think better, think intuitively' (Hamm, 1988, p.99). The Benner view may be said to represent one end of the spectrum in a debate as to whether a valid, independent and objective evaluation of expert performance in the clinical professions is possible. This debate lies behind much of the tension between the 'artistic-intuitive and rational-analytic views of clinical reasoning' (Dowie and Elstein, 1988, p.7). For example, a nursing critic of Benner has raised several questions concerning the application of the Dreyfus model to the development of nursing expertise (English, 1993). Amongst the stated concerns, there is the question of how the model can provide guidance to nurses in becoming experts, other than by working through the stages of skill acquisition, which, by Benner's own admission, does not guarantee the acquisition of expert status. English also questions the acceptability of intuition as the basis of the expert's perception, on the basis of, amongst other things, demands (often from nurses themselves) for more objective measures of clinical performance and outcomes to improve the ability of nurses to demonstrate the value of nursing work, particularly in expensive critical care units, in a political and economic climate which requires health care to be justified, usually in monetary terms.

Information-processing models

Information-processing theory is a theoretical framework that postulates that an individual operates as an information-processing system. From this model, the basic principle which facilitates an understanding of clinical decision making is that of 'limited rationality', i.e. the fact that individuals have limited information-processing capabilities (Newell and Simon, 1972). In terms of clinical reasoning and decision making, the most relevant factor is the relatively limited capacity of short-term memory, which makes it difficult to cope efficiently with the large amount of information that is available about a clinical problem. Effective clinical reasoning and decision making rely on a person's ability to adapt to this short-term memory limitation (Elstein and Bordage, 1988), particularly in complex situations such as critical care.

A strategy used by nurses to conserve the limited information-processing resources in their short-term memory is described by Corcoran (1986a, 1986b). Corcoran noted that, instead of using a systematic approach to planning, most experts were using opportunistic overall approaches in the more complex cases. This was indicated by their propensity to 'jump about pursuing whatever was opportune at a given point in the planning process' (Corcoran, 1986b, p.107). Similarly, Grobe *et al.* (1991, p. 313) found that experienced nurses coped with problems and interventions concurrently rather than linearly, in order to 'reduce cognitive strain'.

Other models

Hughes and Young (1990) used a logical analytical decision model to examine the relationship between the complexity of a task and the consistency of decision making in intensive care nurses. They found that a minority of nurses made decisions which corresponded to those recommended by a decision model and that agreement with the model decreased as the complexity of the task increased. As possible explanations for their findings, the authors suggested that systematic strategies may not work for highly complex problems, or that decision makers may not be able to systematically manipulate complex data without external decision support (such as computer programs based on decision analysis principles). A third alternative, they suggested, is that consistency in decision making could be influenced by other components of the decision task apart from complexity. Given that only slightly more than one-third of the respondents' decision making was consistent with the model even in the least complex task, the possibility remains that there may be limitations in the model as a predictor of the decision-making skills required where there are high levels of complexity and uncertainty. The results reflect the need for decision-making skills which go beyond logical analytical modes.

The social context of critical care was the focus of an ethnographic study by Chase (1995), investigating nurses' perspectives of the influence of social context on clinical judgement. The study involved interviews and participant observation in an open heart surgical unit and a general surgical ICU, for the purpose of obtaining a comparison of judgement processes across units. The study describes how the nurses and physicians were organized into parallel hierarchies, which allowed for checks on clinical judgement both within and across professional lines. Certain rituals characteristic of critical care units (i.e. the nursing report, doctors' rounds and the use of flow sheets) provided a context for a critique on clinical judgement processes. The researcher noted how the clinical judgement process was observed differently for the nurse compared to the physician and that this difference in perspective could lead to conflict. Of particular interest were the circumstances under which nurses sought to convince less experienced physicians to contact senior medical personnel for advice, which occurred in situations where the nurse believed that the resident was unable or unwilling to take action during episodes of patient deterioration. In general, however, communication of matters of judgement was most often shared in casual, open conversations, and when conflicting views occurred nurses and residents were usually able to resolve the issue reasonably amicably.

Promoting quality decision making in critical care nursing

The foregoing discussion suggests that critical care nurses' decision making ranges in complexity from decisions associated with everyday work practices concerning patient care to decisions leading to actions where the patient's life is at risk. Impinging upon this range of decisions is the environment of critical care. This environment of course includes the presence of technologically advanced equipment and the need for moment-by-moment decisions which arises as a consequence of the clinical assessment information much of this equipment provides. The equipment is also used for therapeutic purposes, requiring nursing decisions relating to its control and adjustment (Bucknall and Thomas, 1996a). The environment, however, is not simply dominated by machinery, but is also characterized by complex social, psychological and ethical interactions between nurses and their patients, between nurses and the families and other significant companions of the patients for whom they care, between nurses and their peers, between nurses and medical practitioners, between nurses and other health care workers, and between nurses and their institutional superiors (Chase, 1995; Corcoran-Perry and Graves, 1990; Corley *et al.*, 1993; Jezewski, 1994).

Competent critical care nurses are a commodity not always easy to obtain. Critical care units are often faced with shortages of staff in gross terms and in particular of experienced staff to guide those with less experience through a patient care environment which is often so complex as to overwhelm the inexperienced individual; such bewilderment may not only prevent effective clinical decision making but also make it more likely that the person leaves that environment before being able to develop into an effective member of the team. The ability to apply critical care nursing knowledge, skills and attitudes to patient care requires clinical decision making at all phases of the interaction.

A first step in dealing with these issues is to clarify what constitutes effective decision making and why it is important (Dunn, 1993). To do so demands a recognition that decisions are required in many critical care clinical circumstances, not only during crisis events, but on a day-by-day, moment-by-moment basis. If a novice or other less experienced nurse can appreciate that it is possible to make effective decisions about apparently trivial things, she may be able to gain confidence in her ability to effectively manage decisions requiring the application of greater knowledge and technical skill. Most if not all critical care units conduct orientation periods for new staff as a means towards this end (Dunn, 1992). In addition, preceptorship schemes in which novice staff are placed 'under the wing' of more experienced practitioners for a period of time are commonplace in Australian ICUs. This system provides opportunities to discuss clinical decision making questions at an early stage.

Education for critical care nurses

Clinical reasoning is significantly enhanced by experience and knowledge (Fonteyn, 1998) and by the context in which the reasoning is occurring. According to Higgs and Jones (1995), the various contexts of a clinical problem include: the personal context of the client, the complex and unique context of the clinical problem, the actual clinical setting, the personal and professional frame of reference of the clinician, the broad context of health care delivery, and the complex context of clinical decision making. Kassirer and Kopelman (1991) refer to the *problem space* being the problem solver's representation of the task environment, and argue that attention to context assists clinicians in framing the clinical problem they are addressing. As is evident from the discussion above, the clinical context of critical care nursing is highly complex, problematical and dynamic. It is a world where knowledge and experience combined with a sound understanding of the problem space, are most necessary to effective clinical reasoning and decision making.

So, how should critical care nurses be prepared for this decision-making role? According to Fonteyn (1998), nursing education is placing an increasing emphasis on teaching and assessing clinical thinking as part of a growing recognition among educators of the necessity to improve students' clinical judgement and critical thinking in the face of the knowledge explosion and the age of constant change. Other factors, such as the desire for professional status recognition and professional autonomy, and the expectations of accountability from the public and employers, also highlight the need for graduate nurses to possess sound decision-making skills. In critical care nursing, where nursing autonomy in decision making is relatively high, where decisions need to be made rapidly and accurately and where consequences of decisions are great, the quality of nurses' decision making abilities is even more significant.

Therefore the knowledge and reasoning abilities of nurses learned at undergraduate level (e.g. the ability to make sound nursing care plans for patients and knowledge of a range of clinical conditions and their management) needs further enhancement in preparation for a critical care nursing role. In addition, given the rate of expansion of knowledge, of technological advancement and of changes in medical and nursing management strategies, ongoing education is required for nurses working in critical care. That is, both specialized postgraduate education (e.g. graduate diplomas or masters degrees in critical care nursing) and inservice or continuing education are needed to support quality performance in this demanding field.

Consider the range of knowledge and reasoning skills we would expect of a highly competent critical care nurse. As the person most continuously with the patient in a critical care unit the critical care nurse needs to have knowledge of the clinical management and services available to the patient from all other health professionals including doctors, physiotherapists and other allied health professionals, pharmacists and social workers as well as from the administrative system. The critical care nurse needs excellent knowledge and skills in nursing care, including knowledge of the operation of relevant equipment used in patient care. In relation to clinical reasoning the critical care nurse must be a highly competent reasoner and decision maker, being able to make sound decisions rapidly, with few errors, and must be able to articulate this reasoning to communicate the patient's condition to other team members, to provide a rationale for the nursing care and to provide the link between the many services the patient receives. Further, the critical care nurse may need to be the patient's advocate and the family's (or care givers') primary contact and support.

Strategies to achieve and continue to advance these many complex and demanding skills need to address several key issues. Firstly, although clinical reasoning is a non-visible (thinking) process, reasoning needs to be made conscious and articulated to understand and assess its nature and soundness. Secondly, specialist critical care nurses need to be the principal critics of their own reasoning, and skills in metacognition and critical reflection are essential in the management and quality control of their reasoning. The development of these skills through reflection and peer discussion is strongly advocated. Thirdly, critical care nurses need to acquire knowledge which supports clinical reasoning in clinical practice. In critical care nursing in particular, this includes knowledge beyond that which can be learned from textbooks. Beyond propositional (research and theoretical) knowledge, the critical care nurse needs professional craft knowledge as an essential element of expert practice. [See Higgs and Titchen (1995) for a discussion of forms of knowledge.] Finally, since experience is a key element in the development of expert practice and reflection on experience is necessary to transform experience into learning, learning strategies to enhance critical care nurses' knowledge and clinical reasoning should incorporate reflection on experience and sharing of experience between nurses, in a framework of critical inquiry.

Strategies proposed for the enhancement of clinical reasoning include mind mapping,[2] the use of hypothetical patients and thinking aloud strategies,[3] specific focus on the learning of critical thinking skills,[4] personal reflection on clinical experiences and individual or group exploration of clinical cases. Fonteyn (1998) provides a detailed set of cases for exploration in a chapter titled *Clinical Dilemmas in Critical Care Nursing* in her recent text.

Conclusion

Critical care nursing is associated with a high level of independent decision making relating to the care of seriously ill people in a technologically advanced environment. Research into clinical decision making in nursing has gradually shifted from a focus on the crisis-determined elements of decision making to investigation of the nature of expertise in critical care nursing and of the way in which expertise is demonstrated in terms of quality in decision making. Other approaches have included the use of information-processing theory for the investigation of clinical reasoning and decision making in critical care nursing.

The main influences on critical care nurses and their decision-making ability include their aptitude, level of educational preparation, the type of unit within which they work, the ethos and climate of the work environment, institutional arrangements such as the organization of nursing care, and the documentation requirements which prevail. A crucial element in determining the range of decisions to be made is the environment of critical care. It includes not only the technological aspects of the work, but also the complex social, psychological and ethical interactions which this work demands. An exploration of the characteristics of decision making in intensive care must therefore take into account these diverse and demanding elements. It is our view that an understanding of the

elements of decision-making skill and of the context in which it occurs can be used educationally to promote and improve quality in the decision-making capabilities of critical care nurses.

References

Baumann, A. and Bourbonnais, F. (1982) Nursing decision making in critical care areas. *Journal of Advanced Nursing*, **7**, 435–446.

Benner, P. (1984) *From Novice to Expert: Excellence and Power in Clinical Nursing Practice*. Reading, MA: Addison-Wesley.

Benner, P., Tanner, C. and Chesla, C. (1992) From beginner to expert: Gaining a differentiated clinical world in critical care nursing. *Advances in Nursing Science*, **14**(3), 13–28.

Bourbonnais, F. F. and Baumann, A. (1985) Crisis decision making in coronary care: A replication study. *Nursing Papers: Perspectives in Nursing*, **17**, 4–19.

Bucknall, T. and Thomas, S. (1996a) Clinical decision making in critical care. *Australian Journal of Advanced Nursing*, **13**(2), 10–17.

Bucknall, T. and Thomas, S. (1996b) Critical care nurse satisfaction with levels of involvement in clinical decisions. *Journal of Advanced Nursing*, **23**, 571–577.

Chase, S. K. (1995) The social context of critical care clinical judgement. *Heart and Lung*, **24**, 154–162.

Corcoran, S. A. (1986a) Planning by expert and novice nurses in cases of varying complexity. *Research in Nursing and Health*, **9**, 155–162.

Corcoran, S. A. (1986b) Task complexity and nursing expertise as factors in decision making. *Nursing Research*, **35**, 107–112.

Corcoran-Perry, S. and Graves, J. (1990) Supplemental-information-seeking behaviour of cardiovascular nurses. *Research in Nursing and Health*, **13**, 119–127.

Corley, M. C., Selig, P. and Ferguson, C. (1993) Critical care nurse participation in ethical and work decisions. *Critical Care Nurse*, June, 120–128.

Dowie, J. and Elstein, A. (1988) *Professional Judgement: A Reader in Clinical Decision Making*. Cambridge: Cambridge University Press.

Dreyfus, H. L. and Dreyfus, S. E. (1985) *Mind Over Machine: The Power of Human Intuition and Expertise in the Era of the Computer*. New York: Free Press.

Dunn, S. V. (1992) Orientation: The transition from novice to competent critical care nurse. *Critical Care Nursing Quarterly*, **15**, 69–77.

Dunn, S. V. (1993) Clinical decision making: A primer for preceptors. *Australian Critical Care*, **6**(2), 20–23.

Elstein, A. S. and Bordage, G. (1988) Psychology of clinical reasoning. In *Professional Judgement: A Reader in Clinical Decision Making* (J. Dowie and A. Elstein, eds), pp. 109–129, Cambridge: Cambridge University Press.

English, I. (1993) Intuition as a function of the expert nurse: A critique of Benner's novice to expert model. *Journal of Advanced Nursing*, **18**, 387–393.

---

[2] See Chapter 23 by Cahill and Fonteyn.
[3] See Higgs (1993).
[4] See Fonteyn (1998).

Fonteyn, M. E. (1995) Clinical reasoning in nursing. In *Clinical Reasoning in the Health Professions* (J. Higgs and M. Jones, eds), pp. 60–71. Oxford: Butterworth-Heinemann.

Fonteyn, M. E. (1998) *Thinking Strategies for Nursing Practice*. Philadelphia, PA: Lippincott.

Grobe, S. J., Drew, J. A. and Fonteyn, M. E. (1991) A descriptive analysis of experienced nurses' clinical reasoning during a planning task. *Research in Nursing and Health*, **14**, 305–314.

Hamm, R. M. (1988) Clinical intuition and clinical analysis: Expertise and the cognitive continuum. In *Professional Judgement: A Reader in Clinical Decision Making* (J. Dowie and A. Elstein, eds), pp. 78–105. Cambridge: Cambridge University Press.

Higgs, J. and Jones, M. (1995) Clinical reasoning. In *Clinical Reasoning in the Health Professions* (J. Higgs and M. Jones, eds), pp. 3–23. Oxford: Butterworth-Heinemann.

Higgs, J. and Titchen, A. (1995) Propositional, professional, and personal knowledge in clinical reasoning. In *Clinical Reasoning in the Health Professions* (J. Higgs and M. Jones, eds), pp. 129–146. Oxford: Butterworth-Heinemann.

Hughes, K. K. and Young, W. B. (1990) The relationship between task complexity and decision making consistency. *Research in Nursing and Health*, **13**, 189–197.

Jacobs, C. J. (1990) Orem's self-care model: Is it relevant to patients in intensive care? *Intensive Care Nursing*, **6**, 100–103.

Jezewski, M. A. (1994) Do not resuscitate status: Conflict and culture brokering in critical care units. *Heart and Lung*, **23**, 458–465.

Kassirer, J. and Kopelman, R. (1991) *Learning Clinical Reasoning*. Baltimore, MD: Williams & Wilkins.

McKinley, S. (1997) Critical care nursing. In *Intensive Care Manual* (T. E. Oh, ed.), pp. 33–39. Oxford: Butterworth-Heinemann.

Newell, A. and Simon, H. A. (1972) *Human Problem Solving*. Englewood Cliffs, NJ: Prentice-Hall.

Tanner, C. A. (1987) Teaching clinical judgement. In *Annual Review of Nursing Research*, Vol. 5 (J. J. Fitzpatrick and R. L. Taunton, eds), pp. 153–173. New York: Springer.

Tanner, C. A. Benner, P. A., Chesla C. and Gordon D. R. (1993) The phenomenology of knowing the patient. *Image: Journal of Nursing Scholarship*, **25**, 273–280.

Section Four

Directions for the future

36

Will evidenced-based practice take the reasoning out of practice?

Mark Jones and Joy Higgs

Five years ago, when we were considering future directions for clinical reasoning teaching, research and practice in the first edition of this book, we identified the following potential directions:

- Emergence of a shared field of study (clinical reasoning) across the health professions.
- Further research to investigate the nature of clinical reasoning and expertise with attention to relationships amongst a broad range of variables including clinician characteristics (e.g. knowledge organization, cognitive or reasoning strategies, experience and expertise, values, attitudes, beliefs, roles), client characteristics (with respect to both the person and the problem), practice settings and outcomes (with consideration of perspectives of clients, clinicians, professions, the public and health care financiers).
- Further research to assess the type and frequency of errors that occur and their relationship to contextual variables and both diagnostic and non-diagnostic outcome measures.
- Continued methodological pluralism in the research of clinical reasoning from the more traditional psychometric-based methods to newer developments such as the phenomenological approach, the interpretive approach and research based on traditional experimental psychology. Both artificially designed research conditions and real-life situations are needed.
- Continuing research from an educational perspective to investigate the growth of individuals' knowledge structures, with additional efforts to clarify the level of the various types of knowledge (e.g. propositional, clinical, personal) required in different practice settings.

- Ongoing research into the effectiveness of educational programs, learning approaches, methods and strategies used to teach/facilitate clinical reasoning.
- Clinical reasoning education and practice which go beyond the focus on finding (scientifically) acceptable answer(s), to prepare and enable clinicians to deal with the human dilemmas of decision making, including its controversies (e.g. euthanasia), its conflicts (e.g. clinician/institution differences of values or judgements), its ambiguities and its differences in preferences and perspectives.
- Continued review of curriculum content with greater priority given to enhancing knowledge structure development and accessibility, self-directed learning behaviours, reasoning strategies, educator preparation, teaching strategies, utilization of higher technology, and continued efforts at developing effective and user-friendly methods for assessing clinical reasoning.
- Continued development and use of new technologies and innovative resources such as computer-assisted interactive learning activities, decision support systems, data base knowledge resources and simulated patients to optimize students' clinical reasoning and clinicians' practice.
- Continued experimentation with different methods of assessing clinical reasoning.
- Acknowledgement that future world-wide trends influencing health care such as increasing financial constraints, changing health care settings and greater consumer involvement will require clinicians to adopt broader perspectives

of client management that include greater attention to individual contexts of client problems and greater involvement of clients in the decision-making process.

● Teaching which recognizes that clinicians of the future will benefit from flexibility and breadth of thinking styles and are likely to make greater use of computer-assisted decision support systems to manage the ever increasing growth of knowledge.

Since that time a number of people have made strides in these areas, as is evident in many chapters in this book. However, the major priorities remain much the same. For this reason we have elected to explore one key issue facing those interested in clinical reasoning and clinical practice. This issue is *evidence-based practice*. The trend of increasing public accountability demands confronting the health sector, particularly in the face of decreasing public funds, has placed the need for assurance of quality health care high on the agenda. For many, this priority is interpreted in terms of the need for research and practice to combine in the process of evidence-based practice.

In this chapter we explore the concept of evidence-based practice and critique the definitions applied to this term, and discuss potential consequences of these definitions. Our main arguments can be summarized as follows:

● To base practice on credible evidence, sound reasoning and defensible professional judgement is unarguably the requirement of all professional practitioners.

● It is a narrow definition of evidence-based practice to restrict evidence to the findings of randomized controlled trials (RCTs), or even somewhat more broadly, to 'scientific method' research. This requirement would be unreasonably limiting to both the notion of what should reasonably constitute evidence (and knowledge) and to the scope of professional practice which will result if such evidence is required for all practice interventions. Instead, it is important to recognize the value of knowledge (and evidence) gained from both the human as well as the basic/applied sciences for practice in the health sciences, where the context is human, not merely biological, and where the services which health professionals can offer for the benefit of their clients are not reducible simply to quantifiable terms. To address the spectrum of our clients' needs we must recognize the value of qualitative research and of knowledge beyond empirico-analytical research, particularly professional craft knowledge, which can be derived, tested and supported through experience.

● Central to the notion of being a professional is the use of professional judgement and reasoned decision making. These cognitive processes need to operate in a way that is supported by different ways of knowing and different knowledge generation strategies (including experience as well as research). Such breadth of knowledge is especially important in the grey areas of human services and interactions where certainties and single correct answers are both unavailable and undesirable.

● The notion of provision of best practice which is associated with evidence-based practice needs similarly to be interpreted as being situationally applicable, not absolutely and objectively definable. The intentions and outcomes of best practice in terms of duty of care to provide high quality (relevant) service as well as the capacity to support with credible evidence the choice of services, constitute the key issue, rather than the capacity of health sciences to write 'textbook' prescriptions or recipes for what is best practice.

Professionalism demands applicability, relevance, flexibility and informed judgement, not just rules. Rules and prescriptions belong to pre-professional occupations.

In support of evidence-based practice

The importance of evidenced-based practice cannot be overstated, and is reflected throughout this book where reasoning or evidenced-based thinking and decision making are explored. Practitioners must be accountable for their decisions; patients depend on the health professions to provide care that is effective, efficient and affordable. Acknowledging that the health professions have always attempted to base their decisions and actions on the best available evidence, Sackett *et al.* (1997, p. 5) provide the following arguments for greater weight being given to research findings from select studies that fulfill stringent criteria of quality:

● New types of evidence are now being generated which, when we know and understand them, create frequent, major changes in the way that we care for our patients.

- Although we need (and our patients would benefit from) this new evidence daily, we usually fail to get it.
- As a result, both our up-to-date knowledge and our clinical performance deteriorate with time.
- Trying to overcome this clinical entropy through traditional continuing medical education programs does not improve our clinical performance.
- Evidenced-based medicine provides a different approach to clinical learning that has been shown to keep its practitioners up to date.

Readers are encouraged to review the Sackett *et al.* (1997) text, as the arguments and examples (primarily in the context of medicine) used to support these points are strong.

What constitutes evidence?

A key issue in the evidence-based practice debate is the question, 'what constitutes evidence?' Sackett *et al.* (1997, p. 2) define evidenced-based medicine as '... the conscientious, explicit and judicious use of current best evidence in making decisions about the care of individual patients'. Evidence-based practice represents a paradigm shift in medicine from management decisions based on clinical experience and an understanding of the pathophysiology of disease to an emphasis on research substantiated decisions (Crombie, 1997). If the evidence of evidence-based practice is restricted to information available from select quantitative studies fulfilling stringent criteria (e.g. the RCT), then this paradigm shift has significant consequences in terms of the scope of practice strategies that would be justifiable under the new regime of RCT evidence. For some health professions whose decisions traditionally go beyond pathophysiological considerations, this shift in what is deemed evidence could create very real dilemmas concerning 'credible' practices.

With the surge in demands both from within the health professions and from external funding bodies for more evidence-based practice and RCTs to validate diagnosis or problem identification and management decisions, it is not surprising that practising clinicians often feel somewhat threatened. Practice philosophies and management strategies, grounded in a combination of biomedical rationale, experience and varying amounts and quality of formal investigation, will increasingly be subjected to closer scrutiny. The results from RCTs form *part* of the knowledge available to inform the various players in health care (clinicians, educators, patients and funding bodies) and direct future practice. Clinicians in particular are wary of the political power within the evidence-based practice movement in its often exclusive reliance on RCTs, and they understandably mistrust the potential misuse of results. They question the validity of practice being guided solely by rigid scientifically generated knowledge. They are frustrated when results fail to match their experience and they are hesitant to abandon what has been successful for them.

While the scientific method is one means of generating knowledge, a broader definition of knowledge/evidence is needed when that knowledge is to be used in the assessment and management of clients whose problems can rarely be reduced to precise categorization or prescriptive management. This need for a broader view of knowledge is particularly true of forms of reasoning other than diagnostic reasoning, but also of diagnostic reasoning where the current state of research-validated knowledge is still insufficient to diagnose many patient problems and identify proven management strategies. It is even more important if patient populations are not simply classified along traditional diagnostic criteria but consideration is also given to the contextual dimensions of patient problems where psychosocial factors can significantly interact with the body's various systems, not only in the presentation of illness and dysfunction but also in the recovery process.

Evidence from RCTs and meta-analysis – How sound is it?

The limitations of RCTs and meta-analysis are highlighted in an investigation by Aker *et al.* (1996), who identified five RCTs evaluating the effect of conservative management of mechanical neck pain where the designs and effect size for pain scores were considered sufficiently similar to permit statistical pooling of results of the individual trials. Their pooled effect size for pain reduction occurring between one and four weeks of treatment was −0.6 (95% confidence interval −0.9 to −0.4), indicating a pain reduction equivalent to 16.2 points on a 100-point scale. The authors concluded that the results 'clearly do not support these approaches nor others commonly used in practice today', but added, 'no treatments have been studied in enough detail to assess either efficacy or effectiveness adequately' (Aker *et al.*, 1996, pp. 1295–1296). How then should these results and conclusions be used by those with a vested interest (clinicians, clients, funding bodies)? If the first quote above is used alone, clinicians and clients may abandon these particular management practices and funding bodies may deny these services. If the second quote is also considered all parties may keep an open mind and await further results, in the meantime continuing or avoiding such treatments depending on their perspectives and professional experience.

This meta-analysis highlights some of the difficulties inherent in relying solely on this form of evidence. For example, clinicians wishing to judge whether the results were relevant to their particular patient population would need to examine more closely the individual trials on which the meta-analysis was performed, to see if the patient populations were similar and to discover what specific treatments were used that produced this non-supportive yet inconclusive result. In this case, patients' problems in the five trials varied from acute whiplash to acute or subacute and chronic mechanical disorders and chronic cervical headache, *yet all* conformed to the definition of mechanical neck disorder 'and hence were considered to be clinically similar' (Aker *et al.*, 1996, p. 292).

There are a number of excellent resources to assist the critical appraisal of published research and meta-analyses in particular (e.g. Dixon *et al.*, 1997; Sackett *et al.*, 1997), but for the purposes of this discussion we highlight three potential sources of error clinicians must consider before accepting broad conclusions such as these.

Homogeneity of the sample

Fundamental to establishing the relevance of RCT results to your practice and patient population is the similarity of your patients to those investigated. Questions such as 'Was the patient population well defined?' and 'Was the diagnosis of the condition well defined?' are basic considerations. The trials included in the meta-analysis of Aker *et al.* (1996) varied in their depth of description of the respective populations and diagnostic criteria. Population demographics were not matched, with the sole rationale for considering these particular studies together being the generalization that they all conformed to the diagnosis of mechanical neck disorder and hence were deemed to be clinically similar. Not all the studies provided a clear specification of the diagnostic criteria of mechanical neck disorder. Rather, it appears to be a label adopted by Aker *et al.* (1996), despite the lack of

consistent reporting on the patient populations to justify this decision. The only consistent criterion for inclusion in the meta-analysis appears to be the presence of neck pain, while other discriminators of 'mechanical' versus 'non-mechanical' and potential confounding variables to the effects of treatment such as history, physical findings and psycho-social status were not uniformly included. While mechanical neck pain is often considered one of the more straightforward types of patient problem to manage, it falls along a continuum of presentations from simple acute musculo-skeletal pain to more complex multistructural, multifactorial chronic pain such as can occur following whiplash. In fact, whiplash is increasingly being recognized as much more than a simple mechanical neck disorder (Harding 1998). Jaspers (1998) reported the incidence of post-traumatic stress disorder as at least 25% in traffic accident victims who sustain physical injury. Patients such as these may not be expected to respond to 'mechanical' treatments alone.

Measurement of outcome

Judging the utility of findings from meta-analyses must also involve consideration of the outcomes on which the success of the interventions were based. In the Aker *et al.* (1996) example, outcome measures varied from range of motion and pain scores to the patient's assessment of the global perceived effect measured on a six-point scale. The meta-analysis was restricted to the pain scores transformed to a 100-point scale. Such a narrow definition of improvement reflects a lack of appreciation of the multiple determinants of health and pain in particular. Other measures such as physical impairments, disability assessments of function and quality of life outcomes should also be considered. Beattie and Maher (1997), for example, illustrate a case of a patient whose measures of impairment, including pain intensity and limitation of lumbar motion, failed to improve in response to treatment although the quality of life measure (Roland–Morris Disability Questionnaire) demonstrated significant gains. While this instance may challenge the notion that the benefits were a result of physical changes, it highlights the importance of a broader perspective of health and the measures that reflect it.

Interpretation of the intervention

Clearly the interventions used will also affect the results. Consideration should be given to whether specific, clearly described interventions were being evaluated or, as in the Aker *et al.* (1996) study, whether multiple interventions were grouped together under a heading such as 'conservative management'. The range of treatments used across the pooled studies in this meta-analysis included manipulation, mobilization, exercise, traction, heat, ice, analgesic and education. There was generally no reference to the details of the treatments, the setting in which treatments were provided or the background of staff administering the treatments. Each of these factors represents a confounding variable that could have influenced the results. Further, this lack of detail makes it difficult for the treatments to be replicated and makes the broad negative conclusions from the meta-analysis less meaningful and possibly even negligent.

We are not asserting that the individual studies comprising the meta-analysis were of no value, as some provided more information than others. However, the Aker *et al.* (1996) study highlights some limitations of meta-analysis and RCTs in general. As discussed by Linton (1998), the similarity between patients, setting, type of problem, staff and ability to perform the treatment will influence the applicability of results. We stress here again that we fully endorse the concepts of RCTs and meta-analysis but caution against the blanket acceptance of their findings without critical appraisal.

However, even with better delineation of the patient population, appropriate outcome measures and treatment descriptions, results from a meta-analysis can provide only broad guidelines as to the appropriateness of an intervention for patients with certain commonalities in their presentation. This limitation is acknowledge by Sackett (1997, p. vi) who states, 'without clinical expertise, practice risks becoming tyrannized by evidence, for even excellent external evidence may be inapplicable to or inappropriate for an individual patient'. Clinicians must use their own assessment and reasoning skills to establish the similarity of a given patient to those studied and then administer the treatment appropriately to the unique variances of that patient.

Using a range of evidence to inform evidence-based practice

In taking a broader, more realistic and comprehensive view of evidence-based practice, we define evidence as knowledge derived from a variety of sources that has been subjected to testing and has been found to be credible. We advocate using a range of evidence in support of evidence-based practice and recognizing that the type of knowledge needed will depend upon the context. In some areas of clinical practice (e.g. pathology) the proportion of research-based knowledge used by the decision maker will be very high. In pharmacy, the importance of RCTs will be significant, while the need for experience-based knowledge in dealing with the medication-taking habits or needs of certain groups (e.g. confused elderly people) will also play an important role. In other circumstances, such as the implementation of a home re-education occupational therapy program for a patient returning home after extensive rehabilitation, the value of knowledge deriving from experience is paramount.

Evidence from clinical experience and expertise

The research literature which deals with the nature of clinical expertise acknowledges the importance of experience as well as formal learning in the development of expertise. Sackett *et al.* (1997, p. 2) include clinicians' experience in their definition of evidence:

> The practice of evidence-based medicine means integrating individual clinical expertise with the best available external clinical evidence from systematic research. By individual clinical expertise, we mean the proficiency and judgement that individual clinicians acquire through clinical experience and clinical practice.

Sackett *et al.* (1997) argue that evidenced-based medicine is not 'cook-book' medicine, pointing out that external evidence can inform, but never replace, individual clinical expertise. They stress that clinical expertise is essential in determining whether the external evidence is relevant to an individual patient and, if so, how it should be used in a clinical decision. While they state that evidence-based medicine is not restricted to RCTs and meta-analysis, that is clearly the authors' 'gold standard' and is used throughout the book in descriptions and examples of how to search for external evidence. For example, in reference to asking research questions about therapy, Sackett *et al.* (1997, p. 4) state that '... we should try to avoid the non-experimental approaches, since these routinely lead to false-positive conclusions about efficacy'. In the section on critical appraisal of evidence for validity and importance, again the emphasis is on guidelines to judging the quality of clinical trials. There is no discussion of the reasoning necessary to identify patients appropriate for specific trials or the reasoning associated with the delivery of treatment within those trials. Further, once a management strategy has been supported by the appropriate external evidence, it is clear that skilled reasoning is required, not simply in appraising the validity and importance of the results but also in applying those results to individual patients who may or may not match the specific population under study.

In a focus article of a prominent pain journal, Linton (1998) argues that in the application of evidence-based practice two fallacies exist. The first is particularly relevant to this discussion, and involves attempting to improve quality and enhance practice performance using a narrow scientific approach. The second is the naïve assumption that knowledge produced from RCTs will automatically result in changed practice behaviour. Linton (1998, p. 46) makes the point that 'although the information presented in the name of 'best evidence' may be wise, it fails to capitalize on the vast knowledge generated by experience.'

Evidence and ways of knowing

In Chapter 3 the generation of knowledge through different research approaches, including the scientific method and the constructivist and critical science research approaches, was identified as a key issue in understanding the knowledge basis for practice. It was argued that there is a need to understand the purpose, value and assumptions that shape the act of inquiry as part of understanding and evaluating the knowledge which is derived from inquiry. This holds true for RCTs and other forms of empirico-analytical research, as for interpretive and critical paradigm research.

A number of researchers and scholars have explored the nature and practice of different ways of knowing and producing knowledge[1] (Carper, 1978; Habermas, 1972; Kolb, 1984; Reason and Heron, 1986; Sarter, 1988). Forms of knowledge which are technical, practical, emancipatory, experiential, propositional, empirical, aesthetic, personal, ethical/moral and intellectual/interpretive have been identified and substantiated by these scholars.

Knowledge from all these dimensions of human being and interaction is needed to comprehensively understand clinical problems and formulate sound decisions for quality practice. Placing such practice within the context of evidence-based practice demands of health professionals that the knowledge they employ is credible and defensible, that it is indeed *evidence*. Using the definition of evidence we provided above, it can be seen that the same elements of 'conviction' and 'testing' applied in Chapter 3 to ascertain the validity of knowledge claims are used in the verification of evidence. Evidence suitable as the basis for clinical practice, therefore, is tested, credible knowledge in its various forms.

Sources of evidence: practice needs evidence from both physical and environmental domains

The relationship between the various psychosocial factors in the determination and presentation of our clients' health underscores our argument for a broader perspective of evidence and the need for skilled clinical reasoning to uncover those interactions and establish their relevance to each patient's problem(s). If we consider the client as the centre (not just the object) of the decision-making process, the importance of physical, psychological and environmental dimensions of health, along with the interactions among these dimensions, are highlighted.

A model developed by Gifford (1998) illustrates this process. The model depicts the interactions of the fundamental pathways into and out of the central nervous system that are necessary for survival and to maintain homeostasis. It illustrates contributions and interactions of the different input, processing and output mechanisms to the maintenance of health and the development and continuation of poor health (e.g. pain and dysfunction). In this model, physical and contextual information concerning the person's illness experience (including reference to past experiences) is received and processed by the brain, resulting in activity of output mechanisms (e.g. somatic motor, autonomic, endocrine, immune and descending pain control responses) and in behaviours. Importantly, how the person's health is manifest via these output mechanisms (behaviourally, cognitively, emotionally and physiologically) depends in part on contextual factors within the person's immediate circumstances as well as on past experiences that contribute to the person's beliefs, attitudes,

---

[1] See Chapter 3 for further discussion.

emotions and behaviours. That is, even given the same extent of tissue injury or illness, no two people will have exactly the same presentation, since the way in which they manifest their pain or illness is shaped in part by who they are.

This model can serve as an analogy and blueprint for how the whole health care team and system should operate. All the factors which the client (in body and mind) 'considers' in making health-related (clinical) decisions need to be considered by the team. Hence it is inadequate for health professionals and health care teams simply to focus on physical diagnoses. Managing patients' problems requires understanding of their unique pain or illness experiences. While all input, processing and output mechanisms will be in operation in any state of ill health, they will not all necessarily be dysfunctional (i.e. contributing to the problem and/or counterproductive to recovery). Clinicians must have the necessary knowledge organization and reasoning skills to distinguish between different types of problem, including problems that truly are primarily nociceptive or residing in the tissues, problems which co-exist or may even be dominant in the processing and output systems (e.g. increased levels of tissue sensitivity resulting from prolonged stress), and problems where the issue is much more behavioural or environmental than physical. With this knowledge and reasoning the clinician is able to make sound decisions (for and with the client) which relate to assessment of the complete problem including associated cognitive, behavioural and emotional effects, and appropriate management strategies. Understanding and managing patients' problems requires a broad perspective of the multiple determinants of health and recovery, along with good reasoning skills to apply that knowledge.

Evidence, reasoning and professional judgement

Understanding the nature and credibility of knowledge and evidence is the first part of the application of evidence to practice. Evidence-based practice requires professional judgement and sound reasoning. It is not merely the attachment of evidence as a trigger or input to a recipe book of decision making. Reasoning is needed to evaluate the quality of evidence, to apply evidence to given situations and people's needs, and to cope with situations in which the health professions (as

inexact sciences) have limited answers to cope with the indeterminate areas of practice and knowledge.

Improving practice performance (the goal of evidence-based practice) requires more than access to new knowledge; it requires skills in reasoning to integrate that knowledge into existing knowledge frameworks, including knowing when and how to use that knowledge. That is, application of declarative or propositional knowledge requires professional craft and procedural knowledge. All professions have had histories where protocols or recipe treatments have been advocated when patients clearly did not and still do not always fit the criteria on which the protocol was designed. Patients rarely have unidimensional problems and the impact of psychosocial factors highlighted in the previous section further invalidates the strict application of any protocol. Research-validated knowledge should inform clinicians but cannot be a sole guide. Linton (1998) provides an example where the way in which an early intervention for acute back pain was administered became the difference between a highly successful intervention and one that may have actually increased the problem. Again, this example highlights the importance of professional craft knowledge in the outcome of any intervention. RCTs typically have not considered the way in which treatment is applied, and there has been limited exploration of the influence on outcomes of clinicians' reasoning, not only in reaching a diagnosis but also in relation to interacting with the patient, understanding the patient's unique illness or pain experience, working collaboratively on problem management, resolving ethical dilemmas and predicting future outcomes.

Therefore, while the results of meta-analyses of RCTs will continue to contribute to our body of evidence, clinicians must possess skilled reasoning to utilize that information critically. Such results are unlikely to match the precise presentation of any given patient sufficiently to be useful in a prescriptive manner. These individual discrepancies are particularly significant when clinicians' reasoning extends beyond diagnosis in the traditional sense to incorporate attention to psychosocial issues, including patients' understandings and goals. Most patient problems are multifactorial, often with more than one source of pain or dysfunction and typically with numerous contributing factors.

Administering a treatment in most circumstances requires professional judgement regarding the nature and the context of the problem. Even with a patient similar to those in a reported research study, judging the amount, manner of delivery and progression of patient treatment, be it physical, advice, or other strategies, depends on a host of diagnostic and non-diagnostic variables. Very few 'cures' have been established for the range of problems most health professionals must manage and therefore treatment effects must be continually monitored, providing empirical evidence to inform ongoing management. It is critical that evidence-based practice does not become cook-book practice. It requires proficiency and judgement acquired through clinical experience and clinical practice to make use of the best available evidence. However, proficiency and judgement are more involved than this one line suggests, as demonstrated by each of the health professions featured in this book as they explore the various interactions between clinicians' knowledge organization, cognitive and metacognitive skills, and the contextual factors that contribute to a client's presentation.

Non-experimental evidence is considered subject to bias and to be avoided in the evaluation of therapy (Sackett, 1997). Indeed bias is a well recognized source of reasoning error (Jones, 1992). In Chapter 34 Scott highlights the following three principal causes of reasoning error:

- Faulty perception or elicitation of cues.
- Incomplete factual knowledge (about a disease process or clinical condition).
- Misapplication of known facts to a specific clinical problem.

Clearly, reasoning errors do not stem only from incomplete declarative experimental evidence. For example, faulty perception or elicitation of cues may be related to inadequate knowledge (both experimental and experienced based) of the relevant cues and underdeveloped craft knowledge in recognizing those cues. Similarly, misapplication of known facts to a specific problem relates to incorrect use of heuristics, an example of poor procedural knowledge. Forming the wrong initial concept of the problem (framing error) and failure to generate plausible hypotheses and adequately test them are common errors frequently related to bias. Knowledge of experimental evidence alone will not safeguard against these reasoning errors. Errors of reasoning are best minimized by having a broad organization of declarative, craft and personal knowledge applied through skilled reflective reasoning.

Evidence-based practice does not take the reasoning out of practice, rather evidence-based practice requires advanced reasoning to make the most of the evidence that is available.

Conclusion

In this chapter we have argued for a broader definition of evidence within the concept of evidence-based practice. In particular, there is a need to include and value the evidence from reflective experience alongside research based evidence (from RCTs and other research methodologies) in this broader concept of evidence-based practice. While we fully endorse critical appraisal of current theory and practice, we have argued that evidence-based practice requires skilled clinical reasoning as a valuable means of knowledge acquisition.

References

Aker, P. D., Gross, A. R., Goldsmith, C. H. and Peloso, P. (1996) Conservative management of mechanical neck pain: Systematic overview and meta-analysis. *British Medical Journal*, **313**, 1291–1296.

Beattie, P. and Maher, C. (1997) The role of functional status questionnaires for low back pain. *Australian Journal of Physiotherapy*, **43**, 29–38.

Carper, B. A. (1978) Fundamental patterns of knowing. *Advances in Nursing Science*, **1**, 13–23.

Crombie, I. K. (1997) The limits of evidence-based medicine. *Pain Forum*, **7**, 63–65.

Dixon, R. A., Munro, J. F. and Silcocks, P. B. (eds) (1997) *The Evidence Based Medicine Workbook: Critical Appraisal for Evaluating Clinical Problem Solving*. Oxford: Butterworth-Heinemann.

Gifford, L. (1998) The mature organisms model. In *Topical Issues in Pain. Whiplash: Science and Management, Fear-Avoidance Beliefs and Behaviour* (L. Gifford, ed.), pp. 45–56. Falmouth, UK: Physiotherapy Pain Association Yearbook 1998–1999, NOI Press.

Habermas, J. (1972) *Knowledge and Human Interest*. London: Heinemann.

Harding, V. (1998) Minimising chronicity after whiplash injury. In *Topical Issues in Pain. Whiplash: Science and Management, Fear-Avoidance Beliefs and Behaviour* (L. Gifford, ed.), pp. 105–114. Falmouth, UK: Physiotherapy Pain Association Yearbook 1998–1999, NOI Press.

Jaspers, J. P. C. (1998) Whiplash and post-traumatic stress disorder. *Disability and Rehabilitation*, **20**, 397–404.

Jones, M. A. (1992) Clinical reasoning in manual therapy. *Physical Therapy*, **72**, 875–884.

Kolb, D. A. (1984) *Experiential Learning: Experience as the Source of Learning and Development*. Englewood Cliffs, NJ: Prentice-Hall.

Linton, S. J. (1998) In defence of reason, meta-analysis and beyond in evidence-based practice. *Pain Forum*, **7**, 46–54.

Reason, P. and Heron, J. (1986) Research with people: The paradigm of cooperative experiential enquiry. *Person-Centred Review*, **1**, 457–476.

Sackett, D. L. (1997) Foreword. In *The Evidence Based Medicine Workbook, Critical Appraisal For Evaluating Clinical Problem Solving* (R. A. Dixon, J. F. Munro and P. B. Silcocks, eds), pp. vii–viii. Oxford: Butterworth-Heinemann.

Sackett, D. L., Richardson, W. S., Rosenberg, W. and Haynes, R. B. (1997) *Evidence-Based Medicine: How to Practice and Teach EBM*. New York: Churchill Livingstone.

Sarter, B. (ed.) (1988) *Paths to Knowledge: Innovative Research Methods for Nursing*. New York: National League for Nursing.

Index